MEDICAL MALPRACTICE TITLES FROM WILEY LAW PUBLICATIONS

OBSTETRIC AND NEONATAL MALPRACTICE

LEGAL AND MEDICAL HANDBOOK

SECOND EDITION

VOLUME 1

SUBSCRIPTION NOTICE

This Wiley product is updated on a periodic basis with supplements to reflect important changes in the subject matter. If you purchased this product directly from John Wiley & Sons, Inc., we have already recorded your subscription for this update service.

If, however, you purchased this product from a bookstore and wish to receive (1) the current update at no additional charge, and (2) future updates and revised or related volumes billed separately with a 30-day examination review, please send your name, company name (if applicable), address and the title of the product to:

Supplement Department
John Wiley & Sons, Inc.
One Wiley Drive
Somerset, NJ 08875
1-800-225-5945

For customers outside the United States, please contact the Wiley office nearest you.

Professional and Reference Division
John Wiley & Sons Canada, Ltd.
22 Worcester Road
Rexdale, Ontario M9W 1L1
CANADA
(416) 675-3580
1-800-567-4797
FAX (416) 675-6599

John Wiley & Sons, Ltd.
Baffins Lane
Chichester
West Sussex, PO19 1UD
UNITED KINGDOM
(44) (243) 779777

Jacaranda Wiley Ltd
PRT Division
P.O. Box 174
North Ryde, NSW 2113
AUSTRALIA
(02) 805-1100
FAX (02) 805-1597

John Wiley & Sons (SEA)
  Pte. Ltd.
2 Clementi Loop
#02-01 Jin Xing Distripark
SINGAPORE 0512
4632400
FAX 4634604

OBSTETRIC AND NEONATAL MALPRACTICE
LEGAL AND MEDICAL HANDBOOK
SECOND EDITION
VOLUME 1

MICHAEL D. VOLK

Volk & Montes
El Paso, Texas

Wiley Law Publications
JOHN WILEY & SONS, INC.
New York · Chichester · Brisbane · Toronto · Singapore

Copyright © 1996 by John Wiley & Sons, Inc.

Previous edition published as *Medical Malpractice: Handling Obstetric and Neonatal Cases.*

Library of Congress Cataloging-in-Publication Data

ISBN 0-471-12896-1 (set)
ISBN 0-471-12897-X (vol. 1)
ISBN 0-471-12898-8 (vol. 2)

Printed in the United States of America

10 9 8 7 6 5 4 3 2 1

This book is dedicated to my family: my lovely wife, Rosalina, our children, Michael and David, whom we love so much, my mother, Mary, and my father, Karl. I want to thank my wife and children for all their support and love these past 10 years since the first edition was published. I also want to thank my mother, Mary, for her support and love. She was always there for me and always will be. This book is dedicated to all of them.

PREFACE

The purpose of publishing this second edition in 1996 is the desire to bring current the information set out in the first edition, which was published in 1986. Much has transpired in those 10 years. There is currently an assault on the tort system in the United States, led by the insurance industry, which obviously has a tremendous financial stake in the outcome. The medical industry is facing a managed care crisis that is also led, at least in part, by the insurance industry. Managed care will clearly result in less quality care for patients. I have seen this for many years in every city where I have litigated when the physician was part of an HMO.

The tort system in the United States is still the most fair method to compensate an injured person. That does not mean that the system is perfect, only that there is no better one in existence today.

There are still courageous physicians and nurses who will step forward and testify to the truth in medicolegal cases in the judicial system here. There are still physicians and nurses who will testify to nearly anything to help a colleague in a malpractice case. There are still physicians and nurses who are intimidated into not telling the truth about events that occur to their patients. These things have not changed.

In this second edition, the physicians have been left, for the most part, to write their own chapters without my editing. This is not to say that I agree with all of their comments.

Sadly, my friend and contributor to the first edition, Dr. Benjamin V. Salazar, is deceased. We will miss him and his contributions greatly.

El Paso, Texas   Michael D. Volk
February 1996

ABOUT THE AUTHOR

Michael D. Volk is a partner in the law firm of Volk & Montes in El Paso, Texas, where he practices medicolegal trial law. He is an associate-in-law of the American College of Legal Medicine and a member of the International Society for the Prevention of Iatrogenic Complications. Mr. Volk is a trustee with the Melvin Belli Society and has been recognized in *Who's Who in American Law*. He is a member of the Texas bar, United States Supreme Court, United States District Court for the Western District of Texas, Fifth Circuit Court of Appeals, and Tenth Circuit Court of Appeals. Mr. Volk has written extensively on medicolegal issues.

ABOUT THE CONTRIBUTORS

William Banner, Jr., is board certified in Pediatrics, Critical Care Pediatrics, and Medical Toxicology. He earned his MD degree from the University of Tennessee and a PhD in Pharmacology from the University of Arizona and is a Clinical Associate Professor of the Oklahoma University College of Medicine/ Tulsa and Critical Care Attending at the Children's Hospital at St. Francis in Tulsa. He is currently President of the American Academy of Clinical Toxicology. His areas of interest include pharmacotherapy of pain management, cardiovascular drugs, and poisoning in childhood especially iron, antidepressants, and lead.

Michael S. Cardwell, M.D., is the director of Maternal-Fetal Medicine at St. Vincent Medical Center in Toledo, Ohio. He is actively engaged in the practice of high-risk obstetrics and serves as a medical expert in obstetric malpractice cases. Dr. Cardwell is board-certified in obstetrics-gynecology, maternal-fetal medicine, forensic medicine, legal medicine, and preventive medicine. He received an M.B.A. degree from Bowling Green State University, an M.P.H. degree from St. Louis University, a J.D. degree from the University of Toledo, and an M.D. from Indiana University.

Everett G. Dillman is president of International Business Planners, Inc., in El Paso, Texas. He provides economic, vocational, statistical, business, and financial assistance to defense and plaintiff attorneys in litigation-related matters. He has been active in governmental, business, and financial circles in the Southwest for over 30 years. He has published extensively in both the vocational and economic areas. Mr. Dillman has served on the Advisory Board of the Lubbock division of the Small Business Administration, on the Board of Directors of the National Association of Forensic Economists, and on the Steering Committee for Forensic Rehabilitation of the National Association of Rehabilitation Professionals.

Steven M. Donn, M.D., is a professor of pediatrics, Division of Neonatal-Perinatal Medicine, and the medical director of the Holden Neonatal Intensive Care Unit at the University of Michigan Medical Center in Ann Arbor. He received an undergraduate degree from the University of Michigan and an M.D. from Tulane University. His post-doctoral training in pediatrics occurred at the University of Vermont College of Medicine and sub-specialty training in neonatal-perinatal medicine was at the University of Michigan. Dr. Donn has published extensively in the areas of critically ill newborns. He is a member of numerous professional societies and is listed in *The Best Doctors in America.*

Patricia H. Ellison, M.D., is an adjunct professor in the Department of Pediatrics at the University of Colorado School of Medicine in Denver, Colorado. She completed her medical education at the University of Pittsburgh, two years of general pediatrics at Children's Hospital of Pittsburgh, and three years of neurology at Albany Medical Hospital. Her special interest is the neurologic evaluation of newborns and infants and the neurological outcome after treatment in the neonatal intensive care unit.

Diane Hodgman, C.N.M., M.S.N., is a nurse midwife at Women and Infants' Hospital in Rhode Island, a clinical teaching associate at Brown University School of Medicine, and an adjunct instructor at the University of Rhode Island College of Nursing. She graduated from Columbia University and also served on its faculty. Ms. Hodgman practiced at the University of California San Francisco and was an assistant clinical professor at its School of Medicine. She has contributed to the *Journal of Nurse Midwifery* and the *Journal of Perinatal Neonatal Nursing.*

C. Antonio Jesurun, M.D., is a professor at the Texas Tech University Health Sciences Center, a state-affiliated research teaching facility. A professor with the Department of Pediatrics, Dr. Jesurun instructs medical students and residents in neonatology and perinatology and provides diagnosis and treatment of critical care infants. He was previously an instructor of neonatology at Wayne State University School of Medicine, Hutzel Hospital. Dr. Jesurun received his graduate medical education at Baylor College of Medicine and a B.A. degree in English from the University of Michigan—Ann Arbor.

Thomas G. Kirkhope, M.D., has a private practice in general obstetrics and gynecology in Toledo, Ohio. He is an associate clinical professor at Medical College of Ohio and former chairman and director of medical education for the Department of Obstetrics and Gynecology at The Toledo Hospital. Dr. Kirkhope received an undergraduate degree from John Carroll University, an M.D. from the Medical College of Wisconsin, Milwaukee, and a J.D. degree from the University of Toledo College of Law. He is on the Committee on Accreditation and Education for the Ohio State Medical Association.

Christine Whelan Knapp, C.N.M., M.S., practices nurse midwifery with Plymouth OB/Gyn Associates in Plymouth, Massachusetts. A graduate of the University of Massachusetts at Amherst, Boston University, and State University of New York at Downstate, she was assistant director of Nursing and coordinator of Nurse Midwifery at Brigham and Women's Hospital in Boston. Ms. Knapp has practiced nurse midwifery at USC/Los Angeles County Hospital and at Women and Infants' Hospital in Rhode Island. She co-edited *Perinatal/ Neonatal Nursing—A Clinical Handbook* and *Case Studies in Perinatal Nursing.*

Robert M. Knapp is a board-certified anesthesiologist in practice at the Jordan Hospital in Plymouth, Massachusetts. He is a graduate of the University of Michigan, the University of Health Sciences College of Osteopathic Medicine in Kansas City, and the Suffolk University Law School in Boston. He completed a fellowship in obstetric anesthesia at Brigham and Women's Hospital in Boston, and spent a number of years as director of obstetric anesthesia at the University of Cincinnati. He has written and lectured on legal and risk management issues pertinent to anesthesiology.

Karen Carter Lyon, Ph.D., R.N., C.S., C.N.A.A., is a clinical nurse specialist and certified by the American Nurses Association as a high-risk perinatal nurse. She has over 20 years of experience in the nursing care of mothers and newborns. Dr. Lyon works as an independent consultant in various areas of clinical and administrative nursing. An expert witness on nursing care for both plaintiffs and defendants, she teaches on the faculties of the University of Texas at El Paso and the University of Phoenix. She is an active member of the Texas Nurses Association, American Nurses Association, American Organization of Nurse Executives, Texas League for Nursing, and Sigma Theta Tau.

SUMMARY CONTENTS

DETAILED CONTENTS

Volume 2

Chapter 19 **Neonatal Problems: Etiology and Management**
Steven M. Donn, M.D.

Chapter 21   Complications and Sequelae of Intensive Care: *Primum Non Nocere*
Steven M. Donn, M.D.

CHAPTER 1

OPENING THE FILE
Michael D. Volk

§ 1.1 Introduction

This chapter primarily illustrates the techniques that can be used to open a file, begin the investigation phase, and determine whether a meritorious claim exists. Medical malpractice cases involve a great deal of time and money. Non-meritorious claims should not be litigated. However, the problem often is whether the claim is meritorious. Certain claims are meritorious on their face. If an obstetrician refuses to assess the progress of a mother and child during labor with resulting damage to the mother or child, there may well be merit. However, situations must be thoroughly investigated before a determination can be made as to whether a claim is valid. The investigation stage may require days, weeks, or many months. For instance, prognosis of the potential client (that is, the child) may not be clear for quite sometime. Often counsel must delay litigation to allow the passage of time so that the damages suffered become clearer.

§ 1.2   Defining Malpractice

Malpractice is a physician's failure to meet the standard of care. Many doctors and health care professionals have their own definition of malpractice. Their definitions may involve greedy patients that force them to practice defensive medicine, and contingent-fee ambulance chasers.

Reasonable health-care professionals and attorneys who practice medicolegal law understand that patients are sometimes seriously injured by health-care providers failing to meet the standard of care. These same professionals also understand that actions are sometimes filed that are not meritorious claims, but are more often the result of not understanding the medical facts, rather than malicious intent. If physicians were more willing to honestly evaluate and discuss the medical facts with the attorney, both professions would be better served. One problem is that some physicians are not willing to do so, but subsequently complain when an action is filed.

Any lawyer who deals frequently with malpractice cases knows that a client has a personal perception of what occurred, which may or may not be correct. Some possible scenarios involve the following:

1. The doctor treated me poorly.
2. The doctor disregarded my complaints.
3. The office staff ignored me.
4. The doctor is acting guilty.
5. The doctor apologized to me.
6. Something bad happened to me.
7. My loved one is deceased.
8. Look at my disfigurement or dismemberment.
9. This could not have occurred without malpractice.

One of the most difficult things for a patient to come to grips with is the injury to a part of the body or the death of a loved one. There can be a search for an answer to the question of why. It is incumbent upon counsel to understand that what the client has determined has happened (and the perceived cause) is not always correct. On the other hand, it is uncanny how often non–medically trained people have a sixth sense of what occurred and why. Listen very carefully and analyze the facts, giving due consideration to what the client believes.

The attorney must go beyond these threshold complaints and discover the medical facts. What the client wants to complain about may be totally irrelevant. Most clients do not have medical knowledge. The attorney must skillfully extract the information needed from the client, often in spite of what the client wants to discuss. This is not to imply that counsel should ignore the history given. However, do not be coerced into litigating a frivolous or borderline case.

§ 1.3   Initial Interview

A client contacts an attorney because of a referral from a former client, another lawyer, or advertising. Of course, as skill and competence increase, so do referrals from other lawyers and former clients.

The initial interview should have three or four stages. In the first stage, the secretary records basic information to identify the client and target the problem. The person with whom a client has initial contact should be a pleasant and compassionate staff member. Clients generally have no desire to involve themselves in a lawsuit until forced to as a result of an injury.

The second stage is a more in-depth interview. This can often be done by a law clerk or paralegal. If the office has no law clerk or paralegal, the secretary must get the in-depth information. The necessary information is discussed in § 1.4.

In the third stage, the detailed medical facts are obtained by a combination of the law clerk, secretary, and trial counsel, or (if the attorney is fortunate) by a nurse or physician on staff. A number of nurses have become disenchanted with the rewards and low pay of nursing and search alternate employment. Often they are excellent persons to interview a prospective client and obtain the detailed medical facts. Without comprehensive medical facts and history, most claims cannot be evaluated.

After the initial material is gathered, the attorney responsible for handling the claim gets acquainted with the basic facts and establishes rapport with the client. At that time the attorney can accept the case, reject the case, or agree to gather further information and investigate the matter, with the decision about acceptance or rejection postponed to a later date. Many times, after an initial interview, the attorney will not be able to accept or reject the claim out of hand.

§ 1.4   Necessary Threshold Data

Counsel should have a form that elicits the important basic information. The completed form becomes a permanent part of the file and enables anyone to refer to it at any time. At the beginning of the form an explanation for the client similar to the one that follows should appear:

Please fill out the questionnaire given to you by my office staff. It is essential that you answer as many of the questions as you can. We need to know all of your past and present medical history so that if we represent you, we are not surprised in court. We realize that some of the questions are sensitive, but please understand that we are not trying to embarrass you or pry into your private lives unnecessarily. We need this information to help you. Your answers are confidential.

The form should gather the following information for maternal injury cases:

1. Name
2. Age
3. Address, city, and zip code
4. Home phone
5. Work phone
6. Social security number
7. Means of transportation to this office
8. Date of malpractice
9. Marital status
10. Spouse's name
11. Employment at time of malpractice (if homemaker, number of children if any)
12. If homemaker, average hours of work per week unable to perform
13. Job title and type of work
14. Rate of pay or salary
15. Average hours of work per week at the time of the alleged malpractice
16. Number of hours or days lost from work due to alleged malpractice
17. Amount of wages or salary lost (obtain lost wages affidavit from employer)
18. Whom you want to sue
19. What you feel was done wrong by the doctor
20. What you feel is your present medical condition
21. All physicians, dentists, podiatrists, chiropractors, or health care providers that have ever treated you in your life, including the physicians that treated you for your current problem
22. The date of the beginning of your last known menstrual period
23. Your due date (the date your baby was to be born)
24. The dates and reasons for all visits to your doctor during your pregnancy
25. All medications, including vitamins, that were given to you or prescribed for you by your doctor
26. The dates of any ultrasounds or sonograms that were performed and the reason they were performed

27. The dates of any and all X-rays taken while you were pregnant, where they were taken, and the reason they were ordered

28. Any complications that you know of that occurred during your pregnancy

29. Any medical conditions you were being treated for, either by your obstetrician or family practitioner, or by any other doctor during your pregnancy

30. What is wrong with you now; that is, why you came to see an attorney

31. All expenses incurred because of the malpractice

32. All serious illnesses or medical conditions you have ever had, the date the condition was diagnosed, and the name of the physician

33. Any lawsuits or claims you or your spouse have ever made against anyone for anything

34. Any serious medical conditions that any of your immediate family has or had

35. All medications you are now taking

36. Any medications or drugs prescribed for you at any time in your life

37. If you are complaining about an injury during labor and delivery, a description of when you first went into labor, continuing chronologically with what occurred until your injury

38. All expenses made necessary by the malpractice

39. All conversations with doctor, nurses, or other health-care providers that you feel are relevant to your claim.

For an injury to a child during the prenatal course, labor, and delivery, or in the first six weeks of life (the neonatal period) include the following questions:

1. Name of parents
2. Ages of parents
3. Name of child
4. Age of child
5. Address, city, and zip code
6. Home phone number
7. Work phone number of parents
8. Social security number of parents
9. Social security number of child
10. Mode of transportation to this office
11. Date of malpractice
12. Whom you want to sue
13. Any jobs, job opportunities, or advancement lost because of need to care for child
14. Amount of salary or wages lost because of need to take care of child

15. How much care your child needs per day

16. Any need for occupational or physical therapy, with dates and the name, address, and phone number of the person giving the therapy

17. What you feel was done wrong by the physician

18. When your child was born

19. The date of the beginning of the mother's last known menstrual period

20. Your due date (the date your baby was to be born)

21. The dates and reasons for all visits to your doctor or doctors during your pregnancy

22. All medications, including vitamins, given to you or prescribed for you by your doctor or doctors during your pregnancy

23. The dates of any ultrasounds or sonograms that were performed and the reason they were performed during your pregnancy

24. The dates of any and all X-rays taken while you were pregnant, where they were taken, and the reason they were taken

25. Any complications that occurred during your pregnancy

26. Any medical conditions you were being treated for by your obstetrician family practitioner, or any other doctor during your pregnancy

27. What is wrong with your child now; that is, why you came to see an attorney

28. All expenses incurred because of the malpractice

29. All serious illnesses or medical conditions the mother or father have ever had, the date of diagnosis, and the name of the physician

30. Any lawsuits or claims either parent has ever made against anyone for anything

31. Any serious medical conditions that any of your immediate family has or had, including children with seizures, deformities, and so forth

32. All medications that either parent or the child is now taking

33. Any medication or drugs prescribed for either parent or child

34. If you are complaining about an injury to the child during labor and delivery, a description of when you first went into labor, continuing chronologically with what occurred until the child's injury

35. The pediatrician, neonatologist, or family doctor who treated your child

36. All tests and medical procedures performed on your child up to the present time

37. All doctors your child has seen since birth

38. All hospitals your child has been admitted into since birth, with the date and reason for each admission

39. All outpatient tests performed on your child since birth

40. The doctor's opinion of your child's condition and its cause.

The attorney's office staff can have the client fill out the form at the time of the initial interview or send it in the mail to be filled out and brought to the initial interview. The interviewers should expand on the information while going over the form, writing directly on the form.

§ 1.5   Obtaining Medical Records

Obtaining medical records can sometimes be an art in itself. Many physicians and hospitals do not like to furnish medical records to anyone, especially attorneys. However, in almost every state there is either statutory law or case law that allows a patient, or a person with proper authorization (such as an attorney) to obtain medical records.[1] A sample medical authorization is reproduced as **Appendix 1–1.**

Physicians sometimes destroy or change records; often the best practice is to have the authorization signed by the client and have someone from the office present the authorization and demand the records. If a personal trip is necessary, the authorization must allow the attorney to view and inspect the records. Counsel must impress upon either the physician or the hospital that the records must be turned over immediately. If they refuse to do so, mention that proper demand was made for the records, and further, that if any records are missing or altered, the claim will be made that the physicians refused to furnish the records in order to destroy or alter the records. A letter confirming the refusal to allow inspection and copying should be sent via certified mail immediately. This generally leads to some hard feelings, but sometimes there is no alternative method to protect the client.

A question that often presents itself is whether the attorney should have to pay for a copy of the records. Counsel must be guided by local practice in the state and by any statutory or case law. A reasonable fee for copies is standard. However, hospitals, clinics, and doctors' offices have been known to charge outrageous prices and this must be resisted.

When records are requested, make it clear that *all* the records must be provided. A physician must furnish all the progress notes, copies of any hospital records that were sent to them, insurance forms, correspondence, test results, and the like. The same holds true for the hospital. A complete copy of the entire chart must be provided if requested. Once counsel becomes skilled in examining charts and dealing in malpractice cases, there may be times when the attorney will want to order only a portion of the charts.

---

[1] For instance, see the Texas statute (repealed in 1983 for civil actions by the Texas Rules of Evidence) that states: "A physician shall furnish copies of medical records requested, or a summary or narrative of the records, pursuant to a written consent for release of the information" Tex. Stat. Ann. art. 4495b, § 5.08k (Vernon 1981).

§ 1.6 Necessary Medical Records

The following records should be obtained in a case of maternal injury:

1. Hospital records pertinent to the injury
2. Prenatal records from the delivering doctor
3. Prior medical records, especially any records that deal with a condition that caused the injury or any contributing conditions
4. Outpatient laboratory tests
5. Any ultrasound or X-ray reports
6. Prescriptions written for the patient
7. Postinjury records reflecting the condition.

It is imperative that counsel determine that all the records have been obtained from the physician's office. Physicians might cull out what they do not want the lawyer to see.

If the client is a child, the following information is necessary:

1. All prenatal records from the pregnancy
2. All ultrasound and X-ray reports
3. All prescriptions written for the patient
4. All outpatient laboratory tests
5. The entire chart from labor and delivery
6. The newborn nursery chart or intensive care nursery chart
7. The hospital and medical records from any hospitalizations after the initial hospitalization after birth
8. Any occupational or physical therapy records
9. The medical records of the pediatrician and any other specialist treating the child.

§ 1.7 Interpreting Medical Records

The interpretation of medical records is a most difficult task for an attorney because of the specialized vocabulary and the scribbling by the records' authors. Physicians may disguise what occurred to a patient by glossing over the injury in the typewritten portions of the chart. Often the key to a case is buried in the handwritten notes. The attorney must read every line in the entire chart and become familiar with interpreting handwritten notes.

After all records are obtained, the first task is to put them in order. Sometimes records have been shuffled in an attempt to make them incomprehensible. Hospital records should be arranged in the following order in the maternal chart:

1. Face sheet
2. History and physical
3. Discharge summary
4. Prenatal record
5. Labor and delivery record
6. Physician's progress notes
7. Physician's orders
8. Consultation sheet
9. Radiology records
10. Laboratory records
11. Operative report
12. Vital signs sheet
13. Medication records
14. Nurses' notes.

Records should be arranged in the following order in fetal and newborn charts:

1. All of the maternal chart
2. Face sheet
3. Newborn exam
4. Admitting summary
5. Discharge summary
6. Physician's progress notes
7. Physician's orders
8. Consultation sheets
9. Radiology records
10. Laboratory records
11. Operative reports
12. Vital signs sheets
13. Medication records
14. Nurses' notes.

The best way to learn how to interpret medical records is to read them with a medical dictionary. Medical records should be a chronological history of the care the patient received. It should include any adverse events that affected the condition of the patient. All pertinent information must be included.

A prenatal record, entitled "Medical History," is reproduced as **Appendix 1–2.** Note that it contains the following sections:

1. History of present pregnancy
2. Previous medical history
3. Previous pregnancies
4. Results of physical examination
5. Results of pelvic examination
6. Results of laboratory examinations
7. A summary of the weekly or monthly visits in graph form
8. Physician progress notes of the pregnancy.

There are two blank ultrasound report forms reproduced in **Appendix 1–3.**

The labor record is the chronological recordation of the progress of labor after admission into the hospital and until the mother is taken to the delivery room. Note that it has the following parts:

1. Previous pregnancy history
2. Due date
3. Condition of the mother's membranes (or bag of water) on admission
4. Date and time labor began and the contraction pattern
5. Vital signs
6. Blood pressure
7. Heart rate of the fetus by auscultation or fetal heart rate monitor
8. Where they auscultated or placed the stethoscope on the mother's abdomen to find the fetal heart rate; that is, in what part or quadrant of the mother's abdomen the fetal heart rate was found
9. Results of the initial vaginal exam showing position of the fetus, station of the fetus, presenting part, dilitation, and effacement
10. Last meal
11. Any allergies
12. Mother's blood type.

After the initial history there is a section that continues until the mother is taken to the delivery room. This section is basically divided into:

1. Recordation of time
2. Results of physical examination
3. Contraction pattern

4. Fetal heart tone location and rate, plus any abnormalities of the heart rate
5. Medications
6. Remarks by the nurse or physician.

If the newborn is taken to the intensive care nursery, the following information should be recorded on the flow sheet:

1. Age and weight of the child
2. Temperature, pulse, respirations, blood pressure activity, color, hematocrit, and abdominal circumference
3. Medications and procedures
4. Blood in and blood out
5. Intravenous solutions
6. Feedings
7. Oxygen settings, if any is being given
8. If supplemental oxygen is being supplied to the child, the blood gases and results of any laboratory studies
9. Nurses' progress notes.

§ 1.8 Standard of Care

For a malpractice case to be won, the attorney must prove that the physician's care fell below the applicable standard of care. It is necessary to understand the applicable standard before litigating. Any malpractice case is decided on whether the standard has been met. The standard of care may be divided into four subparts. Each jurisdiction employs either one standard or a combination of standards as follows:

Locality rule. This is the rule whereby a physician must perform according to the standard in the community. For instance, an obstetrician must meet the standard of care and perform medically only according to the standard that other physicians in the local community meet. This is the oldest standard of care, but it is still used in some jurisdictions.[2]

---

[2] "[A] specialist has a duty to possess and exercise that degree of skill and care ordinarily employed, under similar circumstances, by the members of his specialty in good standing, located in the same locality." Loftus v. Hayden, 391 A.2d 749 (Del. 1978). In Florida, there are some conflicting definitions. In an obstetrical malpractice case, the court stated that a "specialist is under a duty to use ordinary skills, means and methods recognized as necessary and customarily followed in the particular type of case according to the standard of those who are qualified by training and experience to perform similar services in the community." Crovella v. Cochrene, 102 So.2d 307 (Fla. Dist. Ct. App. 1958). The locality rule is also followed in the following jurisdictions: Illinois: Livengood v. Howard, 11 Ill. App. 3d 1, 295 N.E.2d 736

Statewide standard. This standard is employed by relatively few jurisdictions. In an Arizona case, the court held that a physician must possess that degree of care and skill possessed and exercised by specialists of good standing in the same speciality throughout the state pursuant to a new malpractice statute.[3] However, there is case law to the contrary in Arizona. In another case, the court held that "the standard of care to be established by the expert testimony is nationwide for specialists and a local one for general practitioners."[4] There may be one other state that follows the statewide rule—Connecticut.[5]

Same or similar community standard. This is a variation of the locality rule, and holds that a physician may testify if he or she is familiar with, and can testify to, the standard of the same or similar community.[6]

(1973); Kentucky: Knapp v. Thornton, 199 Ky. 216, 250 S.W. 853 (1923); Mississippi: Dazet v. Bass, 254 So. 2d 183 (Miss. 1971) (gynecological malpractice); New York: Toth v. Community Hosp., 22 N.Y.2d 255, 229 N.E.2d 368, 292 N.Y.S.2d 440 (1968) (pediatric malpractice case); Oregon: Malila v. Mecham, 187 Or. 330, 211 P.2d 747 (1949); Vermont: Rann v. Twitchell, 82 Vt. 79, 71 A.1045 (1909). In a Washington case, the court announced an unusual hybrid. It stated:

> [A] qualified medical practitioner is held to the standard of care and skill which is expected of the average practitioner in the class to which he belongs, acting in the same or similar circumstances, in an area coextensive with the medical and professional means available in those centers that are readily accessible for appropriate treatment of the patient.

Pederson v. Dumouchel, 72 Wash. 2d 73, 431 P.2d 973, 978 (1967); *see also* Campbell v. Oliva, 424 F.2d 1244 (6th Cir. 1970).

[3] Gaston v. Hunter, 121 Ariz. 33, 588 P.2d 326, 346 (1978).

[4] Pollard v. Goldsmith, 117 Ariz. 363, 572 P.2d 1201, 1203 (1977).

[5] Katsetos v. Nolan, 170 Conn. 637, 368 A.2d 172 (1976).

[6] Poulin v. Zartman, 542 P.2d 251 (Alaska 1975), *on reh'g,* 548 P.2d 1299 (Alaska 1976); Jeanes v. Milner, 428 F.2d 598 (8th Cir. 1970); *but see* Rickett v. Hayes, 256 Ark. 893, 511 S.W.2d 187 (1974), (in which an oral surgeon was held to the standards of the profession generally and not to those of any geographical area); Carmichael v. Reitz, 17 Cal. App. 3d 958, 95 Cal. Rptr. 381 (1971). However, in another California obstetrical case, the court held, "[O]ne who holds himself out as a specialist owes to his patients a duty of possessing that degree of learning and skill ordinarily possessed by specialists of good standing practicing in the same special field and in the same locality and under similar circumstances." Valentine v. Kaiser Found. Hosp., 194 Cal. App. 2d 282, 15 Cal. Rptr. 26 (1961), *disapproved on other grounds sub nom.* Siverson v. Weber, 57 Cal. 2d 834, 372 P.2d 97, 22 Cal. Rptr. 337 (1962). Florida, although using the same community standard in some cases, uses the same or similar community in others. In Schwab v. Tolley, 345 So. 2d 747 (Fla. Dist. Ct. App. 1977), the court held that a specialist must possess and exercise "the skill and diligence of the average practitioner in the same or a similar community." Speer v. United States, 512 F. Supp. 670 (N.D. Tex.), *aff'd,* 675 F.2d 100 (5th Cir. 1981); *but see* Karp v. Colley, 493 F.2d 408 (5th Cir.), *reh'g denied,* 496 F.2d 878 (5th Cir), *cert. denied,* 419 U.S. 845 (1974) (applying nationwide standard); Werster v. Caylor, 231 Ind. 625, 110 N.E.2d 337 (1953), *disapproved on other grounds sub nom.* New York City & SLR v. Henderson, 237 Ind. 456, 146 N.E.2d 531 (1957), *reh'g denied,* 237 Ind. 494, 147 N.E.2d 237 (1958); Halligan v. Cotton, 193 Neb. 331, 227

Nationwide standard of care. This standard of care is a much more liberal rule. With the nationwide standard of care, an expert may testify that the standard is the same throughout the nation and that anyone in the nation in that specialty should be familiar with and meet the standard. A typical definition is that a specialist must exercise the same degree of care, skill, and diligence that a similar specialist in the medical community would exercise in a similar case.[7] In a dental case, an oral surgeon was held to the standard of the profession generally, and not to that of any geographical area.[8] This is clearly the trend.

Minimum fundamental standard of care. There is also a feeling among plaintiff malpractice lawyers that this other category should apply. The expert testifies that any physician would realize that to conduct oneself as the defendant did is a violation of the minimum fundamental standard of care. This is the most liberal rule; an attempt to utilize this standard should be employed in any appropriate case.

N.W.2d 10 (1975); Pharmaseal Lab., Inc. v. Goff, 90 N.M. 753, 568 P.2d 589 (1977); Koury v. Follo, 272 N.C. 366, 158 S.E.2d 548 (1968) (pediatric malpractice case); Belk v. Schweizer, 268 N.C. 50, 149 S.E.2d 565 (1966) (OB-GYN case); Runyon v. Reed, 510 P.2d 943 (Okla. 1973), *but see* Karriman v. Orthopedic Clinic, 516 P.2d 534 (Okla. 1973) (applying nationwide standards); Cavallaro v. Sharp, 84 R.I. 67, 121 A.2d 669 (1956); Brownwell v. Williams, 597 S.W.2d 542 (Tex. Civ. App. 1980); Swan v. Lamb, 584 P.2d 814 (Utah 1978) stating that physicians "who profess to be experts in the field of surgery or medicine are held to the standard of care exercised by experts in the same field in cities of comparable size throughout the medical profession." Hinkle v. Martin, 286 S.E.2d 768 (W. Va. 1979); *but see* Hundley v. Martinez, 151 W. Va. 977, 158 S.E.2d 159 (1967) (applying the nationwide standard).

[7] Early v. Noblin, 380 So. 2d 272 (Ala. 1980).

[8] Rickett v. Hayes, 256 Ark. 893, 511 S.W.2d 187 (1974); "A specialist must exercise that degree of care and skill expected of reasonably competent practitioners in their specialty acting in the same or similar circumstances nationwide." Robbins v. Footer, 553 F.2d 123 (D.C. Cir. 1977); Karp v. Colley, 493 F.2d 408 (5th Cir), *reh'g denied,* 496 F.2d 878 (5th Cir.), *cert denied,* 419 U.S. 845 (1974); McPhee v. Reichel, 461 F.2d 947 (3d Cir. 1972) (obstetrical malpractice); Alexandris v. Jewett, 388 F.2d 829 (1st Cir. 1968) (obstetrical malpractice case); Perin v. Hayne, 210 N.W.2d 609 (Iowa 1973); Simpson v. Davis, 219 Kan. 584, 549 P.2d 950 (1976); Steele v. St. Paul Fire & Marine Ins. Co., 371 So. 2d 843 (La. Ct. App. 1979), *cert denied,* 374 So. 2d 658 (La. 1979) (obstetrical malpractice); Roberts v. Tardif, 417 A.2d 444 (Me. 1980) (obstetrical malpractice case); Shilkret v. Annapolis Emergency Hosp. Ass'n, 276 Md. 187, 349 A.2d 245 (1975) (obstetrical malpractice case); Brune v. Belinkoff, 354 Mass. 102, 235 N.E.2d 793 (1968) (obstetrical malpractice case); Gilmore v. O'Sullivan, 106 Mich. App. 35, 307 N.W.2d 695 (1981); McCollough v. Hutzel Hosp., 88 Mich. App. 235, 267 N.W.2d 569 (1979) (both obstetrical malpractice); Christy v. Faliterman, 288 Minn. 144, 179 N.W.2d 288 (1970); Hart v. Steele, 416 S.W.2d 927 (Mo. 1967); Orcutt v. Miller, 595 P.2d 1191 (Nev. 1979); Fernandez v. Baruch, 52 N.J. 127 244 A.2d 109 (1968); Bruni v. Tatsumi, 46 Ohio St. 2d 127, 346 N.E.2d 673 (1976); Karriman v. Orthopedic Clinic, 516 P.2d 534 (Okla. 1973); Pratt v. Stein, 298 Pa. Super. 92, 444 A.2d 674 (1982); Morrison v. McKillop, 17 Wash. App. 396, 563 P.2d 220 (1977); Shier v. Freedman, 58 Wis. 2d 269, 206 N.W.2d 166, *modified on other grounds & reh'g denied,* 58 Wis. 2d 269, 208 N.W.2d 328 (1973).

§ 1.9 Initial Medical Review

The initial medical review is completed by the person best qualified to do so. If a physician is available, the physician should do it. If a nurse is available, the nurse should do it. If there is no physician or nurse available, the attorney who is handling the case may be able to do the initial review. However, it takes a great deal of experience for an attorney without medical training to be able to do the review. It is preferable to have someone who is medically trained dissect the file. There are medicolegal services that can evaluate the case.[9] The better practice is to find a physician that will consult.

Under no circumstances should the case be pursued without a medical review by someone competent to do so. Frivolous litigation is wrong and must not be undertaken for moral, ethical, and legal reasons. It is not enough to be ignorant of the facts and hide behind that ignorance. The filing of a lawsuit is an emotional experience for the defendant. There must be probable cause to believe that negligence occurred and resulted in damages. Things are not always what they seem to be. A detailed investigation must be done without question in every case.

§ 1.10 Liability

Whether there is liability—part of the two-pronged test of liability and damages—may or may not be determinable in the investigation initial phase. Some cases are clear, and clarity increases as the knowledge of the attorney grows. A basic caveat for all attorneys undertaking the representation of a client in an obstetrical or neonatal case is that the attorney should be very conservative. Do not think that every case is meritorious. In fact, most cases are not meritorious.

If after the initial medical review there is a finding that there probably was negligence, counsel can begin the case. Many lawyers want a report in their files signed by a physician before they begin a case. This is certainly advisable, especially if counsel does not have access to medicolegal help on a routine basis.

Not only must there be liability, but there must also be sufficient damages. Follow the axiom of *de minimis non curat lex*.[10] Medical malpractice cases without substantial damages cannot be litigated. Often, counsel has to advance litigation expenses as well as take a contingency. Small cases result in either losses for the attorney or small rewards. More importantly, clients are not happy with small recoveries.

---

[9] See § 2.2.

[10] "The law does not care for, or take notice of, very small or trifling matters." Black's Law Dictionary 431 (6th ed. 1990).

There is no way to formulate a rule on liability for all cases. The ability to determine whether there is liability comes from experience, the medical review, and a thorough knowledge of the facts. Without these things, there can be no discussion of liability.

§ 1.11 Determining Damages

Litigation expenses can range from $5,000 to more than $100,000. Each attorney has to decide on the minimum value for any case they will litigate. Most experienced medical malpractice lawyers will not litigate any case unless the damages are very substantial. Unfortunately, there is no way to compensate adequately patients who have either had a bad result from medical treatment that was not negligence or have a small claim.

When a client is first interviewed and the initial information is gathered, an analysis should be made of medical bills, out-of-pocket expenses, lost wages, future lost wages, and so forth. This does not have to be done initially by an economist and does not have to be precise. However, an approximate figure should be calculated to determine whether the damages are sufficient to litigate the claim.

§ 1.12 Notice of Claim to the Defendant

Some states require notice to a defendant. A review of the case law before suit is filed is important.

Affording physicians time before litigation to have their carriers evaluate the claim to determine whether settlement discussions will take place is a fine idea. A claim against a professional should be approached in a professional manner. The defendant should be given an opportunity to discuss the claim with the carrier before litigation. Although claims are infrequently settled before suit, counsel can file litigation knowing that a professional approach to resolving the dispute was attempted. Litigation should never be undertaken with any attitude other than a desire to compensate the plaintiff fairly and reasonably. Do not allow clients to vent anger and frustration through the lawsuit, using the attorney as a tool. An approach whereby a physician has 30 or 60 days to discuss the claim with the carrier is appropriate in many circumstances, providing that the statute of limitations is not a problem.

If the physician will be contacted prior to filing suit, a letter should be sent to the physician, by certified mail with return receipt requested, and to the physician's carrier. A sample letter is reproduced in **Appendix 1–5.**

§ 1.13　Attorney as Defendant: Countersuits
by Doctors

In some states, if a malpractice claim is filed and lost or if the case is dismissed, the attorney may be a defendant in an action based upon the filing of a frivolous lawsuit.[11] It is unfortunate that some states do allow countersuits. Disputes should be settled in a courtroom rather than in an alley.

Countersuits are often filed in cases wherein the wrong defendant was sued, there was absolutely no medical evaluation before filing, and the like.

Courts have normally held that unless there are special damages,[12] a defendant in a prior action cannot institute litigation for malicious prosecution or abuse of process.[13] Injury to professional reputation does not give rise to special damages.[14] Moreover, "mere termination of a lawsuit in favor of an adverse party does not mean there was a want of probable cause to believe on a set of stated facts that cause of action did exist."[15]

An attorney should not be intimidated by defense lawyers, insurance carriers, or defendant physicians who state that they are going to file a countersuit. The attorney should do what is right and ethical.

---

[11] The cases have been collected in an excellent annotation entitled *Medical Malpractice Countersuits,* 84 A.L.R.3d 555 (1978). The states that have allowed countersuits are the following: Illinois in 1976 allowed an action in which a physician recovered compensatory and punitive damages, alleging that a lawsuit was filed against the physician and that the attorneys filing it had violated their duty to refrain from willfully and wantonly bringing suit against a person by involving that person in litigation without reasonable cause. Annotated, 84 A.L.R.3d 560. In Nevada, a physician recovered $35,000 compensatory damages and $50,000 punitive damages in a countersuit, alleging that the original malpractice claim was frivolous and that no proper investigation of the merits of the cause of action had been carried out. *Id.* In a Kansas case, a physician was held to state a cause of action for malicious prosecution wherein the physician alleged that the defendant attorney initiated and continued a malpractice case without probable cause and with malice. The case terminated in the physician's favor and the court held that a cause of action was stated. Annotated, 84 A.L.R.3d 46 (1984). A Kentucky court allowed a cause of action for malicious prosecution and the recovery of damages for humiliation, mortification, and loss of reputation. *Id.* Michigan probably would allow a countersuit if it were shown that an attorney had no probable cause to file and continue malpractice litigation. *Id.*

[12] *Special damages* are defined as including an arrest of the person or seizure of property. Dakters v. Shane, 64 Ohio App. 2d 168, 412 N.E.2d 399 (1978).

[13] Annotation, 84 A.L.R.3d 555.

[14] *Id.*

[15] *Id.* at 47.

§ 1.14 Appendix 1–1: Authority to Release Medical or Hospital Records

To:

PATIENT:

PATIENT NUMBER:

ADDRESS:

You are hereby authorized to furnish and release to _____ all information and records requested concerning findings, treatment rendered, and opinions as to my condition. Please do not disclose information to insurance adjusters or other persons without written authority from me. This authority will continue in force until revoked by me in writing. A copy of this authorization is as valid as the original. The purpose of this authorization is for _____ to review and inspect my records so that I may be advised concerning my legal rights.

I hereby give permission to copy, view, photograph, or photostat all of the hospital or office notes and information, including laboratory tests and X-rays, and the receipt of any and all information you have concerning my physical and mental condition, including histories, examinations, tests, treatment, consultations, and opinions and any and all other information available.

Date:

_____
Patient with authority to act for minor; or, if deceased, legal representative

§ 1.15 Appendix 1–2: Medical History Form

PRENATAL RECORD

Hospital					Date	
Pts. Name	Age	Race	Relig.	Country of Birth		Insurance
Address	Phone	Marital Status S M W D Sep.		Years Married		
Name of Father of Child	Age	Ht.	Wt.	Significant disease		
Business Address		Business Phone		Occupation		

FAMILY HISTORY: (Tbc, Hypertension, Heart D., Diabetes, Neuro-Psych., Epilepsy, Allergies, Mult. Births, Congenital Anom.)

MENSTRUAL HISTORY: Onset at		Yrs.	Interval		Days	Duration		Days	Amt.
Months Preg. Attempted	L.M.P.			Normal?			E.D.C.		

PRIOR MEDICAL HISTORY	√ Pos.	Remarks (Include date and time of Rx)	HISTORY SINCE LAST MENSTRUAL PERIOD	√ Pos.	Remarks (Include date and time of Rx)
Kidney Disease			Nausea		
Heart Disease			Vomiting		
Hypertension			Indigestion		
Rheumatic Fever			Constipation		
Tuberculosis			Headache		
Venereal Disease			Bleeding (Specify)		
Gyn. Disorder			Vaginal Discharge		
German Measles			Edema		
Nervous & Mental			Abdominal Pain		
Diabetes			Urinary Complaints		
Thyroid Dysfunction			German Measles		
Phlebitis, Varicosities			Other Virus		
Epilepsy			Radiation (Specify)		
Drug Sensitivity			Accidents		
Allergies			Medications		
Blood Dyscrasia					
Blood Transfusions					
Rh, ABO Sensitivity					
Operations, Accidents					

SUMMARY OF PREVIOUS PREGNANCIES			Full Term		Premature		Abortions			Now Alive		Mult. Births
No.	Year	Place of Confinement	Dur. of Gestation	Dur. of Labor	Type of Delivery	Born A or D	Weight	Maternal		Complications	Child	

Patient's Name: _____ Date of Birth: _____

PHYSICAL EXAMINATION

T.	P.	R.	B.P.	Hgt.	Pres. Wt.	Wt. at L.M.P.

Eyes	Teeth	Thyroid	Throat	Skin

Heart

Lungs

Breasts	Nipples	Tumors

Abdomen   Height of Fundus

Fetal Heart   Presentation and Position

Extremities   Varicosities   Edema

General Body Type

PELVIC EXAMINATION (bi-manual and speculum):

Vulva

Vagina

Perineum

Cervix

Uterus

Adnexae

Rectal Exam.

Diag. Conj.	cm.	Trans. Diam. Outlet	cm.	Shape Sacrum

Arch   Coccyx   S.-S. notch

Ischial Spines

Inlet:	Mid Pelvis:	Outlet:	Prognosis for Delivery:
☐ Adequate	☐ Adequate	☐ Adequate	
☐ Borderline	☐ Borderline	☐ Borderline	
☐ Contracted	☐ Contracted	☐ Contracted	

DATE OF LABORATORY EXAMINATION	FOR SYPHILIS	TYPE	RESULTS
Blood Type and Rh: Patient	Father of Child		
Hemoglobin	Hematocrit or RBC		
Antibody Screen #1	Antibody Screen #2		
Rubella Titer			

Pap Smear:

FACTS OF SPECIAL IMPORTANCE:

Initial Over-all Evaluation of Patient

Sensitivities	Nutritional Status
Type of Del. planned	Anesthesia planned
Physician to call if attending M.D. not available	
M.D. who will attend infant	Is breast feeding planned?
Date	Signed

Name							Hosp.										Hosp. No.		Office No.	

SUBSEQUENT PRENATAL VISITS

Date	Headache	Dizziness	Edema	Nausea & Vomiting	Bleeding	Blood Pressure	Weight	Ht. of Fundus	Position & Presentation	Fetal heart	Albumin	Sugar	Hct.	Weeks	Rx and Remarks	Initials

SYMPTOMS / *Urine* / Ht. Wt. at L.M.P.

Date	Progress Notes & Consultation	Date	Progress Notes & Consultation
Date	Signed		

§ 1.16 Appendix 1–3: Ultrasound Report

An ultrasound report can be useful to counsel, as explained in §§ **1.4**, **1.6**, and **1.7**.

FIRST TRIMESTER STAGE I OBSTETRIC ULTRASOUND REPORT

PATIENT NAME: _____ PATIENT I.D. NO. _____

EXAM DATE: ☐☐ ☐☐ ☐☐   LMP DATE: ☐☐ ☐☐ ☐☐   ☐ UNKNOWN
MO. DAY YEAR   MO. DAY YEAR

SMOKER: ☐ YES ☐ NO

PATIENT AGE: ☐ YRS   RACE: ☐   HEIGHT: ☐ ft. ☐ in.   WEIGHT: ☐ lbs.   G ☐ P ☐☐☐☐
                                                                              F P A L

INDICATION CODE NUMBER: ☐

ESTIMATED CLINICAL DATES: ☐ WEEKS

PREGNANCY LOCATION: ☐ INTRAUTERINE   ☐ ECTOPIC   ☐ UNCERTAIN

FETAL NUMBER: ☐   GESTATIONAL SAC NUMBER: ☐

FETAL ACTIVITY: ☐ HEART   ☐ BODY   ☐ BOTH   ☐ NEITHER

CROWN-RUMP LENGTH: ☐ CENTIMETERS

PELVIC MASS: ☐ NO   ☐ YES (DESCRIBE): _____

_____

UTERUS ANOMALY OR PATHOLOGY: ☐ NO   ☐ YES (DESCRIBE): _____

_____

EXAMINATION TECHNICAL QUALITY: ☐ GOOD   ☐ FAIR   ☐ POOR

ULTRASOUND GESTATIONAL AGE ESTIMATE (WEEKS): ☐

REMARKS: _____

_____

_____
SIGNATURE OF RESPONSIBLE PHYSICIAN

Reprinted with permission of Advanced Technology Laboratories, Inc.

SECOND AND THIRD TRIMESTER STAGE I OBSTETRICAL ULTRASOUND REPORT

PATIENT NAME _____

                                         ☐ INITIAL EXAM

PATIENT I.D. NO _____   ☐ REPEAT EXAM

EXAM DATE: [MO | DAY | YEAR]   LMP DATE: [MO | DAY | YEAR]   UNKNOWN ☐

SMOKER: ☐ YES ☐ NO

PATIENT AGE: [ ] YRS   RACE: [ ]   HEIGHT: [ ] ft. [ ] in.   WEIGHT: [ ] lbs.   G [ ] P [| | |]
                                                                 F   P   A   L

INDICATION CODE NUMBER: [ ]

ESTIMATED CLINICAL DATES: [ ] WEEKS

DESCRIPTIVE DATA SECTION

THE FETUS

Number: ☐ 1 ☐ 2 ☐ 3
Presentation: ☐ VTX ☐ BREECH
            ☐ Transverse ☐ Other

Activity: ☐ Heart ☐ Body
        ☐ Breathing

Gender: ☐ Male ☐ Female
        ☐ Unknown

PELVIC MASS

☐ None Seen
☐ Present (Describe): _____
_____
_____

THE PLACENTA

Location: ☐ Anterior   ☐ Posterior
           ☐ R Lateral   ☐ L Lateral

Height: ☐ Fundal   ☐ High
          ☐ Mid   ☐ Low
          ☐ Marginal Previa
          ☐ Partial Previa
          ☐ Complete Previa

Grade 3: ☐ No   ☐ Yes

UTERUS PATHOLOGY

☐ None Seen
☐ Present (Describe): _____
_____
_____

AMNIOTIC FLUID AMOUNT

☐ Normal
☐ Increased
☐ Decreased

EXAM TECHNICAL QUALITY

☐ Good   ☐ Fair   ☐ Poor

FETAL BLADDER/KIDNEYS

☐ Bladder Only Seen
☐ Kidneys Only Seen
☐ Both Seen
☐ Neither Seen

Abnormal fetal anatomy seen or suspected: ☐ No   ☐ Yes (Describe): _____
Second opinion ultrasound consultation planned: ☐ No   ☐ Yes

MEASUREMENT AND CALCULATION SECTION

BPD [ ] cms   OFD [ ] cms   A-PAD [ ] cms   TAD [ ] cms   FEMUR [ ] cms

Head Circumference [ ] cms   Abdominal Circumference [ ] cms

RESULTS AND INTERPRETATION SECTION

ULTRASOUND AGE ESTIMATE

BPD Weeks = [ ]
Femur Weeks = [ ]
ABD Circ Weeks = [ ]
Head Circ Weeks = [ ]
Average Estimated Gestational Age = [ ]

ULTRASOUND FETAL WEIGHT ESTIMATE

[ ] grams

[ ] lbs/oz

RATIOS

Cephalic Index = [ ] %
Femur/BPD = [ ] %
Head Circ/ Abd. Circ = [ ] %

REMARKS: _____

GESTATIONAL AGE

☐   Good Clinical Dates   ☐ Poor Clinical Dates

WEIGHT FOR DATES

☐ AGA   ☐ LGA   ☐ SGA

_____
Signature of Responsible Physician

1983 ADVANCED TECHNOLOGY LABORATORIES, INC.   C-3182   PRINTED IN USA   9-83

§ 1.17   Appendix 1–4: Sample Report of a C-Section

PATIENT NAME: DATE:

CASE NO.:

SURGEON: ASSISTANT:

OPERATION: Primary Low Transverse C-Section

SPONGE COUNT: Correct

PREOPERATIVE DIAGNOSIS: Failure to progress, with fetal distress.

POSTOPERATIVE DIAGNOSIS: Same

PROCEDURE: The patient was taken to the operating room and placed in the supine position, whereafter the abdomen was prepped and draped in the usual antiseptic fashion, general anesthesia was induced with an endotracheal tube. Following this, a transverse skin incision was made. The fascia was entered sharply, and the fascial incision extended inferiorly and superiorly. The midline was identified. The peritoneum was easily entered. Following this the lower uterine segment was incised, and a low cervical transverse cesarean section was done with delivery of a meconium-stained male infant. The patient was given initial 1 minute Apgar of 5/5 by the pediatrician, Dr. _____, who was in attendance. Following this, the appropriate cord specimen was collected, and the placenta was manually removed. The uterus was explored, and all loose fragments of membrane were removed. The uterine incision itself was closed in two layers with 0 chromic with adequate hemostasis resulting. The peritoneum was closed with 00 chromic. Both tubes and ovaries appeared to be normal, and all, as much as possible, of the loose clot and blood was removed. The anterior peritoneum was closed with 00 chromic, and the fascia was closed with a running, alternating, interlocking of 0 Vicryl. The subcu was approximated with 000 Dexon, and a subcuticular stitch was done with this same suture.

The patient tolerated the procedure well, and was taken to the recovery room alert, awake, with stable vital signs. Estimated blood loss 600 c.c.

§ 1.18   Appendix 1–5: Sample Claim Letter

Dear Dr. _____:

I have been retained by [_____ or the family of _____] to investigate the medical care afforded to [her or their] child.

I want to give you an opportunity to discuss this claim with your insurance carrier and private attorney, or if uninsured, with your attorney.

We are both professionals and should attempt to resolve this dispute in a professional manner.

I would like to have the opportunity to discuss this claim with your insurance company and private attorney or your attorney if you have no insurance.

I would appreciate your response to this letter or the response of your representative. If I do not hear from you or your representative within 30 days, litigation will be commenced.

_____
Signature of attorney

CHAPTER 2

STANDARD MEDICAL RESEARCH TECHNIQUES

Michael D. Volk

§ 2.1 Introduction

Medical malpractice litigation cannot be undertaken unless counsel is prepared to engage in significant amounts of medical research.[1] As in all litigation that has scientific or technical aspects, a thorough knowledge of the subject matter is mandatory.[2] An attorney must not approach this type of litigation without understanding that a great deal of hard work and insightful knowledge of the subject is necessary. This chapter points counsel in the right direction for researching medical techniques.

---

[1] Firestone, *The Physician-Attorney as Co-Counsel,* 20 Trial No. 5, at 77 (May 1984).

[2] Smith, *Medical Malpractice Trial Techniques,* ATLA Masters at Work 385 (1984); Volk, *Cross-Examination of the Medical Expert,* 16 Trial No. 5, at 43 (May 1980).

§ 2.2   Attorney Evaluation Without Assistance

For the attorney who has no experience, or minimal experience, in medicolegal litigation, several questions must be answered at the outset of the case. One of the first questions is how counsel is equipped to handle medical malpractice litigation. An attorney with medical training possesses certain skills that can be valuable, but medical training does not automatically turn an attorney into a medical malpractice litigator. Many fine attorneys without medical training are excellent malpractice lawyers; some attorneys with medical training are not good malpractice lawyers. However, the vast majority of medically trained attorneys, whether doctors or nurses, do reasonably well in medicolegal litigation. The most important factors are a desire to work hard, an understanding of the case and the surrounding operative facts, a genuine desire to assist the client, and the ability to communicate.

Another question is what resources counsel can draw upon to assist in the case, including whether any members of the office staff have medical training, or whether there is a friendly nurse or physician available to assist in putting the case together. The attorney who has no experience in medicolegal litigation, who handles a medical malpractice case very infrequently, and who has no resources to draw upon should seriously consider referring the case or associating an attorney that has medicolegal experience.[3] The client will be best served and the result will probably be far better than if the inexperienced attorney with no resources to draw upon or who only infrequently handles this type of litigation attempts to represent the client alone.

However, an attorney without a medical background can start with certain steps that can be accomplished rather painlessly and inexpensively. Familiarity with a medical library is one of the first steps. Counsel should begin building a medical library in the office and gain access to a nearby, complete medical library.[4] Medical schools or nursing schools usually have fairly comprehensive libraries that can be utilized under most circumstances. A few days in a library reviewing standard texts and journals in obstetrics and neonatology is worthwhile. Note cards can be used to list the textbooks, monographs, and journals available in obstetrics and neonatology. The note cards will be valuable when marshaling the medical literature for a case. Initial screening that is ineffective is the cause of most frivolous malpractice claims.[5] Counsel must be prepared and able to advise *against* litigation if the case is not meritorious.[6] However, the attorney must thoroughly review the case because the "crippled case," as described by Melvin Belli,[7] may not be so crippled after an exhaustive analysis

---

[3] Smith, *Medical Malpractice Trial Techniques,* ATLA Masters at Work 385 (1984).

[4] D. Tennenhouse, Attorneys Medical Deskbook §§ 63–64 (1983).

[5] Richards & Rathbun, *Effective Initial Screening,* 16 Trial No. 5, at 45 (May 1980).

[6] M. Belli, Modern Trial 2d § 3.1 (1982).

[7] *Id.* § 3.21.

of the facts. Conversely, what may seem to the inexperienced malpractice litigator as a meritorious case may prove to be completely nonmeritorious once an in-depth analysis is done. All that glitters is definitely not gold.

Befriending an attorney with significant medical malpractice experience can also be most helpful, although attorneys are wary of other attorneys who always want free advice. The proper way is to associate with experienced counsel in the first few cases so that the client is served and the inexperienced attorney begins to learn. This is a system that can work very well while not harming the client. However, many experienced attorneys want the entire case referred to them, with no interference by the referring lawyer. There is a good argument that experienced counsel do not need to educate any lawyer with a case to refer. An inexperienced attorney who litigates a medical malpractice case with a poor result, because the attorney has done a poor job, invites a legal malpractice case.

One source for contacting lawyers who have handled cases similar to the one being investigated is the Association of Trial Lawyers of America (ATLA) Exchange Service. The address is 1050 31st Street NW, Washington, D.C. 20007, and the phone number is 1-800-424-2725. For a nominal fee, the ATLA Exchange Service will send addresses of other attorneys who have handled similar cases and will do some basic research. Computer research can also be obtained and paid for through the ATLA Exchange Service.

The inexperienced attorney must begin to read medicolegal literature. This can be a frustrating experience for the neophyte but is a valuable source of information, both baseline and specific. The beginner must not expect to understand everything or, at the beginning, much of anything. Counsel should merely attempt to absorb the material, without becoming upset if the medical terminology and concepts are foreign. One should remember the first few weeks in law school when the legal terminology and cases were just as confusing but were eventually mastered.

Probably the best way for the inexperienced attorney to learn is to attend seminars on medicolegal issues and medical malpractice whenever possible. Counsel should contact the American College of Legal Medicine at Suite 412, 213 W. Institute Place, Chicago, Illinois 60610, for a listing of seminars to be held in the future. The American Society of Law and Medicine at 765 Commonwealth Avenue, 16th Floor, Boston, Massachusetts 02215, should also be contacted, as well as ATLA at the address noted above and the appropriate state trial lawyers organization. For those attorneys who are experienced in medical malpractice, particularly in obstetrical and neonatal cases, the above information also holds true.

One must always recognize limitations. Those cases that are evaluated without medical assistance should be very few and far between. This is not to imply that the experienced medicolegal litigator cannot understand whether a case is meritorious, but only that there are certain complex facts to put in the proper perspective in nearly every case that will require the intervention of a medically trained person. Of course, all litigators in obstetrical and neonatal cases must constantly search for new sources of information.

§ 2.3 Medicolegal Services

Many medicolegal services will review records and the other facts of a case as well as assist in discovery. These services, for a fee, will point counsel in the right direction as well as obtain witnesses to testify. There is absolutely nothing wrong with asking for a list of references from attorneys who have used the service or checking out an expert provided by a medicolegal service. A request for the curriculum vitae or biographical information on any witness is certainly proper. Some of these services are very reputable and some are not. One should inquire as to the following:

1. A list of references of other attorneys
2. A list of charges up front for the services rendered
3. What portion of the charges goes to the expert (some medicolegal services pay only a small percentage to the expert and keep the remainder)
4. A copy of any and all advertisements that have been used for their benefit
5. Whether their experts will travel
6. A curriculum vitae of the expert.

There is nothing wrong with the concept of the medicolegal service. However, some unscrupulous operators have kept the vast majority of any fees charged and paid the physician a small portion. This is unfair to the witness and the witness who finds out will be extremely upset.

Some defense lawyers attempt to impeach a witness whose name is given to plaintiff's counsel by a medicolegal service. The questions often asked are: "Are you affiliated with a medical malpractice referral service? Do you accept referrals from a company that obtains medical experts to testify against other doctors? Have you listed your name with a service that advertises for doctors to testify against other doctors?" The important thing is that the witness be well trained, honest, and respected in his or her field, not how the expert's name was obtained by the plaintiff's counsel.

§ 2.4 Computerized Medical Research

The explosion of computer use in modern-day society has also affected medico-legal work. The ability to scan a data bank with thousands of medical subjects, articles, and authors has greatly reduced the amount of time an attorney needs to spend doing medical research. What used to take many hours can now be done by a computer in minutes.

However, computer application to medical research must be approached in the proper manner. The attorney should ask the question: "What is the goal to be reached from the computer research?" Normally, the goal desired is the gathering of medical literature pertinent to the case in point. For instance, in an obstetrical case which concerns the use of pitocin (a drug to strengthen contractions, which is sometimes used to induce labor), a computer search can determine, during the applicable time period, what the medical journals are saying about the use of the drug.

There are basically two ways to search the pertinent medical literature. The first is an author's search. Often, plaintiffs' attorneys will want to check the defendants on the computer to determine whether they have ever written any articles prior to deposing the witness. Those articles can then be obtained and investigated for cross-examination. Attorneys can also use the computer to examine all the articles written by their own experts. More importantly, attorneys can check their opponents' experts on the computer to provide ammunition for cross-examination.

The second method of searching is the subject search. The subject search allows the gathering of medical references on any subject that the computer holds. For example, entering "pitocin" on the computer will obtain a reference for every time the word "pitocin" is mentioned in an article. Of course, the references often will not be helpful, but they have to be sifted through to find the ones that are important to the case. A key word such as "pitocin" is needed for the computer to search the articles.

Most computer services provide foreign medical citations, as well as citations in English, and normally those are difficult to obtain. However, most printouts also indicate if the article is in English or if there is an English abstract to the article.

It is very important that the attorney be selective and prepare the search before running it on a computer and even before logging onto a computer service. One should not use a computer just for the thrill of using it. It is necessary to define what is wanted succinctly.

One valuable use of the computer is to help determine whether a case is meritorious. If the overwhelming majority of the medical literature is against the plaintiff, there is a good chance that the plaintiff will have trouble obtaining expert testimony to support a violation of the standard of care. The standard of care is defined then, in part, by the medical literature.

Any articles that are obtained through computer research should be set up in a filing system for future use.

§ 2.5 —Computer Services

Various computer services can be utilized to do medical research. The National Library of Medicine is located at the Department of Health and Human Services,

National Institute of Health, 8600 Rockville Pike, Bethesda, Maryland 20209. Under some circumstances, a user can get on-line with this computer, but it is relatively difficult to use. It is necessary to be schooled in computer use to be able to utilize the National Library of Medicine data banks.

An alternative is to go to a medical school library and use the National Library of Medicine system.[8] For a small fee, the computer operator can search for the requested information.[9] The Medline system contains the three most recent years of medical literature and is updated monthly. A Medline search is utilized if counsel wants to find out what the current medical data and thought on a subject are. Medlars is the data base that has medical information from 1966 up to the three most recent years, which would, of course, be available through Medline.

Any personal computer with a modem, whether at home or at the office, can also access the data banks. This is a proprietary system. The rates fluctuate depending on the service and time of day but generally are very reasonable. After an hour or two of practice, one can become relatively proficient in the use of the service. These data banks generally cover the same period of time as Medline and Medlars, that is, back to 1966. It can be utilized with an author or term search, and the data banks are being expanded rapidly.

§ 2.6 Standard Journals

There are some standard medical journals with which counsel should become familiar.[10] This does not mean that every issue of every journal has to be read cover-to-cover, but the attorney should be familiar with and use them as sources of information when working on a case, both for direct evidence and for impeachment. Three types of journals are discussed in this section.

First there are the obstetrical journals. Most of these journals should be obtainable at any medical school or nursing school, or from most practitioners. An excellent obstetrical journal to begin with is the *American Journal of Obstetrics and Gynecology.* This is certainly one of the standard journals in the area and covers a wide range of topics. Another standard journal is *Obstetrics and Gynecology.* The *Journal of Reproductive Medicine* also has many topics that are of interest to the medicolegal practitioner. Many physicians in the United States recognize the authority of the *British Journal of Obstetrics and Gynecology.* There are several journals that deal with perinatology, or the study of the perinatal period. The best known of these are *Clinics in Perinatology* and *Seminars in Perinatology. Contemporary Obstetrics-Gynecology* is also an excellent journal. Some lesser-used journals are *Gynecologic and Obstetric*

---

[8] D. Tennenhouse, Attorneys Medical Deskbook § 62 (1983).

[9] Volk, *Cross-Examination of the Medical Expert,* 16 Trial No. 5, at 43 (May 1980).

[10] Smith, *Medical Malpractice Trial Techniques,* ATLA Masters at Work 386 (1984).

Investigation, Obstetrics and Gynecological Survey, and *Surgery—Gynecology and Obstetrics.* The *Journal of Nurse-Midwifery* is a journal that should be used when investigating a case against a registered nurse or certified nurse midwife.

In the areas of neonatology, counsel can obtain information in *Seminars in Perinatology* and *Clinics in Perinatology.* Attorneys should also be familiar with the journals entitled *American Journal of Diseases of Children, Pediatrics, Pediatric Annals, Current Problems in Pediatrics, Archives of Disease in Childhood,* and *Clinical Pediatrics.*

The last group of journals concerns the neurological condition of the neonate, development of the neonate, and the rehabilitation of an ill neonate and child. The journals *Human Genetics* and *Medical Genetics* offer information on congenital anomalies. The journals *Brain* and *Developmental Medicine and Child Neurology* deal with the neurological aspects of the child. The journals *Child Development* and the *Journal of Rehabilitation* discuss, in part, the rehabilitation of the child.

All of these journals are excellent; however, one cannot read everything in every journal. The journals must be scanned for articles pertinent to a particular case or for background information. Most physicians will testify that by the time textbooks are published they are out of date. While this is not altogether true, the admission of "black-letter medicine" is sometimes difficult to obtain in a deposition or a trial. It is much easier to obtain admissions about journals as up-to-date authoritative sources.

§ 2.7 Standard Texts: Obstetrical

There are many excellent texts and more being published each day in the area of obstetrics or maternal-fetal medicine with which counsel must be familiar. The standard text that obstetricians recognize as authoritative is *Williams Obstetrics,* by J.A. Pritchard, M.D., P.C. McDonald, M.D., and N.F. Gant, M.D. (19th ed. 1993). *Williams Obstetrics* discusses the full range of nearly every subject that can come up in obstetrics and is the first book that any lawyer interested in obstetrical cases should purchase. Another excellent beginning place is *Maternal-Fetal Medicine: Principles and Practice,* by R.K. Creasy, M.D., and R. Resnik, M.D. (3rd ed. 1994), a textbook that was first published in 1984 which encompasses early fetal development through the neonatal period. It discusses such important subjects as maternal nutrition, ultrasound, fetal heart rate, the evaluation of fetal maturity, multiple gestations, infections, and the like. Another good text is the *Atlas of Perinatology,* by S. Aladjem, M.D., and D. Vidyasagar, M.D. (1982). Among other things, this text discusses non-stress fetal monitoring, resuscitation of the newborn, birth injuries, and injuries acquired in the neonatal intensive care unit. *Medical Care of the Pregnant Patient,* edited by R.S. Abrams, M.D., and P. Wexler, M.D. (1983), discusses, among other subjects, special problems during pregnancy, antenatal fetal assessment, principles of teratology, and risks of radiation exposure. *Operative Perinatology,* edited by L. Iffy, M.D., and D. Charles, M.D. (2d ed. 1992), discusses surgery on the pregnant patient and the surrounding surgical subjects such as infection control and how to manage surgical procedures during pregnancy. *Complications in Obstetric and Gynecologic Surgery,* edited by G. Schaefer, M.D., and E.A. Graber, M.D. (1981), is a very interesting book that can be utilized in medicolegal cases with excellent chapters discussing the various complications that may occur during surgery. *Clinical Care of the Obstetric Patient,* edited by R.L. Berkowitz, M.D. (1983), discusses, among other things, amniotic fluid embolism, management of hepatic failure in pregnancy, drug intoxication, and anaphylactic shock in the obstetric patient, and includes an excellent chapter on anesthesia for the critical-care obstetric patient. *Complications in Anesthesiology,* edited by F.K. Orkin, M.D., and L. H. Cooperman, M.D. (1983), has a section entitled "Obstetrics, Gynecology and Neonatal" which discusses anesthesia administration to the mother and fetus. Preeclampsia or pregnancy-induced hypertension is the subject of the book, *Preeclampsia: The Hypertensive Disease of Pregnancy,* by I. MacGillivray, M.D. (1983). This book focuses *only* on the subject of preeclampsia or pregnancy-induced hypertension on the mother and fetus. A book on the pathology of the perinatal period is *Perinatal Pathology,* edited by Jonathan S. Wigglesworth, M.D. (1984). This book discusses perinatal death, performance of the perinatal autopsy, and the pathology of the placenta, and contains specific chapters on each organ system of the fetus or neonate.

Antenatal and Neonatal Screening, edited by N.J. Wald (1984), discusses the all-important subject of fetal screening to determine congenital syndromes such as Tay-Sach's Disease and Down's Syndrome. *Genetic Diseases in Pregnancy— Maternal Effects and Fetal Outcome,* edited by J.D. Schulman and G.L. Simpson (1981), also discusses genetic problems during pregnancy and is very detailed. *Congenital Malformations: Notes and Comments,* by J. Warkany, M.D. (1971), is an excellent early book on the causes of congenital malformations and is very detailed. *Genetics and Birth Defects in Clinical Practice,* by M. Feingold, M.D., and H. Pashayan, M.D. (1983), is another text dealing with genetic defects.

The administration of drugs during pregnancy is a subject of great concern because of the potential for harming the fetus. *Drug Therapy in Obstetrics and Gynecology,* edited by W.F. Rayburn and F.P. Zuspan (3d ed. 1992), discusses the full range of drugs used during pregnancy and the neonatal period. *Clinical Pharmacology in Pregnancy—Fundamentals and Rational Pharmacotherapy,* edited by H.P. Kuemmeile, M.D., and K. Brendel, Ph.D. (1984), is also an excellent book discussing all types of drug administration during pregnancy. *Clinical Pharmacology in Obstetrics,* edited by P. Lewis, M.D. (1983), is a good text to begin researching a case dealing with the administration of drugs in an obstetrical patient.

High Risk Pregnancy and Delivery, by F. Arias, M.D., Ph.D. (1984), discusses the identification of the high-risk patient and what to do once the patient is identified. The preface to this book states that the book is written to provide residents, obstetricians, medical students, and nurses with practical information. *The Manual of Gynecologic and Obstetric Emergencies,* by B.Z. Taber, M.D. (2d ed 1984), is an excellent handbook on obstetrical emergencies. *Managing OB-GYN Emergencies,* edited by J.T. Queenan, M.D. (2d ed 1983), not only discusses emergencies in obstetrics but also has a section on anesthetic emergencies. *Modern Management of High Risk Pregnancy,* edited by N.H. Lauersen (1983), covers many topics including fetal monitoring, the prevention and management of prematurity, modern management of premature rupture of membranes, intrapartum fetal monitoring, meconium-stained amniotic fluid, and acid-base fetal monitoring.

Intrauterine Growth Retardation: Pathophysiology and Clinical Management, by C.C. Lin, M.D., and M.I. Evans, M.D. (1984), deals with the specific subject of the growth-retarded fetus during the prenatal period, discussing causes as well as diagnosis and management. *Preterm Birth: Causes, Prevention and Management,* edited by F. Fuchs, M.D., and P.G. Stubblefield, M.D. (1984), discusses the causes of preterm birth, therapy to prevent preterm birth, and the management and outcome of preterm birth.

Fetal Heart Rate Monitoring, by R.K. Freeman and T.J. Garite (2d ed. 1991), is an excellent book on fetal monitoring and should be the first book purchased and consulted when counsel is faced with a fetal monitor strip that needs to be investigated. This book is a necessity for obstetrical cases. *Principles and Practice of Ultrasonography in Obstetrics and Gynecology,* edited by Arthur C. Fleisher, M.D. (4th ed. 1991), is an up-to-date book on the use of ultrasonography in obstetrics.

Standards of Obstetric and Gynecologic Services (1985), by the American College of Obstetricians and Gynecologists (ACOG), is a must for any medicolegal lawyer's library. The ACOG's address is: American College of Obstetricians and Gynecologists, 600 Maryland Avenue, S.W., Washington, D.C. 20004. This book sets out the standards for a board-certified obstetrician practicing modern-day obstetrics.

§ 2.8   —Neonatal and Pediatric

Neonatology, Pathophysiology and Management of the Newborn, edited by G.B. Avery, M.D., Ph.D. (2d ed 1981), is one of the standard textbooks in neonatal medicine and must be considered one of the primary books for an attorney to buy when starting a medical library. The book is divided into 40 chapters and covers transition and stabilization in section three and the newborn infant in section four, and it contains a host of excellent chapters. *Atlas of Procedures in Neonatology,* edited by M. Fletcher, M.D., M.G. McDonald, M.D., and G.B. Avery, M.D., Ph.D. (2d ed. 1993), is an excellent and standard text discussing the whole range of neonatal medicine, including the support of the neonate, monitoring, blood sampling, respiratory care, tube placement, and transfusions, among other topics. This is a good place to start for any attorney handling a neonatal case. Another good basic medical reference is *Nelson's Textbook of Pediatrics,* edited by V.C. Vaughan, III, M.D., R.J. McKay, Jr., M.D., R.E. Behrman, M.D., and W.E. Nelson, M.D. (15th ed. 1996). *Nelson's* does not limit itself to the neonatal period but is a good source book for neonatal and pediatric cases.

Many physicians recognize as authoritative, *Neurology of the Newborn,* by Joseph J. Volpe, M.D. (3d. ed. 1995). Dr. Volpe is a well-recognized pediatric neurologist, and his book includes an excellent chapter on the neurological examination of the newborn as well as four chapters discussing brain injury and intracranial hemorrhage. He also has an excellent chapter on perinatal trauma. A very valuable and authoritative book is *Textbook of Child Neurology,* by J.H. Menkes, M.D. (5th ed. 1995). This is an excellent text with very fine chapters on perinatal trauma, infections of the nervous system, postnatal trauma, and injuries by physical agents and toxic disorders. This book is a must for attorneys to buy for their medical libraries. *Neurologic Infections in Children,* by W.E. Bell, M.D., and W.F. McCormick, M.D. (2d ed 1981), discusses in detail the all-important subject of infections of the newborn and child. The book discusses bacterial infections, viral infections, miscellaneous infections, and neurologic conditions related to inflammatory or infectious disorders. *Neonatal Neurology,* by G.M. Fenichel (3d ed 1995), is a small volume that is quite readable on the subject of neonatal neurology. This well-written book discusses convulsions, hypotonia, asphyxia, trauma, and infectious and metabolic diseases. *Intrauterine Asphyxia and the Developing Fetal Brain,* edited by L. Gluck, M.D. (1977), is based on a conference sponsored by the Department of Pediatrics at the University of California in San Diego and the Institute of Pediatric Service of the Johnson and Johnson baby products company. This book has many excellent contributors and discusses in detail the all-important subject of intrauterine asphyxia.

Practical Neonatal Respiratory Care, edited by R.L. Schreiner and J.A. Kisling (1982), discusses in detail resuscitation, respiratory care, and lung disease in the neonate, including neonatal apnea and hyaline membrane disease.

The Neonate with Congenital Heart Disease, by R.D. Rowe, M.D., R.M. Freedom, M.D., A. Mehrizi, M.D., and K.R. Boom, M.D. (2d ed.1981), is an excellent text for information about congenital heart disease in the neonate. This book discusses the anatomy of the heart and great vessels, physical examination of the newborn with respect to the cardiovascular system, and diseases which have to be promptly treated.

A fine short text has been written by Dr. L.B. Rorke, entitled *Pathology of Perinatal Brain Injury (1982).* Dr. Rorke is a neuropathologist, and this excellent volume discusses the factors relating to brain damage, hemorrhages, and how the brain is vulnerable to hypoxia. *Perinatal and Infant Brain Imaging: Role of Ultrasound and Computed Tomography,* by C.M. Rumack, M.D., and

M.L. Johnson, M.D. (1984), is a well-written text on neonatal brain imaging. Although this is a difficult subject for the attorney to grasp, it is important that counsel become familiar with it. *The Rehabilitation of a Child with a Traumatic Brain Injury,* edited by R.A. Hock, Ph.D. (1984), is an excellent text to help the attorney understand the rehabilitation techniques of and goals for a brain-injured child. While it does not deal specifically with the neonatal intensive care unit, this book can be helpful.

Treatment of Cerebral Palsy and Motor Delay, by S. Levitt (3d ed. 1995), is a volume written by a physiotherapist that discusses how a physiotherapist treats a cerebral palsy victim. The physiotherapist has an important part in the life of every child with cerebral palsy, and the attorney handling these types of cases must understand the physiotherapist's role. *Comprehensive Management of Cerebral Palsy,* edited by G.H. Thompson, M.D., I.L. Rubin, M.D., and R.M. Bilenker, M.D. (1983), is a book dealing with the full range of medical care given to a child with cerebral palsy. The book is broken down into five sections:

1. Coordination of comprehensive care
2. Etiology and prevention
3. Associated dysfunction
4. Therapeutic and surgical management
5. Social, educational, and maturational considerations.

Early Diagnosis and Therapy in Cerebral Palsy: A Primer on Infant Developmental Problems, by A.L. Scherzer and I. Tscharnuter (2d ed. 1990), defines cerebral palsy and discusses the evaluation and differential diagnoses of the cerebral palsy child. There is a chapter on home management and a chapter on treatment, and the last chapter is entitled "Assessment of the Management-Treatment Program."

Assessment of the Newborn: A Guide for the Practitioner, edited by M. Ziar, M.D., T.A. Clarke, M.D., and T.A. Merritt, M.D. (1984), is an excellent text that is divided into four general sections. The first one deals with general considerations of special problems, the second covers initial assessment of the newborn, the third deals with signs and symptoms of neonatal disease, and the fourth is on laboratory aids and the diagnosis of neonatal problems. There are excellent chapters on stabilization of the newborn, feeding, physical examination, birth injuries, and cyanosis.

The Handbook of Neonatal Intensive Care, by G.B. Merenstein, M.D., and S.L. Gardner, R.N. (3d ed. 1993), is a book that has some up-to-date information concerning regionalization and initial nursery care, heat balance (critically important for the neonate), and infections in the neonate. *Emergency Transfer of the High Risk Neonate,* by A. Ferrara, M.D., Ph.D., and A. Harin, M.D. (1980), is one of the few texts which deals strictly with the transfer of the fetus, both in utero and after the child is born. The failure to transfer the neonate can be an important element of some medicolegal cases, and this book is a valuable resource. *Care of the High Risk Neonate,* by M.H. Klaus, M.D., and A.A. Fanaroff, M.D. (4th ed. 1993), is a standard text in the area. This book utilizes a series of case studies that are excellent reading for an attorney because they discuss how treatment of the child should progress for different specific diseases. Each chapter contains at least two case studies. Dr. L.O. Lubchenco is the author of an older standard work entitled *The High Risk Infant* (1976). This is one of the earlier texts to discuss gestational age, the preterm and postterm infant, and the large-for-gestational-age (LGA) and small-for-gestational-age (SGA) infant. Dr. Lubchenco's book is well recognized by most physicians who practice neonatal medicine.

§ 2.9   Employment of a Medically Trained Person

One way for the attorney dealing in obstetrical and neonatal cases to get support is the employment of a medically trained person.[11] This can be direct employment, whereby the person works for the attorney, or it can be a health care provider functioning as a consultant. Compensation of such persons varies with the amount of medical training they have and whether they are employees or consultants. There are basically two classes of persons that can be utilized: physicians and nurses.

Active practitioners are usually too busy to be employed or to consult too frequently. However, counsel can build up contacts with consultants who can be utilized on an infrequent but steady basis. Obviously, the more consultants that counsel has available, the more efficiently cases can be reviewed. At some medical schools, a relatively permanent consultant can be obtained with a set agreement as to how much that consultant should be paid for the work, either by the hour or by the case.

It is an excellent idea to use physicians who are retired or semiretired. Some physicians are fascinated with the legal process, and their rates for the work can be reasonable. They may have a great deal of experience. Any physician can help point the attorney in the right direction by gathering medical literature, framing interrogatory questions and requests to admit, and helping to frame questions to be put to witnesses at depositions or at trial. This physician does not have to be a board-certified obstetrician, pediatrician, or neonatalogist. Many family practitioners and general practitioners have a great deal of experience and knowledge in the area of obstetrical and neonatal medicine. While they may not be the witnesses that would be used at trial, they can be very helpful.

Some attorneys on occasion have used medical students, interns, and residents to help them. Using these persons can be very dangerous since they are not fully trained physicians, but if counsel knows and understands their limitations,

---

[11] Volk, *Cross-Examination of the Medical Expert,* 16 Trial No. 5, at 44 (May 1980).

they can be most helpful. Few of these physicians in training, unless they are financially strapped, would be able to consult on a regular basis because of their work load.

Probably the category of health care professional that is most readily available is the nurse, either a licensed vocational nurse (licensed practical nurse) or registered nurse. Many of these nurses are disgruntled with the medical system because of their low status and bad experiences with patients being harmed by the health-care system. They may be burned out from the rigors of nursing and may be interested in a more leisurely type of work. Often a local nursing school can provide names of interested nurses, either from the faculty or friends of the faculty. It is not unheard of to advertise in the local newspaper's "help wanted" section for a nurse. Nurses are not paid well by hospitals and physicians and often are looking for work that will increase their compensation. Additionally, many nurses feel that they are patient advocates, and helping on meritorious medicolegal claims is a function of patient advocacy. Sometimes counsel will represent a nurse that may be hired or will know a nurse who is interested in working with an attorney. Many nurses with experience in obstetrical nursing, intensive care nursery, and pediatrics can be extremely helpful and can become proficient in evaluating medicolegal cases and assisting in putting the cases together for trial.

The key to utilizing medically trained persons is always to recognize their limitations and their biases. However, any attorney who attempts to review and litigate obstetrical and neonatal cases without the guiding hand of a medically trained person who is qualified and competent is looking for trouble.

CHAPTER 3

NORMAL PREGNANCY

Michael S. Cardwell, M.D.

Thomas G. Kirkhope, M.D.

ANTENATAL DIAGNOSIS

§ 3.1   Signs of Pregnancy

Knowledge of the presence or absence of a pregnancy in a woman is crucial to the proper diagnosis and treatment of all disease processes, whether related to the pregnancy or not. For this reason, any physician who assumes the care of any woman of reproductive age must always consider the possibility that a pregnancy may be present.

Ordinarily the diagnosis of pregnancy is easy to establish. On occasion, however, confusion may occur, especially during the early weeks. Diagnostic signs and symptoms that indicate the presence of pregnancy may be divided into three levels: presumptive evidence (discussed in § 3.2); probable evidence (discussed in § 3.3); and positive evidence (discussed in § 3.4).

§ 3.2   —Presumptive Evidence

Presumptive evidence involves signs and symptoms that are commonly found in pregnancy, but that can be related to other factors. Most are subjective.

Symptoms include:

1. Nausea with or without vomiting—commonly called "morning sickness," although not necessarily present only in the morning
2. Disturbances in urination—generally manifests itself as urinary frequency; usually attributed to the presence of the enlarging uterus resting on the bladder, causing a sensation of bladder fullness
3. Fatigue—a woman's feeling that she could "sleep all the time" despite obtaining what would normally be considered adequate rest
4. Perception of fetal movement by the mother ("quickening")—usually occurs around 18 to 20 weeks' gestation in a first pregnancy; may be earlier in later pregnancies.

Signs include:

1. Amenorrhea (cessation of menses)—despite possibility of occasional vaginal bleeding during pregnancy for various reasons, no regular rhythmic

recurrence of bleeding related to ovulation during pregnancy; can be reason other than pregnancy causing amenorrhea

2. Anatomical changes in the breasts—hormone Prolactin causes the functional milk-producing tissue in the breasts to increase in size and amount in early pregnancy; enlargement usually accompanied by a varying amount of breast tenderness, which tends to subside early in the second trimester

3. Discoloration of the mucosal lining of the vagina—usually observable on pelvic examination early in the pregnancy; not always obvious

4. Increased skin pigmentation—begins early in pregnancy and usually persists to some extent even after the pregnancy is over; may also be seen in women using oral contraceptives.

§ 3.3 —Probable Evidence

Although the following signs are more likely to be associated with pregnancy than with other states, they are not considered diagnostic.

1. Enlargement of the abdomen—takes place at a predictable rate starting at about 12 weeks; measurement of the rate of enlargement provides some evidence about the stage of gestation (see § 3.5)

2. Changes in size, shape, and consistency of the uterus—usually recognizable after 6 weeks' gestation, but possibly obscured by the presence of an obese abdomen, guarding by the patient being examined, or uterine pathology unrelated to pregnancy; ovarian enlargement from various causes sometimes mistaken for uterine enlargement

3. Anatomical changes in the cervix—bluish coloration, increased softness, and possible semblance of being "disconnected" from the uterine fundus on pelvic examination; eversion of the external is also common during pregnancy

4. Braxton Hicks contractions of the uterus—occur usually during the third trimester of pregnancy; can be appreciated by the mother and by the examiner, but are not painful; do not cause dilatation of the cervix as labor contractions do; physiologic function not known

5. "Ballottement"—fetus floating in a fluid medium in the uterus rebounding from sudden mild pressure exerted over the uterus, causing a tap against the examining hand

6. Positive pregnancy test.

A pregnancy test can be conducted on either urine or blood. Biological pregnancy tests utilizing living animals are now rarely used. Immunologic tests are now standard, and are extremely sensitive. All pregnancy tests depend on the presence of a hormone in the blood of the mother, produced by the placenta, called human chorionic gonadotropin (HCG). Some currently available home pregnancy tests can detect a pregnancy even before the first missed menstrual period. Although there are various sources of error for these tests, including various tumors of the reproductive system, their accuracy rate is usually stated as approximately 97 percent.

§ 3.4 —Positive Evidence

The following three signs of pregnancy are considered diagnostic, irrefutable, or "pathognomonic":

1. Identification of fetal heart action
2. Perception of fetal movement by the examiner
3. Real-time ultrasonic examination.

Fetal heart action can be identified by auscultation (listening with the fetoscope or ordinary stethoscope) or by continuous Doppler ultrasound. The fetal heart rate is ordinarily much faster than that of the mother: 120 to 160 beats per minute, as compared with 70 to 80 in the mother. Both maternal and fetal pulses should be counted for accurate comparison. There is no other condition in the human that can produce the presence of a second heart beat heard through the maternal abdominal wall.

After about 20 weeks' gestation, fetal movements can be felt by the examining hand on the maternal abdomen at irregular intervals. Movement may be visible as well as palpable. They may vary in intensity from a faint flutter to brisk movement. Contractions of the intestines or abdominal wall musculature may feel somewhat similar but should not confuse the experienced examiner.

A gestational sac is normally visible within the uterus during ultrasonic examination at five weeks, counting from the first day of the last menstrual period. (It may be even earlier using the trans-vaginal probe.) The body of the embryo itself may not be visible until six weeks' gestation, depending on the sophistication of the ultrasound equipment being used. In most current machines, a fetal heart rate should be visible and measurable utilizing this technique.

§ 3.5 Calculation of Dates

The importance of determining an accurate estimated date of delivery (EDD or EDC) can hardly be overemphasized. Complications may arise in pregnancies that persist beyond term, as well as in those which threaten to terminate early. In addition, modern prenatal care requires careful timing of various diagnostic tests, both routine and specialized. Therefore, the gestational age of the fetus must be known as accurately as possible at every stage of the pregnancy.

The normal duration of pregnancy is 280 days or 40 weeks (duration of pregnancy is not expressed in months), starting from the first day of the last normal menstrual period (LNMP). This calculation is based on the assumption that the average woman ovulates at 14 days following the first day of her LNMP. The extent to which a woman deviates from this "normal" pattern will determine how accurately her EDD may be calculated.

Calculation of the EDD is customarily carried out by application of Naegele's rule: from the date of the first day of the LNMP, subtract three months, then add seven days. For example, a woman whose LNMP is September 1 will in normal circumstances expect to deliver approximately June 8. It is important to emphasize that no rule can determine an EDD with an accuracy of greater than plus or minus two weeks. Therefore, if the woman in the example delivers at any time between May 25 and June 22, she is considered to have delivered at term.

If the LNMP is not known with accuracy, estimated gestational age can be determined by a number of other methods. The most exact of these would be an accurately known date of conception. Unfortunately, this information is rarely available. Other methods include:

1. Measurement of the height of the uterus from the symphysis pubis to the top of the fundus. This is considered a very rough estimate. One rule of thumb states that the height of the fundus measured in centimeters by this method is roughly equal to the gestational age in weeks between 20 and 36 weeks. Accuracy of this method is affected by such things as the thickness of the maternal abdominal wall, the presence of abnormalities of the uterus such as fibroid tumors, the fetal position, the fullness of the maternal bladder, and multiple (for example, twin) gestation.

2. Appearance of audible fetal heart tones. In ordinary circumstances, fetal heart tones become audible by auscultation (stethoscope) by 18 to 20 weeks' gestation. By Doppler ultrasound examination they may be detectable as early as 10 weeks. Accuracy of this method is limited by many factors, including the thickness of the maternal abdominal wall, the position of the fetus, the position of other structures in the maternal pelvis, and so forth.

3. Carefully performed vaginal examination by an experienced clinician in the first trimester. This is considered a reasonably accurate method of confirmation of dates if it agrees with dates as determined by the LNMP. It is subject to the same sources of error as measurement of the fundal height measured abdominally.

4. Measurement of various fetal dimensions by real-time ultrasound. The accuracy of this method varies with the gestational age at which it is performed. (For further discussion of this modality, see § **3.21.**)

In general, a reasonably certain LNMP obtained from the mother, combined with a finding of a first trimester uterus of corresponding size, yields a gestational age and EDD of sufficient accuracy for use in most pregnancies. If doubt exists, or if more exact information is required, real-time ultrasound is ordinarily utilized.

ANTENATAL MANAGEMENT

§ 3.6   Initial Visit

Most obstetricians recommend that the patient be seen for her first prenatal visit as soon as she is reasonably certain she is pregnant. At this visit, the pregnant state is confirmed by examination or by laboratory testing if needed. A careful medical history is obtained, general physical and pelvic examinations are performed, and standard laboratory tests are ordered.[1] If the physician is aware of known or suspected coexistent medical problems, other laboratory work may be ordered, as well as consultation with other specialists, as appropriate.

In the medical history, particular attention is given to the woman's reproductive history, including: number of previous pregnancies and their outcome; history of complications in either mother or child; stillbirths; premature labors; abortions, both spontaneous and induced; periods of infertility; and history of sexually transmitted diseases. Other important factors in the history include: maternal age; tobacco, alcohol, and other drug use; family medical problems; and personal medical problems unrelated to the pregnancy. Employment history may also be important to determine possible exposure to toxic substances or extreme work conditions. A nutritional history should be taken, and if there is doubt about adequate intake, a professional dietitian may provide helpful consultation.

§ 3.7   Routine and Special Laboratory Tests

Commonly accepted laboratory tests in modern obstetric practice[2] involve testing of the patient's blood, urine, or cervix. Tests regarding blood include:

---

[1] American College of Obstetricians and Gynecologists, Committee on Obstetrics: Maternal and Fetal Medicine: Scope of Services for Uncomplicated Obstetric Care, ACOG Committee Opinions No. 79 (1990).

[2] American Academy of Pediatrics and American College of Obstetricians and Gynecologists, Guidelines for Perinatal Care (3d ed. 1992).

1. Hemoglobin or hematocrit—for evidence of anemia or other hematologic disorders
2. ABO and Rh typing—for evidence of ABO and Rh incompatibility
3. Irregular antibodies—evidence of other blood group incompatibilities
4. Serologic test for syphilis—various screening tests acceptable; most commonly used is the Venereal Disease Research Laboratory (VDRL)
5. Rubella antibodies—lifelong immunity; repeat of test not necessary for patient previously shown to be immune to Rubella
6. Hepatitis B virus screen—further testing possibly required if there is a past history of hepatitis of any type
7. Sickle cell disease, if patient is black
8. Human Immunodeficiency Virus—not currently performed routinely in all pregnancies, but usually offered in cases where patient is at high risk (for example, known I.V. drug abusers, sexual partners of I.V. drug abusers, hemophiliacs, and so forth).

Tests involving the urine include:

1. Routine urinalysis
2. Culture, colony count, and sensitivity.

Asymptomatic bacteriuria (presence of pathogenic bacteria in bladder urine) is common in women, whether or not they are pregnant. In pregnancy it does not tend to clear spontaneously, and requires treatment. If the problem is not recognized and eradicated, acute pyelonephritis (infection of the kidneys), which is associated with an increased incidence of premature labor, may result.

Tests involving the cervix include:

1. Neisseria Gonorrheac culture—required by statute in many states; asymptomatic colonization of the cervix by N. Gonorrheae is common; may lead to Ophthalmia Neonatorum (blindness in the newborn) if not discovered and treated during the pregnancy
2. Chlamydia culture—recommended by the Center for Disease Control[3] if the N. Gonorrheae culture is positive
3. Group B Strep culture—Group B Strep associated with a particularly virulent form of pneumonia in some newborns; routine culture not universally agreed upon because some experts feel this is not a cost-effective way to find and treat the disease; treatment of the mother to prevent the disease in the newborn likely to be effective only if carried out during labor

---

[3] Center for Disease Control (1989).

4. Pap smear—no increased risk for cervical cancer in pregnancy, but pap often done at this time simply because the patient is available to be tested.

Other laboratory work is usually obtained later in the pregnancy. Tests performed at 16 weeks include:

1. Serum alpha-fetoprotein[4] (AFP)—now considered standard, to look for the presence of neural tube defects (NTDs) (certain brain or spinal cord defects) in the fetus; possible indication of certain other problems in the fetus from abnormal results on this test; many false positives requiring further investigation

2. "Triple Screen"—a combination of three tests (AFP, Serum Chorionic Gonadotropin, and Serum Estriol) said to be able to show evidence of certain genetic problems as well as NTDs; not universally utilized by all obstetricians

3. Genetic studies—for example, second trimester amniocentesis (removal of amniotic fluid from within the uterus, surrounding the fetus, by needle, for testing), or chorionic villus sampling (biopsy of placental cells) as early as eight weeks gestation; appropriate in certain cases (see § **3.10**).

Tests at 28 weeks include:

1. A standardized blood test for gestational onset diabetes mellitus—most commonly used at present is the "1-hour Glucola screen"; positive result calls for further testing

2. If mother is Rh negative, repeat antibody test for unsensitized Rh-negative patients—tests whether the mother has developed antibodies against her Rh-positive fetus; negative result calls for mother to be given Anti-Rho-D antibody to prevent Rh isoimmunization in the fetus; positive result calls for appropriate workup to evaluate the nature of the isoimmunization

3. Repeat hemoglobin or hematocrit.

Two tests performed at 32 to 36 weeks are:

1. Repeat testing for sexually transmitted disease
2. Repeat hemoglobin and hematocrit measurement.

Other tests, such as those to evaluate thyroid function, although not routine in early pregnancy, may need to be obtained if the history suggests the presence of other problems. Routine real-time ultrasound examinations are not the standard and, as of this writing, are not recommended by the American College of

---

[4] J. Goldberg, Alpha-Fetoprotein, ACOG Technical Bull. No. 154, American College of Obstetricians and Gynecologists (1991).

Obstetricians and Gynecologists (ACOG). Still, they are very commonly performed by most obstetricians and are capable of discovering otherwise unsuspected findings in the fetus. There are, however, many circumstances in which the use of ultrasonography might be considered as the appropriate "standard of care" if problems with the fetus are suspected from the history or during the prenatal course. (See **Appendix 3–1.**)

§ 3.8 Subsequent Prenatal Visits

Prenatal visits after the initial one are usually scheduled four weeks apart. At each visit, weight gain is recorded. Inadequate weight gain in pregnancy is associated with intrauterine growth restriction and low birth weight. Maternal weight gain both before and during pregnancy has an effect on perinatal mortality. Adequate weight gain is therefore considered of great importance, and lack of adequate weight gain calls for appropriate investigation and intervention. Current recommendations for adequate weight gain in normal pregnancy are 25 to 30 pounds over prepregnancy weight. In general, if the mother's diet is adequate, prenatal vitamin supplements are not necessary. Oral iron preparations are recommended, however, since many women are unable to meet the increased iron demands of a developing fetus without compromising their own iron stores.

Caloric requirement depends on several factors, such as patterns of physical activity, prepregnancy weight, and the mother's general health. Inadequate weight gain is associated with increased risk of spontaneous abortion, intrauterine growth restriction, prematurity, and mental retardation. Weight reduction during pregnancy is not recommended.

Exercise, as a rule, is encouraged. There is no evidence that any particular form of exercise, exercise intensity, or specific heart rates resulting from exercise must be avoided. There are, however, some generally accepted guidelines:[5]

1. Regular exercise is preferable to intermittent.
2. Exercise in the supine position should be avoided after the first trimester.
3. Women who are pregnant should stop exercising when fatigued and should not exercise to exhaustion.
4. In the third trimester, exercise which causes loss of balance or risk of trauma to the abdomen should be avoided.
5. Caloric intake should be increased to accommodate the level of exercise.
6. Heat dissipation should be assured by use of adequate fluid intake and wearing of appropriate clothing.
7. Prepregnancy exercise routine should not be resumed completely until four to six weeks postpartum.

---

[5] R. Artal, Exercise During Pregnancy and the Postpartum Period, ACOG Technical Bull. No. 189, American College of Obstetrics and Gynecology (1994).

Other concerns at each prenatal visit include observation and recording of the blood pressure (to look for evidence of toxemia of pregnancy), urinalysis (for evidence of proteinuria and urinary tract infection), timed performance of certain routine tests (see § 3.7), measurement of growth of the fundal height, observation of the fetal heart rate and fetal position, and inquiry into fetal activity and maternal symptoms. As the pregnancy progresses, more frequent visits are scheduled, usually every two weeks from 32 to 36 weeks, and weekly thereafter until delivery.[6] Development of significant symptoms or findings may indicate closer observation by such methods as non-stress testing, repeated ultrasound examinations, or additional laboratory tests.

§ 3.9   Risk Assessment

Certain factors in the mother's medical history or physical condition place the pregnancy at an increased risk for a poor outcome. Several systems have been developed which assign a "score" to these factors in an attempt to predict the likelihood of problems, but most of these have been unsatisfactory. The following is a list of factors recognized by most obstetricians and ACOG[7] as being associated with increased danger to the developing fetus. These factors may necessitate further evaluation, consultation, or referral for a subspecialist's care.

Medical problems that constitute risk factors are:

1. Cardiovascular, renal, collagen, pulmonary, infectious, hepatic, and sexually transmitted diseases
2. Metabolic or endocrine disorders
3. Chronic urinary tract infections
4. Maternal viral, bacterial, or protozoal infections
5. Diabetes mellitus
6. Severe anemia
7. Isoimmune thrombocytopenia
8. Convulsive or neurologic disorders
9. Substance abuse (for example, alcohol, tobacco, illicit drugs, prescribed medications [for example, barbiturates, sedatives])
10. Nutritional disorders, hyperemesis, anorexia.

---

[6] American Academy of Pediatrics, American College of Obstetricians and Gynecologists, Guidelines for Perinatal Care (3d ed. 1992).

[7] American Academy of Pediatrics and American College of Obstetricians and Gynecologists, Guidelines for Perinatal Care (3d ed. 1992).

Obstetric and genetic problems recognized as risk factors include:

1. Poor obstetric history
2. Maternal age under 16 or over 35 years
3. Previous congenital anomalies
4. Multiple gestation
5. Isoimmunization
6. Intrauterine growth restriction
7. Third trimester bleeding
8. Pregnancy-induced hypertension (pre-eclampsia)
9. Uterine structural anomalies
10. Abnormal amniotic fluid volume (oligohydramnios, polyhydramnios)
11. Fetal cardiac arrhythmias
12. Prematurity
13. Breech or transverse lie (intrapartum)
14. Rupture of membranes for a time period longer than 24 hours
15. Chorioamnionitis.

§ 3.10 Genetic Counseling

Ordinary genetic counseling usually may be provided by any well-trained individual: obstetrician, pediatrician, family physician, or member of the genetics team. More complex problems are referred to a geneticist. In every pregnancy, careful inquiry should be made into the patient's medical history and family medical history to search for evidence of genetic problems.

The American College of Obstetricians and Gynecologists recommends genetic studies on the fetus whenever one or more of the following conditions is met:[8]

1. Advanced maternal age—Because of the increased incidence of Down's syndrome and other genetic disorders in older mothers, genetic amniocentesis is offered to mothers who will be age 35 or older at the time of expected delivery.
2. Previous child with chromosomal abnormality—The risk of occurrence of the same or another genetic problem is approximately 1 percent.
3. Parental translocation or inversion—If either parent is known to be a carrier of a genetic abnormality, the offspring is at increased risk.

---

[8] J. Simpson, Antenatal Diagnosis of Genetic Disorders, ACOG Technical Bull. No. 108, American College of Obstetricians and Gynecologists (1987).

4. Neural Tube Defects—certain defects in the brain or spinal cord.

5. Inborn errors of metabolism—At least 200 inborn errors of metabolism can be diagnosed prenatally. Each has a specific inheritance pattern, and it is unlikely that the practicing obstetrician can keep track of all of them. It is therefore recommended that a patient at risk for producing a child with one of these should be seen by a consulting geneticist for advice regarding genetic testing.

6. Other common disorders—Duchenne muscular dystrophy, hemophilia, polycystic kidney disease, sickle cell anemia, alpha- and beta- thalassemia. Increasing numbers of other disorders are continually becoming detectable.

This subject is covered more extensively in **Chapter 4.** (See § **3.19** for a discussion of amniocentesis.)

§ 3.11 Work Outside the Home

The Pregnancy Discrimination Act of 1978 has encouraged and resulted in greater participation of women in the workforce. The United States Supreme Court ruled in 1991 that federal law prohibits employers from excluding women from job categories because they are or might become pregnant. It is estimated that approximately one-half of women of the childbearing age in the United States are employed outside the home. Naeye and Peters[9] noted that pregnant women who were employed had infants whose birthweights were significantly lower than women who were not. Teitelman and co-workers[10] evaluated types of work performed and concluded that women who worked at jobs that required prolonged standing are at greater risk for preterm delivery. This finding was confirmed by Klebanoff and co-workers.[11]

Most physicians feel that any occupation that subjects the pregnant woman to severe physical strain should be avoided. However, a woman with an uncomplicated pregnancy and a normal fetus should be allowed to continue work until the onset of labor if her job presents no greater potential hazards than those encountered in normal daily life in the community or home.[12]

---

[9] R. Naeye & E. Peters, *Working During Pregnancy: Effects on the Fetus,* 69 Pediatrics 724 (1982).

[10] A. Teitelman, L. Welsch, K. Hellenbrand & M. Bracken, *Effect of Maternal Work Activity on Preterm Birth and Low Birthweight,* 131 Am. J. Epidemiol. 104 (1990).

[11] M. Klebanoff, P. Shiono & J. Carey, *The Effect of Physical Activity During Pregnancy on Preterm Delivery and Birthweight,* 163 Am. J. Obstet. Gynecol. 1450 (1990).

[12] American Academy of Pediatrics and American College of Obstetricians and Gynecologists, Guidelines for Perinatal Care (3d ed. 1992).

Women are generally allowed to return to work six weeks after delivery because it is felt that this period is required for her physiologic condition to return to normal. Recommendations, however, are individualized according to the patient's particular circumstances.

§ 3.12 Travel

Travel should not generally be prohibited in pregnancy. Travel in properly pressurized aircraft offers no unusual risk.[13]

When traveling by road, especially if the woman is driving, it is advisable to stop every two to three hours and walk about for some minutes before resuming travel. Pregnant women are encouraged to wear properly positioned safety belts throughout pregnancy while traveling in motor vehicles. The lap-belt portion should be placed under the pregnant woman's abdomen and across her upper thighs. The passenger should adjust her seating position to the belt so that it crosses her shoulder without chafing her neck. The shoulder belt should be positioned between the breasts and should never be slipped off the shoulder because doing so may negate the effectiveness of the entire restraint system. During long trips, the safety belt should be periodically readjusted for comfort and position.

Special problems may arise with regard to long trips, and particularly with respect to international travel. A woman may develop a pregnancy complication at an area remote from facilities that can provide adequate treatment. This possibility should be taken into consideration before embarking.

§ 3.13 Sexual Activity

In general, for healthy women in a normal pregnancy, there is no need to avoid sexual intercourse. In the third trimester, some adjustments in coital position may be advisable for comfort, particularly if the male partner is especially heavy. In the past it was customary to advise couples to avoid intercourse during the last four weeks of pregnancy. There is no evidence that normal relations cause any particular harm in a normal pregnancy, and indeed this advice was probably rarely followed. In fact, trying to abide by the doctor's advice in this regard may cause undue harm to the couple's relationship. There is some theoretical concern that depositing of prostaglandins in the vagina by the male partner may increase the risk of premature labor, but there is no evidence that this actually occurs. On the other hand, whenever spontaneous abortion or

---

[13] F. Cunningham, P. MacDonald, K. Leveno, N. Gant & L. Gilstrap, Williams Obstetrics 262 (19th ed. 1993).

premature labor threatens, or undiagnosed bleeding or rupture of amniotic membranes occurs, coitus should unquestionably be avoided.

§ 3.14 Smoking

Mothers who smoke during pregnancy have infants whose birth weights average less than infants of nonsmokers. Maternal smoking also seems to be related to an increased frequency of perinatal mortality,[14] spontaneous abortion, low birth weight, and placental abruption.[15] The frequency of major birth defects seems not to be affected by smoking.[16]

The other dangers of smoking, however, are well known. Mothers, therefore, are well advised to discontinue smoking for their own health and that of their families, as well as the health of the fetus.

§ 3.15 Alcohol

The effect of alcohol on human pregnancy was first described by Jones in 1973.[17] It has since been confirmed by many other investigators. The so-called Fetal Alcohol Syndrome consists of prenatal and postnatal growth deficiency, mental retardation, behavioral disturbances, and a characteristic facial appearance. Congenital heart defects and brain defects are common. The syndrome is seen in the children of 30 to 40 percent of women who are frank alcoholics.[18]

Alcoholism is described as the ingestion of three or more ounces of absolute alcohol daily throughout the pregnancy. Lesser amounts are associated with less severe manifestations that are referred to as "fetal alcohol effects."[19]

Whether the effects of alcohol linger after the woman stops drinking is unknown. In 1992, one group of researchers presented evidence of an apparent "threshold effect" of alcohol exposure.[20] They reported that 30 percent of

---

[14] U.S. Department of Health and Human Services, Pub. No. (CDC)90-8416, The Health Benefits of Smoking Cessation: A Report of the Surgeon General (1990).

[15] S. Hellerstein & B. Sachs, Smoking and Reproductive Health, ACOG Technical Bull. No. 180, American College of Obstetricians and Gynecologists (1993).

[16] B. Sachs, *The Effect of Smoking on Late Pregnancy Outcome,* 7 Semin Reprod Endocrinol 319 (1989).

[17] K. Jones, D. Smith, C. Ulleland & A. Streissguth, *Patterns of Malformation in Offspring of Chronic Alcoholic Mothers,* 1 Lancet 1267 (1973).

[18] K. Jones, Smith's Recognizable Patterns of Human Malformation (4th ed. 1988).

[19] J. Mills, B. Graubard, E. Harley, G. Rhoads & H. Berendes, *Maternal Alcohol Consumption and Birth Weight: How Much Drinking During Pregnancy Is Safe?,* 252 JAMA 1875 (1984).

[20] J. Jacobson, S. Jacobson, R. Sokol, S. Martier & J. Ager, *Prenatal Alcohol Exposure and Neurobehavioral Function in Infancy: Evidence for Threshold and Differential Vulnerability,* 166 Am. J. Obstet. Gynecol. 346 (1992).

offspring exposed to 14 ounces of absolute alcohol or more near the time of conception or 3.5 ounces or more per day during pregnancy had impaired neurobehavioral functions. In all such studies, dosages are very difficult to verify since one must depend on patients' reporting. Therefore it must be admitted that no safe level for maternal drinking during pregnancy has been established.

§ 3.16   Common Complaints and Treatments

Nausea and vomiting are common complaints in the early part of pregnancy. The symptoms are usually worse in the morning but may persist throughout the day. Both hormonal and psychogenic factors have been implicated. The woman who has this problem is seldom afforded complete relief in spite of attempts at management. Treatment ranges from home remedies, such as herbs and soups, to antiemetics (antivomiting agents). Small but frequent feedings usually help to minimize the problem.

There has been recent controversy over the use of antiemetics in the early part of pregnancy, particularly involving Bendectin. Bendectin is a combination of the antihistaminic doxylamine succinate, and pyridoxine. The drug is no longer used during pregnancy because of the suggestion that it might be teratogenic (capable of inducing birth defects). The medical literature supported its relative safety, but its manufacturer removed it from the market in 1983. Currently trimethobenzamide (Tigan) is often used for nausea and vomiting in pregnancy. It should be emphasized, however, that no antiemetic drug has been proven completely free of effects on the fetus when used in the first trimester.

Headache is another frequent complaint, particularly in early pregnancy. Very often, no cause can be demonstrated. Treatment is largely symptomatic, usually with simple analgesics such as acetaminophen (many brand names, including Tylenol). When headache persists or becomes more severe, a careful investigation for possible etiologies is indicated.

Leukorrhea (chronic white vaginal discharge) during pregnancy is not uncommon. Often, no pathologic factor is encountered. Mucoid secretions from the vagina and cervix may be a contributing factor. However, if the discharge becomes annoying, or if it is accompanied by other symptoms such as itching or "burning," evaluation is called for to rule out an infectious process. Infectious leukorrhea may be due to Candida albicans, a fungus, or Trichomonas vaginalis, a protozoon. Vulvovaginitis (inflammation of the vulva or vagina) caused by Candida is effectively treated by a number of local vaginal preparations in the form of tablets, creams, or ointments. Miconazole (Monistat) and Clotrimazole (Mycelex and Gyne-Lotrimin) are considered safe and effective in the treatment of vaginal candidiasis in pregnancy. These are all now available in low-dosage forms over the counter, and in higher dosages by prescription.

Metronidazole (Flagyl, Protostat, and Metryl) is the orally effective drug of choice for infectious leukorrhea. Both the patient and her sexual partner must be treated in order to achieve optimal results. Observed carcinogenesis (induction of cancers) in rats and mutagenicity (induction of genetic changes) in bacteria have caused this drug to be considered a risk for teratogenesis (causing of birth defects) if used in the first trimester. Therefore it is probably prudent to limit its use to the later weeks of pregnancy. Adequate human studies, however, are lacking.

§ 3.17   Immunizations

The desirability of immunizations in pregnancy depends on the type of vaccine used and the likelihood of exposure of the mother to the infectious process. In general, vaccines which contain live viruses are considered high risk for fetal damage. An extensive list of various types of immunizations appropriate for use in pregnancy was published by ACOG in 1991, and the reader is referred to this publication for further information.[21]

§ 3.18   Antepartum Fetal Surveillance

In the past, the ability to evaluate fetal well-being during gestation was severely limited by inability to gain access to the fetus through the maternal abdominal wall. The only diagnostic tools available to the physician were direct auscultation of the fetal heart with a fetuscope or stethoscope, measurement of the uterine fundal height, and X-ray. All other information about the fetus was gathered indirectly, through observation of the mother.

One of the first tests done directly on the developing fetus was amniocentesis, discussed in § 3.19. More extensive invasion of the amniotic cavity presents increased problems. The human uterus, unlike that of some other animal species, is quite intolerant of such procedures as hysterotomy (opening with a large incision) and quickly goes into premature labor if disturbed too much. Such things as surgery to correct birth defects prior to delivery have progressed slowly because of limited ability to manage this problem.

Other diagnostic methods have developed along with amniocentesis, however. Because they do not require invasion of the uterus, they have quickly become widely used, some almost routinely. It is no longer considered necessary or even desirable to wait until there is definitive evidence of fetal compromise before these methods of evaluation are used. Suspicion or even concern about a complication is all that is required. Thus they are often used in what appear to

---

[21] L. Fehrs, W. Williams, S. Cochi, W. Orenstein & C. Tyler, Immunization During Pregnancy, ACOG Technical Bull. No. 160, American College of Obstetricians and Gynecologists (1991).

be completely normal pregnancies. They may be used individually or in combination with one another to gain more complete information.

§ 3.19 Amniocentesis

In 1961, Liley[22] reported on the use of amniocentesis (the sampling of amniotic fluid from around the fetus by needle for testing) in evaluation and treatment of Rh incompatibility. Complications of the procedure, even in those early days, were minimal, and testing of the amniotic fluid came to be viewed as the first readily available "window" on the developing fetus. The indications for the procedure were quickly broadened to include fetal maturity testing, biochemical testing, genetic testing, and, more recently, alpha-fetoprotein.

Amniocentesis may be performed during the second trimester, usually to obtain fetal cells for genetic testing or the fluid itself for metabolic testing. The ideal time in pregnancy for genetic amniocentesis to be done is 14 to 16 weeks, although it can be done at any time up until term. It should be preceded by genetic counseling. The time required for culturing and reading the cells removed for genetic study is about three weeks.

In high-risk pregnancies, amniocentesis may be performed near term to asses fetal maturity in preparation for delivery. In cases of suspected chorioamnionitis (intrauterine infection), it may be advantageous to obtain amniotic fluid for bacterial culture or stain to confirm the presence of pathogens. Amniocentesis is also still used, sometimes serially, in certain cases of Rh and other incompatibilities. (See **Chapter 4.**)

§ 3.20 Fetal Movement Observation

Women typically first feel the spontaneous movements of the fetus (quickening) between 16 and 20 weeks gestation. After this time fetal movements are perceived more or less constantly throughout the remaining portion of the pregnancy. Many researchers since the early 1970s have reported their observation that decreased fetal movements as pregnancy progresses are associated with an increase in fetal mortality and morbidity. As a result, many systems for regular counting of fetal movements on a daily basis by the mother have been developed. Some are formalized into a scoring system, and the mother is given a card or form on which to record her observations. Others simply recommend to the mother to report any persistent decrease in fetal activity she notices. In all of them, a report of a decrease in perceived fetal movement, particularly in the

---

[22] A. Liley, *Liquor Amnii Analysis in Management of Pregnancy Complicated by Rhesus Sensitization,* 82 Am. J. Obstet. Gynecol. 1359 (1961).

third trimester, calls for further investigation by the clinician, usually by non-stress testing (see § **3.22**).

§ 3.21 Ultrasonography

Diagnostic ultrasonography in obstetrics has improved enormously since its introduction in the late 1950s, and its use has expanded along with this advance in sophistication. As an imaging technique, it has several advantages over X-ray, not the least of which is its apparent lack of side effects. As of this writing, there are no known harmful effects on the fetus, the mother, the sonographic instrument operator, or other patients from ultrasound use in the frequencies and dosages used in present-day diagnostic studies.[23]

The most common indication for the use of diagnostic ultrasound in modern-day obstetrics is determination or verification of fetal age. In this function it is most accurate in the first trimester, at 8 to 14 weeks of gestational age. Other common uses are in the establishment of the intrauterine location of the pregnancy, thus ruling out ectopic (for example, tubal) pregnancy. It is also used in estimation of fetal weight, diagnosis of multiple pregnancy, and as an adjunct in the performance of various procedures such as chorionic villus sampling and amniocentesis.

In 1984, the U.S. Department of Health and Human Services published a list of acceptable indications for diagnostic ultrasound in pregnancy.[24] This list has been accepted by ACOG and distributed to its members for reference. The indications are enumerated in **Appendix 3–1.** According to the recommendations of ACOG, ultrasound studies may be "limited" or "comprehensive" depending on the indication for which they are performed and the skill of the operator. Standards are published for both.[25]

§ 3.22 Antepartum Electronic Fetal
Heart Monitoring

Electronic fetal heart rate monitoring (EFM) may be performed both in the antepartum (during the prenatal course) and in the intrapartum (in labor) period. When used in the antepartum period, only the external or indirect method is appropriate. Two "probes" are applied to the maternal abdomen, and the fetal heart rate and any uterine activity is recorded. There is also a third marking device that is used by the mother to record other events, such as perceived fetal movements. EFM is used in the following antenatal tests:

---

[23] E. Horger III, Ultrasonography in Pregnancy, ACOG Technical Bull. No. 187, American College of Obstetricians and Gynecologists (1993).

[24] National Institutes of Health Pub. No. 84-667 (1984).

[25] *Id.*

The non-stress test (NST).   This test is based on the observation that movement by a normal, well-oxygenated fetus is associated with a transient elevation in its heart rate, referred to as an "acceleration." If the fetus moves, and the movement is perceived by the mother, a mark is made on the EFM recording. Any accompanying heart rate acceleration should be observable on the fetal heart rate (FHR) portion of the recording. If there are a sufficient number of movements accompanied by accelerations of sufficient amplitude and duration, the test is considered "reactive." If the prescribed conditions are not met, it is considered "non-reactive," and if the test is not interpretable because of technical reasons it may be "unsatisfactory." A "non-reactive" reading is considered "non-reassuring," possibly calling for further evaluation of fetal well-being.

The contraction stress test (CST).   Here, the same instrumentation is used, but the observation is of the FHR in relation to uterine activity, that is, uterine contractions. A reading that uterine contractions are occurring at the rate of three in ten minutes, and are associated with late decelerations, is called "positive," a non-reassuring pattern. (See **Chapter 8** for a discussion of types of FHR decelerations.) If no contractions are occurring, the clinician may elect to produce them with an intravenous oxytocin solution (the oxytocin challenge test [OCT]) or by breast stimulation (the nipple stimulation test, which is now not widely used). If no decelerations are seen, the test is interpreted as "negative," which is a reassuring pattern. If decelerations are produced but are not consistent, the result is termed "suspicious." If contractions cannot be produced, the test is considered unsatisfactory. Any result other than negative calls for further evaluation of fetal well-being.

The Biophysical Profile (BPP).   In this test, the EFM is used in combination with ultrasound to produce a "profile" of fetal activity. A scoring system is used in which a reactive NST is given two points. Other parameters of activity are observed and scored over a 30-minute period by ultrasound observation. A maximum score of eight is possible for this portion of the test, so that a perfect score for the combined observations is ten. Any total score of eight or more is considered reassuring. Four to six is suspicious, and below four is non-reassuring.

Amniotic fluid index.   In the third and late second trimesters of pregnancy, diminished placental function may result in decreased perfusion of the fetal kidneys. This reduces the production of fetal urine, which in turn causes a reduction in the amount of amniotic fluid. Amniotic fluid volume assessment, then, represents a means of evaluating placental function. The relative amount of amniotic fluid present can be estimated using real-time ultrasound, and this result, combined with the result of NST, can give a satisfactory estimate of fetal well-being. This method also has the advantage of being less cumbersome than complete BPP assessment.

These tests, or a combination of them, are often used in evaluation of the following fetal problems: intrauterine growth restriction, post-date gestation, decreased fetal movement, oligohydramnios (decreased amount of amniotic fluid), isoimmunization, previous fetal demise, and multiple gestation. Their use may also be appropriate in certain maternal conditions, such as hypertensive disorders, insulin-dependent diabetes mellitus, chronic renal disease, systemic lupus erythematous, cyanotic heart disease, hemoglobinopathies (certain disorders of the oxygen-carrying component of blood), and thyroid disease.[26] These prenatal problems are discussed in **Chapter 4.**

§ 3.23   Chorionic Villus Sampling

Chorionic villus sampling is another test to search for the presence of genetic disease in the fetus. It is performed earlier in pregnancy than genetic amniocentesis (see **§ 3.19**), often as early as eight weeks. This constitutes its chief advantage over amniocentesis, since it enables a much earlier determination of the genetic makeup of the fetus. If therapeutic abortion is to be performed because of the presence of a genetically abnormal fetus, it can be done at a much earlier gestational age, a safer time for the mother.

Under ultrasound control, a probe is inserted into the uterus, through either the cervix or the abdomen, and a sampling of chorionic (placental) tissue is obtained. The cells can be read directly rather than after being cultured, further contributing to the early availability of information on which to base decisions regarding abortion.

§ 3.24   X-Rays in Pregnancy

In modern obstetrics there are few indications for diagnostic radiation. X-ray has been completely replaced by ultrasonography and amniocentesis in determination of fetal maturity. X-ray pelvimetry is rarely indicated, unless there is a reason to suspect a pelvic anomaly (for example, a history of pelvic fracture). On occasion it may be appropriate to obtain a film for an overall view of fetal positions when choosing a mode of delivery in a multiple pregnancy.

Radiologists performing X-ray studies on females at any time during their reproductive years now routinely inquire into the possibility of pregnancy. However, if the fetus has been exposed, perhaps in a patient who was unaware she was pregnant, information must be obtained in order to evaluate the amount of exposure and the gestational age at which it occurred. A determination can then be made about the likelihood of a teratogenic (defect-producing) effect on

---

[26] American College of Obstetricians and Gynecologists, Antepartum Fetal Surveillance, ACOG Technical Bull. No. 188 (1994).

the fetus. The patient is counselled accordingly to give her an opportunity to decide whether the pregnancy is to be continued. In most cases, the amount of radiation exposure to the fetus from ordinary routine X-ray studies is not sufficient to produce significant damage.

§ 3.25 Other Antenatal Testing

The use of certain other antenatal tests, such as periumbilical blood sampling (PUBS) and continuous Doppler ultrasonography, is confined to high-risk pregnancies. They are discussed in **Chapter 4.**

§ 3.26 Appendix 3–1: Indications for Diagnostic Ultrasonography During Pregnancy

The following list is adapted from one compiled by the National Institutes of Health.[27]

Indications for Ultrasonography During Pregnancy

1. Estimation of gestational age for patients with uncertain clinical dates, or verification of dates for patients who are to undergo scheduled elective repeat cesarean delivery, indicated induction of labor, or other elective termination of pregnancy
2. Evaluation of fetal growth
3. Vaginal bleeding of undetermined etiology in pregnancy
4. Determination of fetal presentation
5. Suspected multiple gestation
6. Adjunct to amniocentesis
7. Significant uterine size or clinical dates discrepancy
8. Pelvic mass
9. Suspected hydatidiform mole
10. Adjunct to cervical cerclage placement
11. Suspected ectopic pregnancy
12. Adjunct to special procedures
13. Suspected fetal death
14. Suspected uterine abnormality

---

[27] U.S. Dep't of Health and Human Services, National Institutes of Health Pub. No. 84-667, Diagnostic Ultrasound in Pregnancy (1984).

15. Intrauterine contraceptive device localization
16. Biophysical evaluation for fetal well-being
17. Observation of intrapartum events
18. Suspected polyhydramnios or oligohydramnios
19. Suspected abruptio placentae
20. Adjunct to external version from breech to vertex presentation
21. Estimation of fetal weight or presentation in premature rupture of membranes or premature labor
22. Abnormal serum alpha-fetoprotein value
23. Follow-up observation of identified fetal anomaly
24. Follow-up evaluation of placental location for identified "placenta previa"
25. History of previous congenital anomaly
26. Serial evaluation of fetal growth in multiple gestation
27. Evaluation of fetal condition in late registrants for prenatal care

CHAPTER 4

HIGH-RISK PREGNANCY

Michael S. Cardwell, M.D.

Thomas G. Kirkhope, M.D.

ANTENATAL DIAGNOSIS AND MANAGEMENT

§ 4.1   Identification of the High-Risk Pregnancy

Pregnancy is considered a normal physiologic event in most women. However, using various scoring systems, up to 40 percent of all pregnancies are considered at risk for adverse outcome for either the baby or the mother or both.[1] It is very important to obtain a detailed history of preexisting maternal medical problems and pertinent reproductive history. It is now the standard to use one of the available prenatal record-keeping systems in order to provide a comprehensive initial assessment of the current pregnancy and to have a means to continuously assess the ongoing pregnancy.[2]

Risk factors that place the pregnancy at risk for adverse outcome include major maternal medical problems such as diabetes, hypertension, or heart disease; complications in the current pregnancy, such as preterm labor or preeclampsia; or an identified fetal anomaly. The antenatal course might have been uneventful; however, intrapartum complications such as fetal distress, umbilical cord prolapse, and chorioamnionitis may occur which increase the possibility of an adverse outcome.

§ 4.2   General Principles of Management

Management of the high-risk pregnancy depends on a number of factors: primarily, the maternal and fetal status and the gestational age. The maternal condition is assessed, with any priority of treatment regiments given to her first. After the mother's medical status is ascertained and found to be stable, the fetus is then evaluated. With the advent of fetal electronic monitoring and obstetrical ultrasonography, the physician is now able to assess fetal health better than at any time in the past. Serial studies using the above tools antenatally can help determine if the pregnancy, which may or may not already be at risk, is progressing without complications and if delivery, as in the case of premature gestations, can be postponed without putting the fetus in jeopardy.

Delivery of a mature fetus is, of course, the ideal in any given situation. When there is a question of gestational dates or doubts as to maturity of the fetus when clinical parameters such as menstrual dates or fundal height measurements are not available or are inconsistent, ultrasound or amniocentesis is recommended

---

[1] S.G. Gabbe, J.R. Niebyl, J.L. Simpson, Obstetrics: Normal and Problem Pregnancies (2d ed. 1991).

[2] Currently available prenatal record-keeping systems include the American College of Obstetricians and Gynecologists Prenatal system, the Hollister prenatal system, the Problem-Oriented Perinatal Risk Assessment System (POPRAS), and the Prenatal Care-Systems Approach by Advanced Medical Systems, Inc.

for confirmation of fetal maturity or immaturity. The amniotic fluid obtained via amniocentesis may be sent for fetal pulmonary maturity studies.

The route of delivery, whether vaginal or abdominal, will be dictated by whichever serves the best interests of maternal and fetal health. The decision to perform a cesarean section will be influenced by factors existing at the time the decision to deliver the infant is made. Delivery of a high-risk pregnancy is best accomplished in a setting where facilities, medical and nursing personnel, and expertise in managing potential or emergent situations are available. This may be difficult to accomplish in remote rural areas. However, regionalization of perinatal care has been achieved in many parts of the country, providing an effective transport system by which a mother whose pregnancy is highly complicated is transferred to a facility that is better equipped to handle the problem. An infant born with complications or who develops problems at birth is transferred to a similar facility.

§ 4.3 Regionalization of Perinatal Care

Regionalization of perinatal care indicates an aggregate of steps taken to organize and implement effective systems for the delivery of perinatal services within a geographic area. The goals of regionalization are:

1. A reduction of maternal and perinatal mortality and morbidity rates
2. The provision of equal access to high-quality perinatal care irrespective of geographic location
3. The provision of high-quality perinatal care appropriate to need
4. The organization and improvement of obstetric and neonatal services in a cost-efficient manner.[3]

Regionalization of perinatal care implies that the personnel (principally physicians and nurses) and the facilities themselves are categorized to provide different levels of maternal and neonatal health care. The first level (level I facility) of perinatal care provides services for uncomplicated or minimally complicated pregnant and newborn patients. In this facility, a program for identifying high-risk mothers and neonates must be instituted, and a mechanism should be formulated for consultation, referral, and transfer of such patients to the next appropriate level of hospital care. The hospital must also be able to handle and manage unexpected or unanticipated emergencies and complications until such transfer can be expedited. *Guidelines for Perinatal Care,*[4] published

[3] M.B. Wingate, *Regionalization of perinatal care, in* 2 Principles and Practice of Obstetrics and Perinatology (1981).

[4] American Academy of Pediatrics, American College of Obstetricians and Gynecologists, Guidelines for Perinatal Care (1992).

through the joint efforts of the American Academy of Pediatrics and the American College of Obstetricians and Gynecologists, recommends the following functions of the staff in a level I facility:

1. Risk assessment of all pregnant patients admitted to the obstetric service
2. Management of uncomplicated perinatal care
3. Stabilization of unexpected problems
4. Initiation of maternal and neonatal transports
5. Patient and community education
6. Data collection and evaluation.

The level II (secondary) facility is the core of the regionalization program. This unit provides most of the services in urban and suburban areas, and the great majority of deliveries occur in this level. Most of the problem pregnancies are managed in this facility. A wide range of services, ranging from antepartum to postpartum and neonatal care, is provided by a level II unit with staffing that has skills in multidisciplinary medicine and nursing. However, some seldom seen or unusual problem cases are best referred to a level III (tertiary) facility, which has the most sophisticated resources as far as personnel, equipment, expertise, and experience are concerned. The functions of a level II facility include all the functions of a level I facility, plus:

1. Diagnosis and treatment of selected high-risk pregnancies and neonatal problems
2. Initiation and acceptance of maternal-fetal and neonatal transports
3. Education of allied health personnel
4. Residency education and affiliation with teaching centers.

A level III facility provides care for normal mothers and neonates in its geographic area and also serves as a referral and consultation center for the perinatal region. This unit must be equipped and staffed to provide services at the level of an intensive care unit on a 24-hour basis. This is where problem cases for both level I and II units are referred for best management. A level III or regional perinatal center's functions include all the functions of level I and II facilities, plus:

1. Diagnosis and treatment of all perinatal problems
2. Acceptance and direction of maternal-fetal and neonatal transports
3. Research and outcome surveillance
4. Graduate and postgraduate education
5. System management.

The health care providers caring for high risk pregnant patients are under a "duty to refer" when medically indicated.[5] The transfer of obstetrical patients is regulated by a federal law called the Emergency Medical Treatment and Active Labor Act (EMTALA).[6] The law was enacted to prevent the dumping of patients, especially obstetrical patients. The interested reader is referred to the recent article by Cardwell covering obstetrical transfers.[7]

§ 4.4 Specific Management

Specific management of any disorder in pregnancy will depend on the underlying cause, gestational age, and other factors as discussed in § 4.2. Conservative or temporizing measures are instituted to gain more maturity for the fetus unless parameters of fetal health indicate that further intrauterine life would be detrimental or if maternal health would be compromised by continuing the pregnancy. Use of specific medications, as well as use of laboratory tests, radiographic or sonographic tests, or other procedures, will depend on indications and assessment of risks and benefits. Delivery of the fetus is indicated if evidence is shown that the fetus continues to deteriorate in health. If termination of an early pregnancy becomes an acceptable or desired option for the patient but this option cannot be provided at the original facility, appropriate referral to another physician or facility that can offer counseling or the procedure itself is extended to the patient. Discussion of postpartum contraception or sterilization is also recommended during early pregnancy to help the patient wisely select the method that she will be comfortable with after delivery.

§ 4.5 Amniocentesis

Amniocentesis, a procedure to obtain fluid from the amniotic sac, may be utilized as part of fetal surveillance in high-risk pregnancies. Amniocentesis for genetic studies is now a common procedure in referral centers or antenatal testing units. Genetic amniocentesis is generally done between 15 and 20 weeks of gestation for the following indications:

1. Advanced maternal age (over 35 years)
2. Abnormal triple test or maternal serum alpha-fetoprotein results
3. Prior fetus or infant with chromosomal abnormality

---

[5] Richardson, Rosoff & McMenamin, *Referral Practices and Health Care Costs: The Dilemma of High Risk Obstetrics,* 6 J. Legal Med. 427 (1985).

[6] Pub. L. No. 99-272, § 9121 (codified as amended at 42 U.S.C. § 1395dd).

[7] M.S. Cardwell, *Transfer of Obstetric Patients under EMTALA,* 16 J. Legal Med. 357 (1995).

4. A recurrent genetic disorder diagnosable with prenatal testing

5. Fetal anomalies discovered on ultrasonography.

The patient should have genetic counseling before the procedure. If the mother is Rh negative, she may be a candidate for Rhogam injection following the procedure. When amniocentesis is performed at any time during pregnancy, a careful ultrasonographic assessment of the pregnancy should first be performed. Another technique, chorionic villi sampling (CVS) may be offered to selected patients as an alternative to genetic amniocentesis. CVS is usually performed between 9 and 12 weeks of gestation.

In other high-risk pregnancies (for example, pregnancies complicated by diabetes, hypertension, intrauterine growth restriction, or premature labor) amniocentesis may be of value to help determine fetal lung maturity and, thus, appropriate timing for delivery. Obviously, in cases of urgent fetal indications, like severe fetal distress, where delivery is the only option, amniocentesis becomes unnecessary. In cases of suspected chorioamnionitis, or intrauterine infection, amniocentesis may be performed to obtain fluid for bacterial culture and confirm the presence or absence of pathogens.

§ 4.6 Ultrasound

Ultrasound use in obstetrics had its beginnings in the late 1950s and early 1960s. Its most common application in present-day obstetrics is determination of gestational age. The normal gestational sac is first visible by ultrasound between the fourth and fifth week after the last menstrual period. The size of the gestational sac increases at a rapid rate from the fourth to the tenth postmenstrual week. If a followup study is done seven to ten days after the first ultrasound, a demonstration of appropriate growth constitutes a most reliable sign of a viable pregnancy.[8]

The most accurate ultrasonic parameter of gestational age is measurement of crown-rump length (CRL). From the sixth to the twelfth postmenstrual week, the embryo is at a stage of rapid growth. While determining the CRL, the sonographer can observe fetal cardiac activity. The biparietal diameter (BPD) can be measured as early as the twelfth postmenstrual week. Early in pregnancy, the BPD growth rate is much more rapid than after 30 weeks. Accuracy of determining gestational age using the BPD late in pregnancy is much less than if serial studies are done every 3 to 4 weeks between 15 and 30 weeks of gestation. This is particularly important to remember when intrauterine growth restriction is suspected on clinical grounds. Other ultrasonic measurements to help determine gestational age are fetal femur length, head circumference, and abdominal circumference. Other applications of ultrasound in obstetrics include

[8] J.P. McGahan & M. Porto, Diagnostic Obstetrical Ultrasound (1994).

fetal assessment using biophysical profile, estimations of fetal weight, diagnosis of multiple pregnancy, growth retardation, and fetal anomalies, as an adjunct in performing amniocentesis, diagnosis of placental location and abnormalities, and diagnosis of fetal death.

SPECIFIC OBSTETRIC PROBLEMS

§ 4.7 Pregnancy-Induced Hypertension and Other Hypertensive Disorders

Hypertension, when it complicates pregnancy, remains a major common cause of maternal and fetal mortality and morbidity. It is associated with about 12 percent of all maternal deaths occurring in the United States and is a leading cause of preterm delivery.[9] There are four criteria for the diagnosis of hypertension in a pregnant woman:[10]

1. A sustained rise of 30 millimeters of mercury (mmHg) or more in systolic blood pressure (BP)
2. A sustained rise of 15 mmHg or more in diastolic BP
3. A sustained systolic BP of 140 mmHg or more
4. A sustained diastolic BP of 90 mmHg or more.

Sustained means on at least two different occasions at least six hours apart.

The present classification of hypertensive disorders in pregnancy as outlined by the American College of Obstetricians and Gynecologists (ACOG) is:

I. Pregnancy-induced hypertension
  A. Preeclampsia
    1. Mild
    2. Severe
  B. Eclampsia
II. Chronic hypertension preceding pregnancy (any etiology)
III. Chronic hypertension (any etiology) with superimposed pregnancy-induced hypertension
  A. Superimposed preeclampsia
  B. Superimposed eclampsia

---

[9] R.W. Rochat, et al., *Maternal Mortality in the United States: Report from the Maternal Mortality Collaborative,* 79 Obstet. Gynecol. 91 (1988).

[10] American College of Obstetricians and Gynecologists, ACOG Technical Bull. No. 91, Management of Preeclampsia (1986).

The diagnosis of preeclampsia is made by the appearance of increased blood pressure accompanied by proteinuria or edema, or both. *Proteinuria* is defined as the presence of 300mg or more of protein in a 24-hour urine collection or a protein concentration of one gram or more per liter in at least two random urine specimens collected 6 hours or more apart. Edema, which may be present in normal pregnant women in the form of ankle or lower leg swelling, becomes a manifestation of preeclampsia if it accompanies hypertension, especially when generalized and reflecting excessive weight gain of greater than five pounds in one week.

Eclampsia is the occurrence of convulsions in a patient with preeclampsia. *Chronic hypertension* is defined as hypertension that is present and observed prior to pregnancy or that is diagnosed before 20 weeks of pregnancy. Preeclampsia or eclampsia may be superimposed on chronic hypertension. The diagnosis is made on the basis of a rise in blood pressure (30 mmHg systolic and 15 mmHg diastolic), together with proteinuria or generalized edema, or both. Transient hypertension indicates development of hypertension during pregnancy or in the first 24 hours postpartum in a previously normotensive woman when there is no other evidence of preeclampsia, such as proteinuria or generalized edema.

Preeclampsia has mild and severe forms. Severe preeclampsia is diagnosed when one or more of the following manifestations is present:[11]

1. Blood pressure of 160 mmHg or more systolic, or 110 mmHg or more diastolic, recorded on at least two occasions at least six hours apart, with the patient at bedrest

2. Proteinuria of five grams or more in 24 hours (more than three or four grams on semiqualitative examination)

3. Oliguria (400 to 500 ml or less in 24 hours)

4. Cerebral or visual disturbances such as altered consciousness, headache, scotomata, or blurred vision

5. Epigastric pain or right upper quadrant pain

6. Pulmonary edema or cyanosis

7. Impaired liver function of unclear etiology

8. Thrombocytopenia.

The usual sequence of the appearance of manifestations in preeclampsia is edema, followed by a rise in blood pressure and proteinuria; however, any order of appearance may be seen.[12] In addition to the clinical features of preeclampsia, some major changes as shown by laboratory studies may further indicate the severity of the disease and may influence the approach to management. Laboratory parameters that are known to be useful in diagnosing and managing preeclampsia include:

---

[11] *Id.*

[12] G. Cunningham, P. MacDonald & N. Gant, Williams Obstetrics (19th ed. 1993).

1. Hematologic: reduction in plasma volume may be indicated by a rapid rise in hematocrit. The hematocrit is not usually elevated in mild preeclampsia but may be extremely high in severe preeclampsia because of marked hemoconcentration.

2. Renal function studies: uric acid clearance and serum uric acid levels are sensitive and useful indicators of renal involvement in preeclampsia. In addition, determination of serum creatinine and creatinine clearance, as well as blood urea nitrogen and urea clearance, is very helpful in management.

3. Coagulation factors: reduction in serial platelet counts (thrombocytopenia) when approaching critical levels as well as changes in coagulation factors (for example, diminishing fibrinogen levels) or increasing titers of fibrin degradation products will certainly influence management.

4. Liver function tests, for example, determination of serum glutamic oxaloacetic transaminase, serum glutamic pyruvic transaminase, and lactic acid dehydrogenase.

The management of preeclampsia is influenced principally by the following factors: severity of the disease, the maternal and fetal status, availability of expertise, and hospital resources. Once a diagnosis of preeclampsia is made, hospitalization may be indicated. However, it may be acceptable to manage in the outpatient setting the patient with uncomplicated, mild hypertension who is without additional signs or symptoms and who is judged to be compliant. Recommendations will include bedrest, particularly in left lateral recumbency, and appropriate nutrition. Frequent visits to the office or clinic are indicated (at least twice a week) for monitoring of blood pressure, weight gain or loss, new symptoms, and degree of proteinuria. The office visits may be supplemented by home visits through a visiting nurses association competent in obstetrics. Antenatal testing of the fetus is done when indicated. Twice weekly non-stress testing with weekly biophysical profiles may be indicated. Hospitalization becomes mandatory when the blood pressure increases further or other complications appear.

Termination of pregnancy or delivery of the infant is the only definitive treatment of preeclampsia. While this is always appropriate therapy for the mother, it may not always be applicable for the fetus who may be grossly premature. In the mildly preeclamptic woman, for example, whose fetus is still immature but in whom fetal health assessment does not reflect any distress or compromise, options other than delivery may be considered as long as the mother remains stable and no signs of worsening are evident, the fetus is not in any kind of distress, and further intrauterine life is not detrimental to the fetus. On the other hand, in the case of severe preeclampsia, especially if there is rapid deterioration of hematologic, renal, and coagulation parameters, delivery becomes urgent for maternal indications, regardless of gestational age. Following are some general principles of management:

1. The prevention of convulsions is of utmost importance. Magnesium sulfate ($MgSO_4$) is the mainstay therapy in severe cases. $MgSO_4$ is given usually as an intravenous infusion prior to delivery during labor while stabilizing the patient's condition.

2. Antihypertensive agents are not routinely given in preeclampsia. However, therapy may be indicated in women in whom the blood pressure has risen so high that intracranial hemorrhage may occur. Diastolic blood pressure over 110 mmHg is often an indication for antihypertensives. Hydralazine, which is a direct vasodilator, is the most widely used agent to lower blood pressure in severe preeclampsia. Care must be given when administering antihypertensive therapy to the undelivered mother since abrupt lowering of the maternal blood pressure may precipitate placental insufficiency.

3. Diuretics are generally contraindicated because these patients already have decreased plasma volume and further depletion of volume may have a deleterious effect on the fetus.

4. Induction of labor may be safely carried out with amniotomy (rupture of membranes) if the cervix is favorable, or pitocin stimulation of labor, or both. However, in a patient with a rapidly deteriorating course, expeditious delivery via cesarean section may be indicated.

In the case of the patient with chronic hypertension in pregnancy, management is just as careful and aggressive. Most patients in this classification have mild chronic hypertension. However, studies of these patients have also shown increased perinatal mortality, preterm deliveries, intrauterine growth retardation, and antepartum and intrapartum fetal distress.[13] Initial workup of these patients may include an electrocardiogram, a serum chemistry profile (SMA-20), urine culture, and creatinine clearance if the serum creatinine is elevated.

Antihypertensive agents, such as alpha-methyldopa (Aldomet), have become part of the management of chronic hypertension in pregnancy. Frequent office visits (every one to two weeks) are recommended. Monitoring of the following is done during each visit: blood pressure, maternal weight, uterine growth, fetal movements, and proteinuria. Ultrasound studies are indicated for assessing fetal growth. Antenatal fetal surveillance is done whenever indicated but usually routinely by 28 to 30 weeks of gestation. A large majority of patients will deliver vaginally at term. Cesarean section is performed for obstetric indications such as fetal distress.

§ 4.8 Diabetes Mellitus

Diabetes mellitus may be defined as a state of carbohydrate intolerance that results from inadequate secretion of insulin or ineffective insulin action. There

---

[13] R.K. Creasy, R. Resnik, Maternal-Fetal Medicine, Principles and Practice (1994).

is an altered metabolism of carbohydrates, protein, and fats. In pregnancy, this altered metabolic state can progressively become worse because of the metabolic changes induced by pregnancy itself. Patients who have latent or subclinical diabetes may become overtly diabetic during pregnancy, or their predisposition to diabetes may be uncovered first when they become pregnant.

Diagnosis

The detection of diabetes in pregnancy begins with the history during the initial visit and clinical manifestations or clues. Important historical factors include a family history of diabetes, previous stillbirth, an infant with congenital malformation, neonatal death from birth trauma, and previous infant weighing 4000 grams or more. The presence of hypertension, obesity, and glycosuria should alert the physician to consider early diabetes screening in the patient.

The standard of care is now to perform screening on all pregnant patients for diabetes.[14] The patient is given 50 grams of glucose orally followed by determination of blood sugar one hour later. The patient need not be fasting for this evaluation. Screening is usually performed between 24 and 28 weeks unless historical risk factors are present which would mandate earlier screening. Values over 140 mg/dl for plasma determinations are considered abnormal. Any abnormal value requires further evaluation by performing a three-hour glucose tolerance test (GTT). If the GTT is abnormal, diabetes is then suspected. **Table 4–1** includes the ranges of normal values. If two values are above the normal limits, the criteria are met for gestational diabetes.

Table 4–1

Three-hour Glucose Tolerance Test

Fasting	105
One hour	190
Two hours	165
Three hours	145

Classification

In 1949, White first proposed a classification based on the patient's age at onset of diabetes, the duration of the diabetes, and the presence or absence of vascular complications.[15] White updated the classification in 1978.[16] The classification has been widely applied and is as follows:

---

[14] American College of Obstetricians and Gynecologists, ACOG Technical Bull. No. 200, Diabetes and Pregnancy (1994).

[15] White, *Pregnancy Complicating Diabetes,* 7 Am. J. Med. 609 (1949).

[16] White, *Classification of Obstetric Diabetes,* 130 Am. J. Obstetric Gynecology (1978).

Class A: Comprises about 90 percent of all patients with diabetes seen by the obstetrician. The diagnosis is based upon a GTT that is abnormal but fasting glucose levels are normal. Patients with Class A diabetes require no insulin. Glucose levels are normalized by dietary regulation. The risk of intrauterine fetal demise is low but still greater than a nondiabetic.

Class B: Onset of diabetes after age 20 and less than 10 years in duration. There are no vascular complications.

Class C: Onset of diabetes between 10 and 19 years, or diabetes has been present for 10 to 19 years. There is no vascular disease as in Class B.

Class D: Onset before age 10 or duration for 20 years or more. A subclassification is as follows: (1) patients who have diabetes before age 10; (2) patients who have had diabetes longer than 20 years; (3) patients with benign retinopathy; (4) patients with calcified leg vessels; and (5) patients with associated hypertension.

Class E: Requires the presence of pelvic calcifications and is no longer used as a diagnosis.

Class F: Diabetes with nephropathy with proteinuria and decreased creatinine clearance.

Class H: Diabetic patients with arteriosclerosis, including coronary artery disease.

Class R: Associated with proliferative retinopathy.

Other classifications have been applied, some of which are already used for nonruminant diabetics. However, the White classification remains the most widely used in managing obstetric patients.

Management

Insulin-dependent diabetics are best managed by a maternal-fetal medicine specialist (perinatologist) with the assistance of a diabetic care team composed of a diabetic education nurse, perinatal dietitian, perinatal nurse, retinologist, and other ancillary personnel. Delivery should be accomplished in an institution with a neonatal intensive care nursery. Class A diabetics may be managed by an obstetrician who is familiar with the treatment plan. The obstetrician and the local facility must have resources that will allow for optimal antepartum fetal health surveillance.

Class A.   As long as fasting glucose levels remain normal, these patients rarely have perinatal deaths. Exceptions include women who had a previous stillbirth or whose previous pregnancy was complicated by preeclampsia, or who required insulin in a previous pregnancy but now fit a Class A diagnosis.

Management consists of strict dietary control to supply an adequate number of calories for pregnancy at the same time achieving normal glucose levels. The obstetrician should see the patient every two weeks until 36 weeks and weekly thereafter. Home glucose monitoring should be used. Optimally, the patient should check her blood sugars five times a day: fasting, two hours postprandial, and at bedtime. The fasting levels should be μ105mg/dl and the two-hour and bedtime values should be μ120mg/dl. The patient should frequently check her urine for glucose and acetone. If the fasting glucose level becomes abnormal, the patient is reclassified as Class B and is then at risk for the increased perinatal complications associated with it. These patients will usually require insulin therapy. Class A patients should not go postterm. Delivery at 37 to 38 weeks (term) is recommended.

Classes B to R.   Fasting blood sugar levels should be maintained near μ105mg/dl and two-hour postprandial levels at μ120mg/dl. Together with dietary regulation, insulin injections, both regular and long-acting, are used to control sugar levels. Early in pregnancy, the following should be performed: chemistry profile, creatinine clearance, and baseline ultrasound examination. A retinal evaluation is recommended after the first visit. Glucose monitoring equipment is now available for patients to use in their homes to facilitate frequent blood sugar determinations. When blood sugar levels are very difficult to control, or if hypertension or pyelonephritis develop, the patient should be hospitalized for better management.

Antepartum fetal surveillance (non-stress tests and biophysical profiles) is usually started at 28 to 32 weeks, and earlier in the more severe classes of diabetics. Serial ultrasound studies will help assess fetal growth and can help to detect the presence of gross congenital anomalies. In the presence of complications, like deteriorating renal function or rising blood pressure, delivery should be considered. The timing of delivery is important, especially among the more severe classes, and is influenced by the age of gestation and status of fetal health. In the absence of deteriorating fetoplacental function, delivery is usually delayed until a lecithin-sphingomyelin (L/S) ratio of at least 2.0 in amniotic fluid analysis has been demonstrated. Other factors influencing the timing of delivery are the presence of maternal complications and the degree of metabolic control of the diabetes. The route of delivery is influenced by the fetal status, condition of the cervix (whether or not favorable for induction of labor), and presence or absence of maternal complications. If other complicating obstetric conditions are present, such as fetopelvic disproportion, abnormal placental location, or fetal growth retardation, delivery by cesarean section may be necessary.

Control of diabetes during pregnancy and thereafter is of utmost importance. The possible adverse effects on the mother include increased likelihood of operative intervention, increased tendency for preeclampsia-eclampsia, increased possibility for infection, and postpartum hemorrhage. Adverse effects in the fetus and newborn infant include increased perinatal morbidity and mortality and increased possibility of congenital anomalies.

§ 4.9 Preterm Labor and Premature Rupture of Membranes

Preterm labor is the occurrence of regular uterine contractions with accompanying changes in the cervix prior to the completion of 37 weeks of gestation (less than 259 days from the last menstrual period).[17] In most cases, the exact cause or causes of preterm or premature labor are not known. Predisposing factors to labor before term include:

1. Spontaneous rupture of membranes
2. Incompetent cervix or uterine anomalies
3. Abruptio placenta and placenta previa
4. Urinary tract infection
5. Uterine overdistention as in hydramnios (excessive amniotic fluid) or multiple pregnancy
6. Fetal anomalies
7. Previous preterm delivery
8. Maternal behavior factors such as smoking, alcohol consumption, or illicit drug use
9. Infection etiologies such as chorioamnionitis.

Because of the higher incidence of perinatal morbidity and mortality among preterm infants compared to term, management of preterm labor requires skill and expertise among both the obstetric and pediatric staff. The patient with preterm labor is best managed in a hospital facility with a neonatal intensive care unit if suppression of labor is not successful and delivery becomes imminent.

The patient whose pregnancy may be complicated by preterm labor may be recognized even before labor begins. Factors known to be associated with preterm labor and delivery should be investigated in every obstetric patient. These include the following:[18]

1. Age less than 18 years or more than 40 years
2. Single
3. Low prepregnant weight

---

[17] American College of Obstetricians and Gynecologists, ACOG Technical Bull. No. 206, Preterm Labor (1995).

[18] *Id.*

4. Poor weight gain or weight loss during pregnancy

5. Smoker

6. Multifetal pregnancy

7. Previous spontaneous abortions or terminations in midtrimesters

8. Urinary tract infection during pregnancy

9. Previous preterm delivery

10. Uterine irritability during current pregnancy

11. Previous stillbirth or neonatal death.

Once a diagnosis of preterm labor is made, it must be determined, before any attempt to arrest it, whether prolongation of intrauterine life is likely to benefit or harm the fetus or the mother. If there is no contraindication for prolongation of fetal life, suppression of labor may be attempted. The currently acceptable regimen for suppression of preterm labor includes: hospitalization, hydration, sedation, and bedrest. If uterine activity persists or intensifies, administration of a tocolytic agent may be necessary. A betamimetic agent such as Terbutaline or Ritodrine may be used. These drugs are not without potential side effects. In the mother, tachycardia, hypotension, chest tightness or pain, vomiting, headaches, fever, and hallucinations have been observed. Pulmonary edema and death have been reported. Maternal metabolic effects of the drug include hyperglycemia (which explains the need for cautious use among diabetics), hypokalemia, lacticacidosis, and ketoacidosis.

Rapidly replacing the betamimetics as the drug of choice for tocolysis is intravenous magnesium sulfate. Magnesium sulfate, well-known for its important role in the management of preeclampsia and eclampsia (see § 4.7), has also been employed in the treatment of preterm labor. Magnesium sulfate provides a possible alternative to betamimetics in situations where severe maternal side effects secondary to betamimetics are not desirable.

Premature Rupture of the Membranes

Premature rupture of the membranes (PROM) is defined as rupture of membranes prior to onset of labor, regardless of age of gestation.[19] It occurs in about 10 percent of all deliveries. In most instances, the cause of the PROM is not understood. Diagnosis is usually made based on history, clinical findings, and simple laboratory tests.

When spontaneous PROM occurs at term, labor will occur within 24 hours after rupture in about 90 percent of patients. The latent period, which is the time from membrane rupture to onset of labor, has been found to be longer among patients with PROM occurring prior to term.

---

[19] American College of Obstetricians and Gynecologists, ACOG Technical Bull. No. 115, Premature Rupture of Membranes (1988).

The complications associated with PROM are those related to infection (maternal or fetal/neonatal) or delivery of a premature infant. Maternal infectious morbidity rises even more if delivery is by cesarean section. Fetal/neonatal infection after PROM is inversely related to the gestational age at the time of rupture and the latent period.

Management of premature rupture of the membranes is influenced by the following:

1. Presence or absence of infection: If chorioamnionitis is clinically evident (fever, maternal tachycardia, uterine irritability, positive Gram's stain of amniotic fluid for bacteria, positive bacterial culture of amniotic fluid), the patient should be delivered. If there is no evidence of infection, a period of observation may be beneficial for both the mother and the fetus. In the mother, spontaneous labor may ensue, or the cervix may ripen, making it more favorable for induction of labor later. In the fetus whose gestation is remote from term, acceleration of pulmonary maturity may occur if expectant management is carried out for days.

2. Gestational age: If the fetus is at term or near term (34 to 38 weeks), delivery is accomplished. If the cervix is unfavorable, cervical ripening agents such as prostaglandin may be used. As mentioned, the majority of patients will go into spontaneous labor within 24 hours when PROM occurs at term. If no labor occurs, induction is started if the cervix is favorable. If the fetus is very remote from term, especially if grossly premature, the mother should first be transferred to a tertiary facility. As long as infection is not evident, the obstetrician will generally choose to temporize until an indication to deliver the fetus arises (infection, signs of fetal distress, active labor). However, recent studies suggest that aggressive management, that is, oxytocin stimulation, at 30 weeks or greater in PROM result in neonatal outcomes as favorable as conservative management.[20] It is advisable to consider giving glucocorticoids to the mother in this situation to help accelerate pulmonary maturity in the premature infant.[21] Suppression of premature labor in the presence of PROM, particularly in the grossly premature infant, may sometimes be considered, if only to buy time for the administered glucocorticoids to achieve their effect on the fetal pulmonary system.

3. Fetal status: The presence of signs of fetal distress requires delivery. Ultrasound evaluation is extremely helpful in assessing fetal health and fetal status with regard to presentation (especially if breech or transverse lie), presence of congenital anomalies, or even a previously unsuspected multiple pregnancy.

[20] S. Cox, K. Leveno, *Intentional Delivery versus Expectant Management with Preterm Ruptured Membranes at 30–34 weeks' Gestation,* 86 Obstet. Gynecol. 875–79 (1995).

[21] National Institutes of Health, Effects of Corticosteroids for Fetal Maturation on Perinatal Outcomes (1994).

§ 4.10   Postdatism and Postmaturity

A pregnancy becomes postterm if it exceeds 42 weeks based on the patient's last known menstrual period (LNMP). The term "postdatism" has been used interchangeably with "prolonged pregnancy" and "postterm pregnancy." The latter is the currently preferred terminology used by most authors. The term "postmaturity" is now designated to mean a complication of intrauterine growth restriction or disturbance in fetal growth associated with postterm pregnancy. Some authors apply the term "dysmaturity" to refer to postmature infants.

The management of postterm pregnancy is based on the following:

1. Reliability of dates: Based on LNMP or other clinical parameters, fetal age dating is usually not difficult to determine. If the menstrual dates are unreliable, and there is a discrepancy between uterine size and menstrual dates, ultrasonographic measurements of fetal growth parameters are required for more reliable assessment of fetal age.
2. Favorability of the cervix for induction of labor.
3. Status of fetal health: Non-stress testing with biophysical profile testing, if indicated, may help determine if immediate delivery is desirable or expectant management is still feasible.
4. Sonographic evidence of placental aging, volume of amniotic fluid, presence or absence of congenital anomalies, fetal presentation (especially if breech or transverse lie).

Once the decision to deliver the postterm patient has been made, care must be taken regarding the potential problems that can accompany labor and delivery, such as intrapartum fetal distress, birth trauma (especially macrosomic or large babies), and meconium aspiration syndrome (MAS). To help prevent MAS, the pharynx of the infant must be aspirated with a DeLee suction tube even before the first breathing effort of the infant, as soon as the head is out of the vaginal introitus or in the open uterus in the case of cesarean section. The pediatrician, if present, may later decide to do endotracheal aspiration if meconium was initially aspirated.

§ 4.11   Intrauterine Growth Restriction

In general, a newborn infant is termed growth-restricted, or small for gestational age (SGA), if the weight at birth falls below the tenth percentile for the infant's gestational age. Factors that have been associated with or are known to predispose to intrauterine growth restriction (IUGR) include: small maternal build or size, poor maternal weight gain during pregnancy, use of illicit drugs, cigarette smoking, chronic alcoholism, fetal infections, congenital malformations, previous IUGR, multiple pregnancy, maternal anemia, chronic renal or vascular disease, and abnormalities of placenta and cord.

The diagnosis of IUGR is made on the basis of historical risk factors, if any, that predispose to the condition, and careful correlation of uterine growth with gestational age during the patient's visits. Ultrasonographic measurements of various parameters of fetal growth can detect growth lag when serially performed.

The management of the growth-restricted fetus depends on the fetal status and age of gestation, and the presence of maternal factors that may have predisposed to the IUGR. In the case of the severely growth-restricted fetus with accompanying signs of fetal distress (poor biophysical profile, nonreactive non-stress test, or positive contraction stress test), delivery is the only option. In the presence of an unfavorable cervix, or if prolonged labor is anticipated, cesarean section may be the better choice for delivery to prevent further stressing the fetus with forces of uterine contractions and the potential problem of intrapartum hypoxia.

§ 4.12 Bleeding During First Half of Pregnancy

Any episode of bleeding at any time during pregnancy should be reported to the physician. During the first 20 weeks, bleeding may be due to abortion, ectopic pregnancy, or hydatidiform mole. Other less important causes are local lesions of the cervix like polyps or cervicitis. The bleeding may or may not be accompanied by severe cramps or pain.

Abortion

Abortion, either spontaneous (commonly called *miscarriage*) or induced, is the termination of pregnancy before 20 weeks of gestation. Chromosomal abnormality in the developing embryo has been cited as the most common cause of spontaneous abortion, especially if the abortion occurs in the early weeks of pregnancy.[22] There are two common clinical types of abortion that are frequently encountered: threatened and incomplete.

Threatened.   This is characterized by occurrence of vaginal bleeding, which may be in the form of spotting or actual scanty flow. The patient may have pelvic cramps or actual pain. The pregnancy remains intact and the cervix has not dilated. The management is primarily symptomatic. The patient is given analgesics for discomfort, bedrest is recommended, and work stoppage is advisable.

Incomplete.   In general, bleeding is heavier, there is more pelvic discomfort or pain, and passage of products of conception becomes evident. Either the fetus,

---

[22] G. Cunningham, P. MacDonald & N. Gant, Williams Obstetrics (19th ed. 1993).

placenta, or both may be expelled, together or separately. Once this is evident, and the abortion is confirmed by an open or dilated cervix, completion of abortion by curettage is recommended. A curettage will completely evacuate the uterus, thus preventing postabortal hemorrhage from retained placental fragments if the abortion was not complete. It is important to send all specimens obtained, whether at the office during examination or at the time of curettage, for histopathologic examination to ascertain the presence or absence of placenta. It is also important to determine the patient's blood type and Rh factor to see if she is a candidate for postcurettage administration of RhoGam

Ectopic Pregnancy

The fertilized egg normally implants in the endometrium lining the uterine cavity. Ectopic pregnancy is implantation anywhere else. Tubal pregnancy, or pregnancy growing in the fallopian tube, is the most common type of ectopic pregnancy. The principal complication of tubal pregnancy is related to the degree of intraperitoneal bleeding that follows rupture of the tube or abortion of the pregnancy through the tube.

Prior to either tubal abortion or rupture, the clinical manifestations of a tubal pregnancy vary from patient to patient. A history of amenorrhea, morning sickness, breast tenderness, and other features of normal pregnancy may be presented by the woman. She may complain of vague low abdominal pains. She may initially consult the physician because of vaginal spotting or actual bleeding. Sometimes there is no history of amenorrhea. When tubal rupture has occurred, the patient presents with varying degrees of hypotension and vasomotor disturbances, if not actual shock. A history of preceding vertigo or syncope is not uncommon. There may be evidence of acute abdomen tenderness with rebound, rigidity of the muscle wall, and absent bowel sounds. Pelvic examination reveals severe tenderness of the cervix, especially on motion, the vaginal cul-de-sac may be bulging and tender, the uterus may be palpable and also tender, and an adnexal mass may or may not be present. The differential diagnosis includes salpingitis (pelvic inflammatory disease), threatened or incomplete abortion of an intrauterine pregnancy, acute appendicitis, and twisted ovarian cyst.

Diagnosis and management of ectopic pregnancy depends on where the pregnancy is located and whether there has been rupture. In the unruptured tubal pregnancy, there may be very few and vague symptoms. The physician must always be "ectopic-conscious." A woman presenting with irregular vaginal bleeding with pelvic pain, especially if there is a history of amenorrhea and other signs of pregnancy, should be investigated for the possibility of extrauterine pregnancy. A radioimmunoassay test for beta human chorionic gonadotropin (HCG) (blood pregnancy test) is most sensitive and can detect even the low levels of HCG in ectopic pregnancy. In recent years, sonography has become a most important tool in the diagnostic approach to ectopic pregnancy.

In the presence of a positive pregnancy test and a gestational sac in the uterus by sonography, it is unlikely that an ectopic pregnancy coexists. If the pregnancy test is positive but no intrauterine pregnancy is demonstrated on sonography, ectopic pregnancy becomes suspect.

If suspicion for ectopic pregnancy is strong, time should not be wasted to confirm it. A diagnostic laparoscopy is most helpful; however, it requires an experienced operator and refined equipment, and sometimes unnecessary delay. Occasionally, the tube with the ectopic pregnancy may be visualized as normal if the gestation is very early. If any doubt persists as to diagnosis, a laparotomy should be performed. If a tubal pregnancy is found, depending on whether rupture has occurred, and depending on the experience and skills of the surgeon, the affected tube may be removed. Alternatively, only the pregnancy may be removed and the fallopian tube conserved, especially if the woman is of low parity and has expressed a desire to retain her reproductive capability.

Any woman who is Rh negative with negative antibody screen and with her reproductive capability retained should receive RhoGam to protect against isoimmunization.

Hydatidiform Mole

Hydatidiform mole is a benign neoplastic degeneration of the chorionic villi of the placenta in the absence of a live fetus. It has clinical features suggestive of a pregnancy, except for the presence of a live pregnancy. Rare cases of hydatidiform mole coexisting with a live fetus have been reported.

Hydatidiform mole presents with clinical features suggestive of pregnancy, such as amenorrhea, morning sickness, uterine enlargement, and positive pregnancy test. The uterus may enlarge faster than expected for dates. The physician may first suspect the presence of hydatidiform mole if fetal heart beats are not detected by Doppler by the twelfth week of gestation. The woman may consult because of on-and-off vaginal bleeding. Ultrasonography will be most helpful at this time. In the case of a molar degeneration of the pregnancy, no gestational sac or fetus is demonstrated. Quantitative measurements of HCG are helpful in the diagnosis and treatment.

The treatment for hydatidiform mole consists of two stages: first, uterine evacuation of the mole, and second, careful followup for detection of malignant change. Uterine evacuation of the mole can be achieved by simple curettage, suction or aspiration curettage, oxytocin or prostaglandin administration, hysterotomy, or hysterectomy. The last is reserved for the elderly woman who has completed her family or who does not desire further childbearing. Women over 40 years of age and of high parity are better treated with hysterectomy because of the increased occurrence of malignant degeneration in these age and parity groups.

A careful followup of the patient after molar evacuation is extremely important. The emphasis is on frequent determinations of HCG titers during the first month and subsequently until negative titers are obtained. The HCG level should progressively fall. If the titers are not falling or are rising again, appropriate consultation and further investigation to rule out malignant change are necessary.

Another pregnancy is discouraged for at least one year following a molar pregnancy. Oral contraceptives are permissible and will not interfere with the followup pregnancy tests.

§ 4.13 Bleeding During Second Half of Pregnancy

During the second half of pregnancy, placenta previa and abruptio placenta constitute the most common major causes of bleeding. Particularly after 28 weeks of gestation, when survival of the fetus is a realistic possibility, appropriate and skilled management can help lower the maternal and perinatal morbidity and mortality.

Placenta Previa

In placenta previa, the placenta is located over the internal os of the cervix. There are several types of placenta previa, depending on their location in the lower segment of the uterus. The most important is the total type, with the internal os being covered completely by the placenta. This type is most prone to developing severe degrees of hemorrhage.

The possibility of placenta previa must be considered in any pregnant patient who has a bleeding episode after the twentieth week of gestation. With more skilled sonologists and sonographers and with the availability of ultrasonography even in small communities, the diagnosis of placenta previa is made earlier and more accurately, thus facilitating appropriate perinatal management and possibly preventing catastrophic bleeding. Pelvic examination of the patient with vaginal bleeding at this stage of pregnancy must never be performed unless placenta previa has been ruled out by sonography.

The management of placenta previa depends on the amount of bleeding and age of gestation. In addition, the type of placenta previa and the mother's parity can influence the treatment. In general, the more remote the fetus is from term, the more conservative the management is. Transfer to a tertiary level facility is recommended, especially if the fetus is premature. Cesarean section is the delivery route of choice in the patient with total placenta previa when delivery has to be accomplished for maternal (profuse bleeding) or fetal (fetal distress) indications. However, even if total placenta previa is confirmed, as long as no indication for delivery arises and the pregnancy is remote from term, expectant management is recommended while waiting for fetal pulmonary maturity or until delivery becomes necessary. Glucocorticoids may be considered for the mother to accelerate fetal lung maturity if the fetus is between 24 and 34 weeks.

Vaginal delivery may be considered in the types of placenta previa that are partial or incomplete as long as the patient is in a facility where cesarean section can be performed immediately if necessary, where blood bank resources are existing, and where a neonatal intensive care unit is available.

Abruptio Placenta

Abruptio placenta refers to the premature separation of the normally implanted placenta. Clinically, the patient may present with one or more of the following features: vaginal bleeding (scanty or profuse), rigid and tender uterus, absent fetal heart tones (which does not necessarily indicate that the fetus is dead), varying degrees of hypovolemia, and coagulopathy. The clinical picture will depend on the degree of abruption.

Diagnosis of abruptio placenta is based mainly on clinical grounds and the exclusion of placenta previa. There are associated factors that may predispose to abruptio placenta.[23] Among these, high parity, elevated intrapartum blood pressure, and previous history of abruption seem to have the greatest association.

The management of abruptio placenta will depend on both maternal and fetal status at the time diagnosis is made. Profuse bleeding, especially if accompanied by shock, requires immediate and aggressive therapy with the aim to correct the hypovolemia and restore effective maternal circulation. Blood must be available in large quantities to replace the hemorrhage. Renal failure and disseminated intravascular clotting are two important complications that may follow massive placental abruption.

Plans for delivery of the fetus are made if the patient continues to manifest either external or internal bleeding, or both. Amniotomy may hasten labor and delivery especially if the fetus is at term or near term. Oxytocin may be helpful in enhancing uterine contractions and thus improving labor, but care must be observed in that oxytocin may aggravate the hypertonus that may exist because of the abruption. Internal fetal and uterine monitors must be applied when feasible for better assessment and planning of delivery. If the fetus shows signs of distress and delivery is not expected soon, cesarean section becomes the treatment of choice.

§ 4.14 Multiple Gestation

Multiple gestation may result from fertilization of a single ovum that subsequently divides into two similar structures, or from fertilization of more than one ovum. Twins are the most common type of multifetal pregnancy and are called either monozygotic (single-ovum or identical) or dizygotic (double-ovum or fraternal). Dizygotic twins are more common than monozygotic twins. The

---

[23] G. Cunningham, P. MacDonald & N. Gant, Williams Obstetrics (19th ed. 1993).

incidence of delivery of dizygotic twins is influenced by heredity, race, age of the mother, parity, and use of "fertility drugs," whereas that of monozygotic twins is not. With the increasing use of fertility drugs, such as gonadotropins and clomiphene, for induction of ovulation, the incidence of twin pregnancies increases.

The presence of twin pregnancy increases perinatal morbidity and mortality. The following are known complications that occur more frequently with multiple pregnancy:[24]

1. Abortion
2. Low birth weight, either from prematurity or growth restriction
3. Congenital anomalies
4. Twin-Twin transfusion
5. Pregnancy-induced or aggravated hypertension
6. Difficult or complicated labor, from abnormal fetal presentation or ineffective or premature labor
7. Maternal anemia
8. Abruptio placenta or placenta previa
9. Postpartum hemorrhage from uterine atony
10. Umbilical cord accidents
11. Hydramnios.

The diagnosis of multiple fetuses is often difficult during early pregnancy and is usually not suspected. Often multiple pregnancies are not diagnosed until labor or even during delivery. The family history and history of use of fertility drugs should alert the physician to the possibility. At about midpregnancy or later, a discrepancy in dates and uterine size, when the uterus is much larger than is expected for the gestational age, requires evaluation by ultrasound. At any time during pregnancy, however, when multiple pregnancy is suspected, confirmation by ultrasound is necessary since early diagnosis will modify the conduct of prenatal care and can help prevent many of the complications that are associated with multiple pregnancy. Because of the complications of multiple pregnancy during labor and delivery, the pregnant woman must be advised that labor and delivery might be necessary at a tertiary facility.

The conduct of prenatal care in multiple pregnancy is geared toward the following objectives:

1. Prevent delivery of grossly premature infants
2. Identify if fetal growth restriction occurs and, if so, accomplish delivery before intrauterine death occurs
3. Prevent or avoid trauma to the fetuses during labor and delivery

---

[24] R. Creasy & R. Resnik, Maternal-Fetal Medicine, Principles and Practice, (3d ed. 1994).

4. Prevent or manage maternal complications

5. Provide adequate and expert neonatal care from birth.

Once a diagnosis of multiple pregnancy is made, appropriate and frequent counseling is provided the patient. The following aspects of prenatal care are also emphasized:

Diet. Nutritional support to the mother must be increased. The mother must at least meet standards in weight gain.

Bedrest. It has been shown that ample bedrest (and avoidance of strenuous work load) can result in increased birth weights for the fetuses, decreased frequency of hypertensive disorders, and lowered perinatal mortality.

Intrauterine fetal growth restriction (see § **4.11**) may occur in one or both fetuses in a twin pregnancy (or one or all in other multiple pregnancies). Maternal nutrition should be adequate, ample bedrest is advisable, and serial ultrasound studies every four weeks between 20 and 36 weeks of gestation are recommended. Ultrasonography gives additional information on the estimated fetal weights, any detectable anomaly, the amount of amniotic fluid, and, of importance just prior to delivery, the fetal presentation.

During labor, the presentation of the fetuses is ascertained by ultrasonography. There has been an increasing use of cesarean section among pregnancies, the most common indication being a presentation other than cephalic by one or both fetuses. Other important indications for cesarean section are complicated labor, hypertension, fetal distress, and prolapse of the cord. If vaginal delivery is decided upon, a physician experienced in vaginal maneuvers, especially for a second twin, should be present, as well as one who is able to perform an immediate cesarean section should the need arise. Many of the complications, such as fetal trauma and trauma to the maternal genital tract from difficult delivery, would be avoided if cesarean section were performed in many multiple pregnancies. In any case, every step in the management, including risks and possible sequelae, should be discussed with the patient and her family.

§ 4.15   Rh Isoimmunization

After the discovery of the Rh system by Landsteiner in 1940, more became known about erythroblastosis fetalis, in which continuous destruction of fetal red blood cells occurring during intrauterine life led to severe anemia and cardiac failure in the fetus, resulting in death. About 97 percent of all cases of erythroblastosis felatis are caused by maternal immunization against the Rh (D) antigen present in the fetal red cells. There are other fetal antigens such as C, c, E, e, K, h, Fy^a (Duffy), M, and Jk^a (Kidd), but are much less common. The most common cause of maternal Rh isoimmunization is the passage of fetal Rh-positive red cells into the bloodstream of Rh-negative mothers during pregnancy or delivery. The mother then develops an immune response in the form of Rh antibodies that can pass through the placenta (rarely during the first pregnancy when the immune response was triggered, thus sparing the first infant from fetal hemolysis) and which can affect future pregnancies.

Maternal isoimmunization can also result from transfusion of Rh-positive blood to an Rh-negative woman, or from sensitization of an Rh-negative woman by a pregnancy presumably with an Rh-positive fetus but which pregnancy did not progress to viability, for example, abortion or ectopic pregnancy.

During routine prenatal screening, antibodies that cross the placenta and adversely affect the fetus can be detected. Screening for such antibodies should be a routine determination together with the other tests requested on the initial visit, even if the patient is a primigravida. When an antibody, particularly one that may lead to fetal anemia from hemolysis, is detected, an initial titer should be determined.

The management of the Rh-sensitized pregnancy is geared toward the detection of the degree of hemolysis that may be existing and the effect on fetal health as pregnancy progresses. With increasing hemolysis of the fetal red cells, more bilirubin is produced and this is reflected in the amniotic fluid. Amniocentesis has become the mainstay of management of the Rh-sensitized pregnancy. The amniotic fluid is sent for spectrophotometric analysis to determine delta OD (optical density) 450 bilirubin values. The time to do the initial amniocentesis depends on the obstetrical history (previous sensitized infants and their perinatal outcomes, such as need for exchange transfusions, any stillbirths, or neonatal deaths). The earliest time would be at about 20 weeks of gestation if previous history dictates an earlier assessment. More realistically, an initial amniocentesis is done between 24 to 28 weeks, especially if the previous sensitized pregnancy or pregnancies had excellent perinatal outcomes.

Subsequent amniocentesis is done depending on the initial delta OD 450 values. A common method used to time subsequent amniocentesis is that based on the work of Liley, wherein the value and subsequent values also determined by amniocentesis are plotted and their positions on three different zones (1, 2, and 3, representing unaffected or mildly affected, moderately affected, and severely affected fetuses) are determined.[25] If the values show deterioration, the obstetrician will decide whether urgent delivery is required to prevent fetal demise or whether waiting another week to repeat amniocentesis is acceptable rather than risk delivery of a grossly premature fetus with very little chance of survival outside the uterus.

The plan for delivery is thus dictated by the delta OD values. Induction of labor is recommended if the cervix is ripe and favorable. Cesarean section is

---

[25] Liley, *Liguor Amnii Analysis in Management of Pregnancy Complicated by Rhesus Sensitization,* 82 Am. J. Obstetric Gynecology 1359 (1961).

indicated, especially if fetal assessment using non-stress tests or contraction stress tests shows a severely compromised fetus. If expectant management, as allowed by acceptable delta OD values, is the course taken, a determination of the L/S ratio is also requested from the amniotic fluid taken during the amniocentesis performed near term. When fetal pulmonary maturity is reached, the pregnancy is terminated.

Because of the complexity of counseling, frequent amniocentesis, interpretation of results, and determination of appropriate timing of delivery, it is highly recommended that pregnant patients with Rh isoimmunization be managed by a team highly experienced in this problem. The team should include an experienced obstetrician, if not a perinatologist, and a neonatologist, both of whom can avail themselves of resources in a tertiary facility.

The Rh-negative pregnant patient with no antibodies should have repeat antibody screening at 28 weeks. She becomes a candidate for administration of Rh-immune globulin (RhoGam) at 28 weeks (unless the baby's father is known to be Rh-negative as well) and again after delivery if the baby is Rh-positive.

Administration of RhoGam to eligible patients has drastically reduced the incidence of Rh isoimmunization. RhoGam is a solution containing immunoglobulin G (IgG) anti-Rho (D) for use in Rh negative individuals exposed to Rh positive red cells. Candidates for RhoGam administration are Rh-negative women who have or had:

1. Threatened abortion
2. Incomplete abortion completed by curettage
3. Termination of pregnancy
4. Ectopic pregnancy
5. Genetic amniocentesis at 16 to 18 weeks gestation
6. Abdominal trauma in the second or third trimester
7. Amniocentesis done in the third trimester
8. Inadvertent recent administration of Rh-positive blood.

As stated previously, antepartum prophylaxis with RhoGam is now recommended at 28 weeks gestation in all Rh-negative unsensitized (negative antibody screen) patients, to be repeated after delivery within 72 hours postpartum if the baby is Rh-positive. In case of doubt, whether the patient should receive extra doses of RhoGam, particularly when feto-maternal bleed is deemed excessive, testing for the presence of fetal red cells in the maternal blood is available and proportionate doses of RhoGam may be deemed necessary depending on the result. A consultation with a perinatologist is often helpful.

§ 4.16 Maternal Infections: TORCH

The so-called TORCH group of maternal infections that can cross the placental barrier and produce adverse effects on the fetus include the following etiologic organisms:

T: Toxoplasma gondii (causes toxoplasmosis)

O: Others, that include treponema pallidum (causes syphilis)

R: Rubella

C: Cytomegaloviruses

H: Herpes simplex virus types I and II.

Toxoplasmosis

Toxoplasmosis may be acquired by consuming raw or undercooked meat of infected animals or by contact with parasites (toxoplasma gondii) from the feces of an infected cat. Cats acquire toxoplasmosis by eating infected mice or other animals. The parasite cysts (the latent form) are found only in cats. The infected patient who has clinical features of the disease will commonly manifest lymphadenopathy (usually cervical) and symptoms of the "flu." Diagnosis may be confirmed by detection of IgG antibodies by different tests, such as indirect fluorescent-antibody test, Sabin-Feldman dye test, indirect hemagglutination inhibition test, and complement fixation test. Serial titer determination may be necessary to diagnose acute infection.

Most infants with congenital toxoplasmosis do not have clinical manifestations. Of those with clinical signs, the following are common: chorioretinitis, abnormal spinal fluid, anemia, enlarged spleen, fever, and jaundice. Convulsions and vomiting are less common. Acute primary toxoplasmosis in pregnancy has also been associated with fetal growth retardation, premature infants, and abortion.

To prevent toxoplasmosis in pregnancy, the patient is advised to have little or no contact with cats, not to handle cat litter, or to avoid eating undercooked meat. In those women with confirmed toxoplasmosis in the first trimester, counseling regarding the risk of serious congenital infection and consideration for termination of pregnancy must be offered. Actual treatment with drugs should be in consultation with or by a physician who has expertise in infectious diseases.

Rubella

Rubella, also known as German measles, is usually a mild illness characterized by fever, joint pain, a transient erythematous rash, and postauricular or suboccipital lymphadenopathy. The cause is a virus. The clinical diagnosis is often confused with other illnesses that manifest a rash and fever. To confirm the infection, antibody testing is available.

Overall, the risk of rubella infection transmitted to the fetus is generally quoted at about 20 percent when the mother acquires the infection during the first trimester, with the highest risk at 50 percent in the first month to about 10 percent by the third month. The most common congenital anomalies are cataracts, patent ductus arteriosus, and deafness.

Prevention of rubella by vaccination of rubella-susceptible women of reproductive age has been advocated. It is recommended that pregnancy be avoided for at least three months after vaccination. Thus, the immediate postpartum period seems to be the best time period to vaccinate women, if their prenatal testing for rubella showed no immunity.

Cytomegalovirus

Cytomegalovirus (CMV) causes cytomegalic inclusion disease, previously thought a rare type of intrauterine infection, but which recent studies have identified as a common etiologic agent. Asymptomatic CMV infection and excretion is commonly found in pregnancy. Its incidence is highest among young, unmarried primiparas with low socio-economic and educational status. The fetus may be infected transplacentally, as it passes through the infected birth canal, through ingestion of infected milk, or by oral-to-oral contact with its mother. Congenital infections may occur following either primary or recurrent infection in the mother. Congenital infections have been reported in consecutive pregnancies. CMV is a sexually transmitted disease, and women may acquire the infection during pregnancy from infected partners.

Diagnosis of CMV infection in the mother on clinical manifestations alone is difficult because over 90 percent are asymptomatic and those who have symptoms have nonspecific "flu-like" complaints. The best way to detect the presence of CMV infection is by isolating the virus. Antibody titers may be requested to help diagnose primary infection.

Most congenitally infected infants do not manifest signs of infection at birth. Those who survive the infection subsequently manifest characteristic findings like mental retardation, chorioretinitis, cerebral calcifications, and microcephaly or hydrocephaly. Other infected neonates manifest jaundice, thrombocytopenia, hepatosplenomegaly, and optic atrophy.

There is no known treatment for CMV infections. Symptomatic treatment of flu-like complaints is given. Counseling is directed toward informing patients of the risk of congenital infection, the potential for birth defects, and possibility of recurrences. Consideration for termination of pregnancy is discussed with the patient if primary CMV infection is documented during the first half of pregnancy.

Herpes

The herpes simplex virus may cause infection in the adult, the neonate, or, rarely, the fetus. The mode of transmission is generally through sexual contact. Two types, herpes simplex virus type I (HSV-1) and type II (HSV-2) are recognized. It is now known that either type can cause infections in the mouth, skin, and genitalia. The major problem in obstetrics is neonatal herpes infection which is acquired perinatally from an infected, lower genital tract of the mother, most often during vaginal delivery. Among women with genital herpes at term, there is a 50 percent risk of the neonate acquiring the infection when delivered vaginally if the infection is primary.[26] Among infected neonates, about 50 percent will have serious sequelae, including death.

Diagnosis of herpes is best confirmed by viral culture of the genital lesion. In the case of a patient with previous history of herpes but no recurrences during pregnancy, vaginal delivery may be anticipated. A genital lesion or reoccurrence at term is an indication for cesarean section.

Other Maternal Infections

Syphilis is a chronic infectious disease caused by the spirochete treponema pallidum. Transmission is through sexual contact. It has long been recognized that maternal syphilis infection can be transferred transplacentally and thus can result in fetal and neonatal infection. Stillbirths, premature births, congenital malformations, and active infection at birth are recognized sequelae of congenital infection. The risk of syphilis to the fetus is now known to exist throughout pregnancy. It was believed in the past that the spirochetes crossed the placenta after 16 weeks of gestation, but recent work has shown that treponema pallidum can be transferred transplacentally as early as six weeks of gestation to infect the fetus.

The most specific method to diagnose syphilis is by dark-field examination of fresh specimens from the lesions of infected persons. This will demonstrate treponema pallidum. In the absence of lesions, nonspecific serologic testing is performed routinely on pregnant patients as part of the initial prenatal laboratory profile. Positive serology results should be tested further with treponema-specific tests for confirmation.

Treatment of the mother is with penicillin as the initial drug of choice. In the pregnant woman who is allergic to penicillin, tetracycline is not an acceptable alternate, as in the nonpregnant patient. Erythromycin base or erythromycin stearate, but not erythromycin estolate, may be used as alternate therapy. Followup with serial quantitative Venereal Disease Research Laboratory

---

[26] American College of Obstetricians and Gynecologists, ACOG Technical Bull. No. 122, Perinatal Herpes Simplex Virus Infections (1988).

(VDRL) titers monthly is recommended during pregnancy, and those with a fourfold rise in titers should be retreated.

The infant with congenital syphilis should be treated if maternal treatment was inadequate, if the drug given was unknown, if the drugs used were other than penicillin, or if adequate followup of the infant will be difficult if not impossible. A spinal fluid analysis should be performed prior to treatment.

Gonorrhea is caused by neisseria gonorrhoeae. The mode of transmission is usually through sexual contact, and both male and female are affected. The primary site of involvement is the genito-urinary tract. Maternal infection with gonorrhea during pregnancy has been associated with an increased incidence of premature rupture of membranes, preterm delivery, chorioamnionitis, neonatal sepsis, and postpartum maternal infection.

The diagnosis of gonorrhea in the pregnant patient is by culture using a selective medium for neisseria gonorrhoeae, obtaining adequate specimens from the endocervix. In patients with history of oral-genital contact, cultures should also be obtained from the tonsillar area and from the pharynx behind the uvula. Treatment in pregnancy is mainly with cephalosporins, and in case of allergy to cephalosporins, spectinomycin or Rocephin are acceptable alternates. In addition, the sexual partner or partners should also be examined, cultured, and treated.

Gonococcal ophthalmitis in the neonate can be prevented by the use of silver nitrate 1 percent or ophthalmic ointments or drops containing tetracycline or erythromycin. Actual ophthalmic infection in the neonate is treated mainly with intravenous penicillin.

§ 4.17　Cardiac

The diagnosis of heart disease in pregnancy is based on the presence of one or more of the following:[27]

1. A diastolic, presystolic, or continuous heart murmur
2. Unequivocal cardiac enlargement
3. A loud, harsh, systolic murmur, especially if associated with a thrill
4. Severe arrhythmia.

The New York Heart Association has provided a classification which helps assess the functional capacity of the heart. The classification is as follows:

Class I: Asymptomatic patients with heart disease and no limitation of physical activity.

Class II: Patients have slight limitation of activity and become symptomatic with ordinary physical activity.

---

[27] J. Metcalfe, J.H. McAnulty, & K. Ueland, Heart Disease and Pregnancy (1986).

Class III: Patients have marked limitation of physical activity and are symptomatic with less than ordinary activity.

Class IV: Patients are symptomatic even at rest.

The management of the pregnant patient with heart disease is based on her functional classification. Excessive weight gain, anemia, and abnormal fluid retention should be prevented. Ample bedrest, control of activity and stress, and management of hypertension if it occurs are important aspects of care. During labor, relief from pain and anxiety is equally important. Delivery should be accomplished vaginally unless an obstetric indication for cesarean section arises. Operative vaginal delivery may help shorten the second stage. Continuous epidural anesthesia may be utilized for pain relief during labor, but care must be taken that hypotension does not occur. The management during pregnancy, labor, and delivery requires the assistance in consultation of a cardiologist who can help monitor the cardiac status of the mother and treat any sudden cardiac complications, especially in the more severe classes (III and IV). During the postpartum period, the patient should receive counseling regarding future pregnancies and appropriate contraceptive or sterilization advice.

§ 4.18 Renal

There are two major types of renal problems that may arise during pregnancy: asymptomatic bacteriuria and acute pyelonephritis.

Asymptomatic Bacteriuria

Infections of the urinary tract constitute the major urinary complication in pregnancy. Asymptomatic bacteriuria, which is the presence of active, multiplying bacteria within the urinary tract without symptoms of a urinary infection, can develop into an acute symptomatic state. During pregnancy, progression to acute pyelonephritis occurs in up to 40 percent of affected women.

It is recommended that pregnant patients with asymptomatic bacteriuria be treated aggressively. The choice of the drug is based on the antibiotic sensitivity of the cultured organism. Initial therapy of choice may be sulfonamides or nitrofurantoin derivatives. Other antibiotics, such as ampicillin or cephalosporins, may be used later if recurrences arise or patients become symptomatic.

Acute Pyelonephritis

Bacterial infection that ascends from the bladder to the kidneys develops into acute pyelonephritis, the most common renal complication of pregnancy. The onset of clinical manifestations is usually abrupt. There is sudden development of fever, chills, and pain in one or both lumbar regions. There may be accompanying nausea and vomiting. Temperatures may vary from 34°C to 40°C. There is marked tenderness of one or both costovertebral angles. E. coli is the most common organism isolated in the urine and blood.

Treatment of acute pyelonephritis is best carried out initially at the hospital until clinical improvement is observed. Signs of bacterial shock (gram-negative septicemia) such as hypotension, low or absent urinary output, and marked fall in body temperature demand prompt and aggressive management. Intravenous antibiotic therapy is instituted, and the choice of antibiotic prior to the report of urine culture and sensitivity will depend on the obstetrician's experience. Ampicillin or cephalosporins are excellent initial choices.

Careful followup during pregnancy and postpartum with repeat urine cultures is important. Reinfection is possible, and prolonged treatment may be necessary. If there are recurrences, intravenous pyelogram may be considered about three months postpartum, when the pregnancy-induced changes in the urinary tract have subsided.

§ 4.19 Neurologic

The effect of pregnancy on epilepsy and epileptic convulsions is variable and unpredictable. Epilepsy may manifest for the first time at or immediately after pregnancy. A major concern in the management of epilepsy in pregnancy is the possibility that some anticonvulsant drugs are potentially teratogenic. The disease itself is associated with an increased risk of fetal anomalies.

The drugs most commonly noted as teratogenic are valproic acid (Depakene) and, to a lesser extent, phenytoin (Dilantin). Both drugs are known to cross the placenta. Trimethadione is another drug incriminated in producing fetal malformations. The management of epilepsy in pregnancy requires extensive counseling and discussion of the disease, its association by itself with congenital malformations, and the choice of anticonvulsant which the obstetrician feels comfortable with as dictated by experience and what the literature says.

§ 4.20 Disseminated Intravascular Coagulation

Disseminated intravascular coagulation (DIC) or consumptive coagulopathy has been associated with some obstetric conditions, among them abruptio placenta, sepsis, missed abortion, intrauterine fetal demise, and amniotic fluid embolism. The initiating process that leads to widespread clotting is the entry of thromboplastins into the circulation from the site of placental injury resulting in depletion of clotting factors (fibrinogen, platelets, factor VIII). The end result is uncontrollable bleeding.

The diagnosis is entertained after correlating the history and recent obstetric events. Laboratory determination of clotting factors can confirm the presence of a coagulopathy but not the degree of severity. Treatment is directed towards removing the initiating process (for example, delivery of placenta in placental abruption) and replacement of clotting factors with blood replacement products like fresh frozen plasma or cryoprecipitate, since fresh whole blood is difficult to obtain. Packed red blood cells are used to replace lost red blood cells.

§ 4.21 Perinatal Group B Streptococcal Infections

Perinatal Group B Streptococcal (GBS) infections are very serious yet potentially preventable. It is estimated that approximately 7,000 to 8,000 cases of neonatal GBS infections occur each year.[28] Many of the neonates die from this serious infection or have permanent serious neurological sequelae. Several protocols are available to the treating physician. However, the trend now is to treat all known GBS maternal carriers intrapartum or treat prophylactically intrapartum when certain risk factors are present such as:[29]

1. Preterm labor (less than 37 weeks)
2. Premature rupture of membranes (less than 37 weeks)
3. Prolonged rupture of membranes (more than 12 hours)
4. Prior sibling affected by GBS
5. Maternal fever
6. Other risk factors such as multiple pelvic exams or internal monitoring.

Intravenous administration of two grams of ampicillin every six hours is recommended. In penicillin-allergic individuals, 600mg of Clindamycin administered intravenously every six to eight hours is recommended.

---

[28] 59 Fed. Reg. 64, 764–73 (1994).

[29] American College of Obstetricians and Gynecologists, ACOG Technical Bull. No. 170, Group B Streptococcal Infections in Pregnancy (1992).

CHAPTER 5

MEDICATIONS AND THE EFFECTS ON THE FETUS

William Banner, Jr., M.D., Ph.D.

§ 5.1 Introduction

Drugs administered through the course of pregnancy may have deleterious effects on the outcome of the fetus. This fact has led to numerous liability claims throughout the world, particularly following the tragic discovery that thalidomide could cause fetal developmental abnormalities, or so-called teratogenic effects (from Greek, meaning monster maker). Few issues are as likely to produce hot emotional responses, particularly between plaintiff's attorneys and physicians, as those involving the effects of drugs on the fetus.

The two primary issues in this type of litigation are causality and fault.[1] Causality is dependent upon the interpretation of scientific data by a lay jury guided by a variety of scientific experts. In some cases, scientific standards of causality using statistical degrees of proof have not been an issue. The dreaded question, "Can you tell me that this could not have caused this problem?," is viewed by physicians as an attempt to subvert the innocent until proven guilty approach. Physicians consider themselves honor-bound to scientific standards of cause and effect. It is not surprising that the rather specious argument of *post hoc ergo propter hoc,* meaning "that which comes before causes that which follows it," is viewed by many physicians as the attorney's attempt to establish unfounded causality in which no scientific evidence exists. Based on current scientific methodology, even with large population samples, it may be extremely difficult to infer causality of a drug to produce a teratogenic effect (an abnormality of the fetus). There are, however, some scientifically well-founded principles upon which to exclude causality. Ethical litigation includes an understanding of these principles of exclusion to prevent specious litigation. For example, a patient who is found to have an extra chromosome present, as with Down's syndrome (mongolism), can be excluded from causation on a scientific basis by administration of a drug during the pregnancy. All of the scientific evidence and understanding of the development of Down's syndrome indicates that the excess chromosome must be derived from an abnormality of the original germ cells. Thus, once the egg and sperm have joined and begun to undergo division, it is not deemed scientifically possible that an event could occur that would produce an excess of chromosomal material in all the cells of the body at one time.

The concept of fault in the area of fetal drug effects is assuming an increasing role in the decision-making processes of physicians and the pharmaceutical manufacturers. The decision to offer drug therapy during pregnancy is being weighted more heavily to assuring benefit. This is a sound approach; that is, use drug therapies only to preserve the life of the mother and fetus. However, modern therapeutics allows the treatment of many relatively non-life-threatening complaints that may nevertheless alter the lifestyle or degree of suffering of the patient. The risks of these therapies are often unknown because of the lack of sufficient information to discriminate appropriately teratogenic drugs from nonteratogenic drugs.

Only under rare circumstances can the real risks and benefits of therapy be discussed with patients in order to allow them truly to make an informed decision regarding the initiation of medication. Fault has, therefore, forced drug companies to make statements intended to discourage drug therapy during pregnancy in the absence of sufficient data to make a rational decision. Under these circumstances, the medical profession is forced to accept the responsibility

---

[1] E. Deutsch, *Legal and Juridical Considerations in Administering Drugs in Pregnancy, in* Clinical Pharmacology in Pregnancy 179–82 (H. Kuemmerle, M.D. ed., 1984).

for the decision to initiate therapy. The unfortunate tendency is for drug manufacturers to view the pressure of litigation as forcing the withdrawal of drugs
from use in pregnancy and pediatrics because of the high-liability potential. In a
different environment, this pressure might necessitate more postmarketing surveillance and greater data gathering to substantiate the effects of drugs on the
fetus. At this point, the gathering of such data might be regarded as negative
because of the liability associated with the clear establishment of causality. This
is particularly difficult when many lawsuits have not depended upon causality in
terms of the scientific standards accepted by most physicians and pharmaceutical manufacturers. Until clear standards of causality can be established, both
physicians and manufacturers are in the position of accepting liability in the
absence of data. Thus, the medical profession is left with a shrinking formulary
of approved drugs for use in pregnancy at a time when the number of prescription drugs available is rapidly expanding.

The purpose of this chapter is to review the basic events in fetal development,
particularly to understand the methods used in evaluating the teratogenic potential of drugs and the concept of exclusionary causality.

§ 5.2   Stages of Fetal Growth

From a toxicologic standpoint, the process of forming the fetus and giving birth
is divided into several periods. The first is the preconception period in which the
sperm and egg are formed. The second state is fetogenesis, during which a
fertilized egg goes from a single cell to multicellular organism. The third phase
is growth. The fourth stage is the perinatal period, or that period immediately
surrounding the birth of the baby.

§ 5.3   —Preconception

The effect of drugs on the sperm, egg, and fertilized egg until the time of
implantation and division is a poorly understood phenomenon. It is at this period
that one-half the genetic material (chromosomes) from the father and one-half
the genetic material from the mother are placed into respective containers (the
sperm and the egg, or *ovum*). Following the introduction of the sperm into the
egg, a complete genetic complement of chromosomes is once again present.
During this critical time, division of the chromosomal material in the sperm and
egg and inclusion or exclusion of chromosomal material may result in severe
deformities such as Down's syndrome (mongolism). This process is described in
detail in reference texts.[2] The normal complement of chromosomes includes 46
structures bearing genetic material, with two of these being sex chromosomes

---

[2] J.S. Thompson & M.W. Thompson, Genetics in Medicine (1973).

(x- or y-shaped). These chromosomes are derived from the mother (23) and from the father (23). In the case of Down's syndrome, one of the donors contributes 24 chromosomes with a duplication of the 21st chromosome. This results in three chromosomes of the 21st type, or *trisomy 21*. Once the sperm and egg have joined to form a single cell with an extra chromosome, all cell lines descended from that single cell contain an extra chromosome. In rare instances, the extra chromosomal material may be present only after the first or second division of the original fertilized egg, in which case, only those cells descended from the abnormal cell have the abnormal chromosomes. Thus, for an abnormality to occur in which the cells of the body contain an extra chromosome, such as in Down's syndrome, the only time at which a drug could be implicated would be prior to or at the time of fertilization. Thus, drugs that are taken following *implantation* (the attachment of the fetal cells to the wall of the uterus), which occurs approximately six days following release of the egg, cannot be construed as having produced an abnormality involving a chromosomal alteration. By 40 to 50 hours after the release of the egg from the ovary, fertilization has generally occurred and the resulting fertilized egg has divided into four cells.

In a similar manner, a large number of genetic disorders that are not manifested by chromosomal abnormalities but are passed on from the parent may be related to a defect in the genetic material that was present in the parent or a defect that occurs prior to fertilization. For example, Hurler's syndrome is a deficiency of a specific enzyme involved in the metabolism of mucopolysaccharides (complex sugars). This enzyme is normally coded in the genetic material from each parent. Absence of the genetic code in one parent does not result in any clinical symptomatology, but that person will have one abnormal gene in all of the cells of the body. If, however, both parents have one chromosome lacking the proper code of this enzyme, then one out of four offspring (by simple probability) may receive the two chromosomes—one from each parent—without the proper enzyme. This pattern of inheritance is termed *autosomal recessive*. In order for a drug to cause a disorder such as Hurler's syndrome from otherwise normal parents, a drug would have to affect simultaneously two chromosomes, one in each parent, in exactly the same location where the sequence for this enzyme is stored. This is beyond any recognized concept of the effects of drugs on chromosomes. Thus, from a scientific standpoint, it is impossible to establish causality between an ingested drug, even one ingested at the time of fertilization, and a disorder such as Hurler's syndrome in which two separate chromosomes have exactly the same lesion in all the cells of the body.

Other inherited disorders require only that one chromosome from either parent be affected by the genetic defect in order for an abnormal infant to be born. This is called an *autosomal dominant* trait. In these situations, the parent is frequently affected by the same disorder, or a spontaneous single change in the chromosomal material takes place in either the sperm or the egg of the parent, resulting in the disorder of the child. While it is conceivable that a drug could be associated with a single chromosomal alteration, to date, very little information concerning this type of drug effect is known. Smith's work is a useful resource in determining the inheritance pattern of a particular trait or syndrome.[3]

Literature on the effect of drugs prior to conception can be divided into works on effects on the male germ cell or sperm, and those on the female egg or ovum. The effects of drugs on the sperm have become a matter of investigation only recently. No convincing data exist to support a relationship between a single drug and birth defects in human children by this mechanism. As has been reviewed by Hill, animal studies have demonstrated that substances such as lead, morphine, and methadone, if taken by the male prior to mating, may have an effect on the number of offspring and their weight.[4] Other studies have suggested that caffeine, smoking, and anesthetic gases may affect the birth-weight of infants when the male is exposed. In addition to direct effects on the infant, some animal studies have suggested that there may be a predominance of females in litters that are affected by drugs such as caffeine. The difficulties of isolating a single agent given to the male prior to conception as having any relationship to the outcome of an offspring in the human should be obvious. This difficulty is typified by the controversy over the effects of Agent Orange on veterans and their offspring. The published study failed to show any association in Vietnam veterans but was sufficiently weak in design that it was unlikely to have found an effect if it did exist.[5]

The female germ cell is in a resting state in the ovary until the process of ovulation occurs. Very little data have been accumulated, but with limited data available, it appears that this resting cell, prior to ovulation, is relatively resistant to the effects of chemicals.[6] In addition, since the cell may spend many years in a resting state in the ovary prior to ovulation (rather than being continually replaced as the male sperm is), any postulated drug effects in the preconception period could conceivably be from any point in the female's life, rather than just the immediate period prior to ovulation and conception. Thus, there does not appear to be any way to postulate a relationship between drug exposure several weeks prior to ovulation and the ultimate outcome of the fetus. The concept that drugs such as LSD would have a permanent effect on human female reproduction, as was touted in the 1960s, has not turned out to be scientifically supportable.

---

[3] D.W. Smith, Recognizable Patterns of Human Malformation (1982).

[4] Hill & Kleinberg, *Effects of Drugs and Chemicals on the Fetus and Newborn,* 59 Mayo Clinic Proc. 707 (1984).

[5] Erickson et al., *Vietnam Veterans Risk for Fathering Babies with Birth Defects,* 252 JAMA 903 (1984).

[6] Hill & Kleinberg, *Effects of Drugs and Chemicals on the Fetus and Newborn,* 59 Mayo Clinic Proc. 707 (1984).

§ 5.4 —Fetogenesis

After ovulation, and with the introduction of the sperm, the fertilized egg is called an *embryo*. At this point, the cells begin to undergo division. Any alteration in the genetic material of this single embryonic cell could conceivably produce an effect on the genetic material in all the cells of the body. Past the third to fourth day of conception, this duplication has already begun; any abnormality in the genetic material of all the cells of the body cannot possibly be attributed to any process that happens following this period. In general, it is believed that effects on the embryo due to radiation or drugs cause a spontaneous lack of viability and embryonic wastage. Indeed, there are no convincing data for specific syndromes being produced at this early stage of development.

Somewhere around the second week of pregnancy, the embryo begins to differentiate into discrete organ systems as opposed to a collection of very similar cells. It is during organogenesis that most of the reports on drug teratogenesis have been focused. It is important to recognize that this period may occur at a time when the female does not yet recognize that pregnancy has occurred and may be exposing herself to a variety of agents, including such common things as ethanol, caffeine, and nicotine. Beginning with organ systems, such as the heart and brain at 18 days postconception, this period of differentiation is the most critical for specific organ system abnormalities. In general, this period can be said to last until approximately the 12th week of gestation, leading to the suggestion that the first trimester is most critical in drug-induced teratogenesis. For example, the extremities appear to undergo differentiation and formation from the 24th to 36th days of life. Thus, exposure to an agent such as thalidomide would be most likely to produce an abnormality if the exposure occurred within that critical time period. Exposures in the last trimester of pregnancy when differentiation has already occurred would be unlikely to produce any effects on limb development. It is also useful to understand these critical periods of specific organ differentiation to appreciate how a single drug can produce varied malformations depending upon the time when it was administered. Thus, an agent may be administered early in the embryonic period and produce primarily an effect on the heart. However, the same drug administered later in the embryonic period would produce an effect on the genital tract.

§ 5.5 —Period of Growth

As the pregnancy progresses beyond the embryonic period to the fetal period, organogenesis is generally believed to be complete. The organ systems have been formed and are undergoing a process of growth. During this period, an effect of a drug will be primarily to decrease the amount of growth occurring.

This appears to have a global effect on growth, as with fetal phenytoin syndrome (phenytoin is an anticonvulsant) and fetal alcohol syndrome in which intra-uterine growth retardation is the primary feature.

The concept of critical periods of development is the key to understanding the effects of a drug on the fetus. During preconception and the immediate embryonic phases, drugs are likely to result in a spontaneous abortion rather than a deformed child. In addition, since this is a critical period for establishing the transmission of genetic material, any postulated drug effect causing a genetic disease or chromosomal abnormality would have to be based in this very early part of the pregnancy. Few data exist to support drug effects during this time period. From about the 15th day of pregnancy through the 12th to 15th week is the critical period of organ development and differentiation of tissue. It is at this time that a developing child is most sensitive to drug effects, and that drug effects such as those due to thalidomide are most prominent. The final period of pregnancy from 15 weeks onward is characterized by drug effects on growth or maladaptation in the immediate period prior to delivery. An example of a maladaptation is the effect of indomethacin to produce pulmonary hypertension if given immediately prior to the delivery. See **Chapter 10.**

§ 5.6 Methods of Assessment

There are three approaches to evaluating drugs for possible teratogenicity. In the first case, the drug is shown to be capable of producing a teratogenic effect in animal models. This is perhaps the weakest evidence for evaluating drugs or chemicals for human teratogenic effects, but may be the only information or method available. The second approach is to use human data to identify an association between an outcome and an ingested medication or chemical. There are many difficulties associated with either retrospective or prospective studies of human populations in attempting to establish a cause and effect relationship between medication and a possible effect on the fetus. In the third case, a mechanism may be identified by which drug produces a specific teratogenic event. This is the strongest evidence linking a drug to an effect, particularly if the effect is an extension of the drug's known pharmacologic properties. It is exceedingly rare for mechanisms of drug teratogenicity to be established, and the medical profession is frequently left with less than ideal information upon which to base clinical opinions.

§ 5.7 —Bacterial Testing

The crudest method of assessment of teratogenic risk is the use of bacteria to demonstrate mutagenicity. These studies generally observe the mutation rate for a given piece of genetic information in bacteria. Bacteria normally undergo a spontaneous rate of mutation; any increase in this rate of mutation can be associated with the effects of added material or radiation. The Ames test, which is the classic test of bacterial mutagenicity, is carried out by starting with bacteria that has a specific enzyme deficiency.[7] For example, certain strains of bacteria may require histidine, the amino acid, to grow successfully in culture. When a number of bacteria are placed on culture media lacking in histidine, the large majority will die. Only those bacteria that are able to undergo mutation will survive. They survive by mutating to form an enzyme that allows them to convert other amino acids into histidine. Out of millions of bacteria placed, only a small fraction undergo this change, grow and multiply on the culture plate, and can be counted. This mutation occurs because of any number of factors in the environment. If a chemical is added to the bacteria prior to placement on the histidine-deficient media and a large increase in the number of spontaneous mutations occurs, this increase may be attributed to the effect of the chemical. It is a far step from this simple screening procedure to the demonstration of birth defects, but this has been used by some as a test for the ability of a chemical to produce events that are associated with teratogenicity and *carcinogenicity* (cancer causing).

§ 5.8 —Animal Testing

Testing for teratogenicity and carcinogenicity in animal models has probably received the most ridicule from the general public. The notion that tremendous doses of cyclamates can produce cancer or birth defects in a rat does not excite the public because of the notion that they would be unable to consume equivalent amounts and, therefore, would not be at similar risks. Actually, the dose-response relationship is probably not the major problem in animal testing for teratogenic effects. Rather, many species of animals are extremely different in the way their offspring are affected by drugs. Because of the marked differences in susceptibility, placental structure, and detoxification mechanisms (as in the liver), it is extremely difficult and dangerous to imply a relationship between animal studies and human experience. It has been well demonstrated that drugs producing teratogenesis in animal species may be perfectly safe in humans. Conversely, drugs that are nonteratogenic in animals may produce major effects in the pregnant human female. What is the purpose, then, of animal testing? The major benefit of animal testing lies in the possibility of identifying specific mechanisms by which defects occur in order to attempt to extrapolate those to the human condition. In addition, despite the fact that safety in animals is no guarantee of safety in humans, the demonstration that a given drug produces a large number of birth defects in several different animal species, including some primate species, should suggest that a high degree of caution be observed before administering the drug to pregnant women.

---

[7] B.N. Ames, *The Detection of Chemical Mutagens with Enteric Bacteria, in* Chemical Mutagen 267–82 (A. Hollaender ed., 1971).

§ 5.9   —Methods of Assessment in Humans

The weakest (but yet the most common) form of reported teratogenicity is the case or clinical report. Nothing is more frustrating to the scientist than reading a case report in which a baby was delivered with a known genetic defect, and in retrospect the pregnancy was associated with therapy with five or six drugs, one of which has been singled out as the provocative agent in producing the spectrum of abnormalities. This classic "post hoc ergo propter hoc" form of logic may produce more harm than any possible benefit. In contrast, case reports of specific and unusual malformations following administration of an uncommon drug in a large series of patients may prompt appropriate retrospective surveys of large populations to detect whether a true teratogenic event is occurring. For example, the identification of phenytoin (Dilantin) as a specific teratogen producing the fetal hydantoin syndrome (or fetal phenytoin syndrome) was largely based on case reports of particular facial abnormalities, poor growth, and cardiac defects observed by geneticists over a period of many years.[8] Even now, the association of anticonvulsant drug treatment with these abnormalities is difficult to establish solely on the basis of population studies as to cause and effect.[9] In a similar fashion, the first reports of fetal alcohol syndrome came from case reports of a series of children with very similar facial appearance. A further example is the effect of coumadin on fetal development. In this case, the failure of development of cartilage, particularly in the nose, and the unusual appearance of the bones in children of mothers treated with coumadin, is an example of an unusual drug producing unusual effects, and was identified solely on the basis of clinical case reports.[10] Given the small number of women receiving coumadin during pregnancy, it is unlikely that population surveys would be able to support such a relationship. Thus, while a case report can be extremely misleading, it may be a source of support for a cause-and-effect relationship when the drug is unusual and the effects observed are unusual.

Another type of human assessment method is the monitoring of birth defects. Many countries, including the United States, have ongoing surveillance procedures to identify sudden increases in teratogenic events. While occasionally helpful in identifying increases in the number of birth defects, these types of surveys are extremely expensive to maintain and may suffer from changes in physicians, the reporting habits, and definitions of birth defects. The major value of population surveys is to suggest the need for further study to identify whether real epidemiologic data exist to establish a cause-and-effect relationship. The use of population surveys has led to some rather spectacular examples

---

[8] D.W. Smith, Recognizable Patterns of Human Malformation (1982).

[9] D. Janz et al., Epilepsy, Pregnancy and the Child (D. Janz, M.D., ed., 1982).

[10] Kort & Cassel, *An Appraisal of Warfarin Therapy During Pregnancy,* 60 S. Afr. Med. J. 578 (1981); Hirsh et al., *Fetal Effects of Coumadin Administered During Pregnancy,* 36 Blood 623 (1970).

of mass hysteria. In Tucson, Arizona, the discovery that the city water supply contained trace elements of a chlorinated hydrocarbon compound led to the suggestion that this was associated with an increase in the number of birth defects reported from the Tucson area over a period of several years. It attracted a great deal of media attention and increased sales of bottled water although there was no established causal link. In fact, any increase in birth defects may simply have been related to increasing densities of physicians, awareness of birth defects, and awareness of reporting procedures.

Retrospective studies to assess teratogenic effects in humans are performed by asking patients with a specific birth defect to recall the factors of pregnancy, including medication that may have influenced the birth defect. By finding a matched control with the same ethnic background and geographic location (and numerous other variables), and asking similar series of questions of a control patient, an attempt is made to demonstrate that the birth defect is associated with administration of a certain medication during the pregnancy. One obvious problem with this is termed *recall bias*. For example, mothers of abnormal children may be more likely to remember, in the course of their soul-searching following the births, what medications were used during the pregnancy. This makes retrospective studies extremely dangerous to attempt to interpret, and only with large samples, good records, and good matching of control patients can any sort of useful information be derived.

A prospective, randomized study is the classic scientific method by which a trained scientist draws conclusions as to cause-and-effect relationships. Unfortunately, assessing the effects of a drug on pregnancy in which the incidence of an abnormality may be extremely low could be a time-consuming and laborious process. Trying to discern a teratogenic effect that may occur in only one out of 1000 to one out of 2000 pregnancies and attribute that defect to a specific drug may require population sizes of 50,000 to 100,000 patients to be studied. This necessitates a multicenter clinical trial. In addition to the difficulties of managing a study of this size, ethical considerations of exposing a group of pregnant women to a drug in order to observe a possible increase in malformations is questionable.

§ 5.10   —Mechanistic Assessment

Deriving a mechanism by which a teratogenic effect may occur involves a collaboration of animal and clinical studies. For example, the treatment of a pregnant female with tetracycline has been associated with yellow, poorly developed teeth. This effect has been mechanistically traced to the binding of tetracycline to calcium-rich organs, such as bones and teeth. Unfortunately, it is extremely rare to find a well-worked-out mechanism for a teratogenic effect. More commonly, what is left is a mechanism in animals or the test tube that might theoretically produce a lesion in the human offspring, although no substantial proof can be offered for this. Often, the strength of this theoretical assessment mandates that a drug not be used during pregnancy, and thus, it is never discovered whether the effect actually does occur. Medicine, and in particular obstetrics, is full of admonishments not to give certain categories of drugs because they produce specific effects in the fetus on a theoretical basis, although no hard data to support the concept may be present.

No single test can positively identify a drug that is capable of producing a teratogenic effect in newborns. For a further review, refer to Hawkins[11] and Stern.[12] Animal testing and bacterial models of mutagenesis could suggest drugs that have a high potential to produce genetic abnormalities, while clinical reports of unusual deformities associated with infrequently used drugs may be supportive evidence to define a teratogenic effect. Epidemiologic studies, both retrospectively and prospectively, are extremely difficult to manage in terms of the large patient populations required to draw conclusions. However, they remain the closest thing to scientific data that is available for the evaluation of many drugs. Finally, while the most ideal circumstance is the determination of a mechanism of action of a drug affecting the fetus, this remains an extremely unusual method to determine teratogenic effects. In fact, this approach has contributed more to folklore by having physicians not using drugs on theoretical grounds, when no evidence exists to support fully the mechanism of action that has been proposed.

§ 5.11   Drug Access to the Fetus

A secondary consideration in the toxicology of drugs in the fetus is whether the drug can reach the fetus to exert an adverse effect. In the past, the placenta was believed to constitute a barrier to drugs, and to act as a protective mechanism to obviate the effects of maternally administered medications. With increasing recognition of the characteristics of the placenta, it is known that this is not the case. The placenta is designed to allow transport of nutritional materials and oxygen to the fetus, and serves only to exclude very large structures such as red blood cells and large proteins. Even some large immunoglobulin particles are able to cross the placenta from mother to child. For most drugs, the very fact that they are able to cross membranes (such as those of the gastrointestinal tract) and be absorbed into the system suggests that they are of sufficiently small size and have solubility characteristics that make them available to the fetus. The placenta may also act as a site of active transport of some substances, and has been demonstrated to be metabolically active (that is, it contains enzymes that can

---

[11] D.F. Hawkins, *Problems in the Assessment of Drug-Induced Effects on the Developing Fetus,* *in* Clinical Pharmacology in Pregnancy 229–34 (H. Kuemmerle, M.D., ed.).

[12] Stern, *In Vivo Assessment of the Teratogenic Potential of Drugs in Humans,* 58 Obstetrics & Gynecology 35 (1981).

transform drugs). The significance of this from a medicolegal standpoint is only that the notion of the placenta as a barrier to all toxins is invalid and misleading.

Another contributor to the effects of drugs on the fetus is change in maternal metabolism. During pregnancy, the mother experiences changes in serum proteins that may bind to drugs and changes in her own baseline metabolic rate. Thus, drugs that normally tend to distribute in the blood may have greater serum or tissue concentrations during pregnancy, and drugs that may be readily removed from the maternal circulation under normal circumstances may achieve higher concentrations during pregnancy. The implication for this kinetic change in terms of drug effects on the fetus is that mothers receiving drugs that may be readily monitored in plasma should be reevaluated after pregnancy has occurred. By monitoring drug levels during pregnancy, high concentrations or low concentrations can be avoided in order to minimize the risk of side effects or maternal diseases on the fetus. For example, phenytoin is a drug used to treat seizure disorders. Without careful monitoring, the concentration could increase or decrease during pregnancy. If the serum concentration decreases, the patient might experience an increase in seizure activity that may have an adverse effect of the fetus. In contrast, if concentrations are allowed to increase, it may increase the risk of fetal phenytoin syndrome resulting in dysmorphic changes in the infant. Drug level monitoring during pregnancy is important in view of the axiom that all medications given to a pregnant female should be used at the lowest effective concentration.

The placenta is not an effective barrier against drug entry into the fetus and should not be considered as such. The altered metabolism of drugs by the fetus may actually increase the concentration of certain metabolites in the fetal compartment. In addition, the altered metabolic state of the mother during the pregnancy should also be kept in mind to optimize control of disease and avoid toxicity.

§ 5.12   Criteria for Associating Cause and Effect

The association of drug use during pregnancy and subsequent effects on the fetus is an area that causes considerable consternation. The evidence for associating cause and effect may fall into several different categories. The strongest of these is the isolation of a mode of action. If the underlying mechanism of a fetal deformity can be ascertained, this is the strongest evidence of drug involvement. An example would be the recognition that tetracycline can deposit in bones and teeth of the developing fetus, resulting in a yellow discoloration of the secondary teeth.

The strongest form of *exclusionary data* (data supporting a disassociation of cause and effect) are those involving the timing of administration. Thus, a drug administered following the first four days of pregnancy (before the pregnancy is even recognized) cannot be associated with an outcome such as a chromosomal abnormality in which the genetic material in all the cells of the body is altered. Weaker but still useful data involve extremely unusual abnormalities associated with the administration of relatively unusual drugs. These type of data, such as the association of coumadin administration with fetal cartilage abnormalities, provide a basis for association between cause and effect. Much weaker and more elusive is the association of a relatively common abnormality and a relatively commonly administered drug. For example, an abnormality such as cleft palate occurs with such frequency in the population that it may be extremely difficult to support any cause and effect relationship with a drug producing this abnormality. Similarly, drugs that are administered to a large segment of the pregnant population, such as the antiemetics (drugs that decrease vomiting), are always subject to many epidemiologic study difficulties like recall bias. By far the weakest of criteria for associating cause and effect is the isolated case report.

All parents who have had a child with abnormalities consider at various points that either they, the deity, or some external chemical or radiologic influence were responsible for their child's abnormality. It is the responsibility of the legal profession to undertake litigation only under circumstances in which a reasonable cause and effect relationship can be established. Recent litigation involving Bendectin is an example of a situation in which an extremely commonly used drug was purported to be associated with several dysmorphic features. This began as isolated case reports that had little scientific basis.[13] Epidemiologic data based on large cohorts of patients receiving the drug failed to support any association between Bendectin and birth defects.[14]

In the case of *Farkas v. Saary*,[15] the plaintiff brought a medical malpractice action against her obstetrician claiming that microphthalmia, a defect of the eye, was caused in her infant son by the doctor's prescription of progesterone to prevent a miscarriage during the first trimester of pregnancy. The defendant doctor moved for summary judgment based upon the fact that Food and Drug Administration guidelines, which required warnings about the risk of the use of progesterone during pregnancy, did not list any effect related to vision as a hazard associated with the drug. The defendant also presented the affidavits of medical experts stating that there is no medical basis for the claim that the child's defect was related to the mother's use of progesterone. The plaintiff presented the affidavit of an expert who stated that it was "contraindicated to use

---

[13] Mellor, *Letter: Fetal Malformation after Debendox Treatment in Early Pregnancy*, 1 Brit. Med. J. 1055 (1978).

[14] Bracken, *Bendectin (Debendox) and Congenital Diaphragmatic Hernia*, 1 Lancet 586 (Mar. 12, 1983); Cordero et al., *Is Bendectin a Teratogen?*, 245 JAMA 2307 (1981); Michaells et al., *Prospective Study of Suspected Associations Between Certain Drugs Administered During Early Pregnancy and Congenital Malformations*, 27 Teratology 57 (1983); Mitchell et al., *Birth Defects Related to Bendectin Use in Pregnancy*, 245 JAMA 2311 (1981); Morelock et al., *Bendectin and Fetal Development*, Am. J. Obstetrics Gynecology 209 (Jan. 15, 1982); Brent, *Editorial: The Bendectin Saga: Another American Tragedy*, 23 Teratology 283 (1983).

[15] 594 N.Y.S.2d 195 (App. Div. 1993).

progesterone to maintain a pregnancy . . . ." It asserted that progesterone is "associated with fetal malformations in . . . the special senses (including the eyes)."

The appellate division found that there was a triable issue of fact as to whether the plaintiff's use of progesterone caused the defect and affirmed the trial court's denial of summary judgment.

§ 5.13   Risk versus Benefit

In all cases of litigation on drug effects on the fetus, a key (and often over-looked) factor is the primary motivation of physicians in using a given therapy. Physicians are trained to weigh relative risks against merits or potential benefits of a procedure to a patient. In the case of maternal drug effects, it is often unclear with whom the primary responsibility of the physician lies—whether it is to the mother or the child. It is rare that a drug is used during pregnancy to protect the life of the mother when it may pose a danger to the fetus. In the current moral climate some might even argue that the fetus has an equal right to survival, and that any drug therapy that might adversely affect it should not be considered, even to protect the life of the mother. Fortunately, this attitude is not preva-lent. Unfortunately, somewhere between protecting the life of the mother and avoiding minor inconveniences of symptoms such as a mild cold, lies a vast gray area in which the potential risks and benefits are relatively difficult to weigh. In circumstances in which the disease itself may influence fetal outcome, it is relatively easy to justify drug therapy. For example, propranolol, a beta receptor blocking agent, is used in the treatment of hypertension in the mother. Severe maternal hypertension has been demonstrated to have an adverse effect on both mother and fetus, and may result in fetal demise. The treatment of hypertension with propranolol has been demonstrated to be effective and to prevent serious deleterious effects on the fetus. The use of this drug is not without some risks. As demonstrated in animal models as well as some human epidemiologic data, it appears that higher concentrations of propranolol may have an effect on the growth of the fetus resulting in a relatively small-for-gestational-age infant. Despite this risk, many physicians feel that the benefits of drug therapy out-weigh the risks (see **Chapter 10**).

The official position of the American Academy of Pediatrics and the Ameri-can College of Obstetrics and Gynecology is that perinatal drug exposure should be kept to a minimum, consistent with good medical practice, and that the lowest effective dose be employed. In the current legal climate it is prudent on the part of physicians to assume that any and all drugs used during pregnancy may have potential effects on the fetus. Informed consent of the mother should include that fact. Further information should include whether the drug therapy will protect the life of the mother or fetus, whether the disease process itself will be reversed (or whether symptoms will merely be ameliorated), and whether symptom amelioration will have a potential positive effect on mother or fetus. In addition, any data available concerning the effects of the drug on the fetus may be reviewed.

It does not seem useful in an informed consent setting to include isolated clinical case reports or weak epidemiologic data as part of the informed consent process. In addition, the *Physicians Desk Reference,* a collection of listings on various drugs made available by the drug companies, includes recommendations on drug usage in pregnancy. Many recommendations fall into Category C and simply state that a compound may have some teratogenic potential and should be used only when benefits outweigh risks. This kind of information is too limited, thus relatively useless. Category summaries follow.

Category A. Controlled studies in women fail to demonstrate a risk to the fetus in the first trimester (with no evidence of a risk in later trimesters), and the possibility of fetal harm appears remote.

Category B. Either animal reproduction studies have not demonstrated a fetal risk (but there are no controlled studies in pregnant women), or animal reproduction studies have shown an adverse effect (other than a decrease in fertility) that was not confirmed in controlled studies in women in the first trimester (and furthermore, there is no evidence of a risk in later trimesters).

Category C. Either studies in animals have revealed adverse effects on the fetus (teratogenic or embryocidal or other) and there are no controlled studies in woman, or studies in women and animals are not available. Drugs should be given only if the potential benefit justifies the potential risk to the fetus.

Category D. There is positive evidence of human fetal risk, but the benefits from use in pregnant women may be acceptable despite the risk (for example, if the drug is needed in a life-threatening situation or for a serious disease for which safer drugs cannot be used or are ineffective).

Category X. Studies in animals or human beings have demonstrated fetal abnormalities or there is evidence of fetal risk based on human experience, or both. The risk of the use of the drug in pregnant women clearly outweighs any possible benefit. The drug is contraindicated in women who are or may become pregnant. For further specifics on drugs, the reader is referred to several general works on drugs in pregnancy.[16]

---

[16] O.P Heinonen et al., Birth Defects and Drugs in Pregnancy (1992); T.H. Shepard, Catalog of Teratogenic Agents (1980); G.G. Briggs et al., Drugs in Pregnancy and Lactation (1983).

CHAPTER 6

COMPLAINT AND PAPER DISCOVERY IN A PRENATAL INJURY CASE

Michael D. Volk

§ 6.1   Introduction

Any chapter on pleading must necessarily be that—pleadings. There is no good way to explain how to plead a lawsuit and draft paper discovery. The best way to present a chapter on pleadings is to fill the chapter with representative pleadings.

The one thing that is necessary in all pleading and paper discovery is to make sure that it is done properly. For instance, a sloppy interrogatory can allow an evasive answer. Because of this there is, by necessity, a need to have standard sets of paper discovery to avoid mistakes. However, do not be afraid to individualize discovery for any particular case.

§ 6.2　Goals of the Complaint

The complaint or pleading that begins suit is probably the first formal document that counsel for the defendant physician will see. The insurance carrier may have a settlement brochure or other correspondence concerning the claim, but the complaint starts formally the process. It may also be that the defendant physician has never seen a formal complaint before. For that and other reasons, the initial pleadings must be concise.

Avoid pleading the facts with specificity. Tell a chronological story of what occurred. The pleading should be general, but with enough information to allow the defendants to know what they are being accused of. Avoid inflammatory language unless the situation particularly calls for it. When the defendant's conduct is particularly outrageous, it may be wise not to initially plead punitive or exemplary damages. When discovery has commenced, firm up the facts and then plead damages.

§ 6.3　Sample Complaint: Fetal Injury from Failure to Monitor Rh Incompatibility

PLAINTIFFS' ORIGINAL PETITION TO THE HONORABLE JUDGE OF SAID COURT:

Now come the Plaintiffs, ＿＿＿＿＿＿ and his wife, ＿＿＿＿＿＿, individually and as next friends of ＿＿＿＿＿＿, and complaining of ＿＿＿＿＿＿, M.D. Plaintiffs would respectfully show the court and jury the following:

I.

Plaintiffs are residents of ＿＿＿＿＿＿ County, state of ＿＿＿＿＿＿. ＿＿＿＿＿＿, M.D. is a physician, practicing obstetrics and gynecology in ＿＿＿＿＿＿ county. Service of process will be had upon him at his office in ＿＿＿＿＿＿ county, state of ＿＿＿＿＿＿. All acts complained of herein occurred within ＿＿＿＿＿＿ county.

II.

Plaintiffs have fully satisfied the presuit requirements of § ＿＿＿ of ＿＿＿＿＿＿ code of ＿＿＿＿＿＿ the state of ＿＿＿＿＿＿.

III.

Prior to July 9, 1990, plaintiffs had contracted with defendant ＿＿＿＿＿＿, M.D. for prenatal care and delivery of their child. On July 9, 1990, plaintiff ＿＿＿＿＿＿

delivered a full-term baby girl. That child's name is _____. Plaintiff _____ was Rh negative; _____, child, was Rh positive and the Coombs tests was negative.

IV.

_____, M.D. was negligent and careless in the treatment of plaintiffs on July 9, 1990, and prior thereto, in the following acts of commission or omission in that said _____, M.D.:

1. Failed to diagnose the potential for Rh incompatibility in the instant pregnancy

2. Failed to properly treat plaintiff and her subsequent children, by administering Rhogam to her

3. Failed to warn plaintiffs of the danger of sensitization if Rhogam was not administered

4. Failed to warn plaintiffs of the dangers that sensitization would result in harming future children conceived by plaintiffs

5. Failed to seek appropriate consultation.

V.

In 1991, Plaintiff _____ was pregnant again. She once again contracted with _____, M.D. to deliver her baby. On March 6, 1992, plaintiff _____ delivered a second baby girl, whose name is _____. That child was diagnosed as having hemolytic disease due to Rh factor and spent 20 days in an intensive care nursery, undergoing an exchange transfusion.

VI

_____, M.D. was negligent and careless in treatment of plaintiffs in the following acts of commission or omission in that said defendant, during the entire pregnancy and delivery of March 6, 1992:

1. Failed to diagnose Rh incompatibility

2. Failed to warn plaintiffs about the dangers of severe incompatibility if plaintiff _____ should become pregnant again in the future

3. Failed to discuss with plaintiffs the possibility or the advisability of some type of sterilization procedure to prevent subsequent pregnancies

4. Failed to seek appropriate consultation.

VII.

Plaintiff _____ became pregnant again and delivered the child, the subject of this lawsuit, on August 15, 1995. This child's name is _____.

VIII.

_____, M.D. was negligent and careless in treatment of plaintiffs in the following acts of commission or omission in that said defendant, before and during the pregnancy delivered on August 15, 1995:

1. Failed to counsel plaintiffs at an appropriate time so that they could decide whether or not the pregnancy should be terminated

2. Failed to timely detect the Rh incompatibility of the fetus, _____

3. Failed to timely treat the Rh incompatibility of the fetus by intrauterine transfusions

4. Failed to timely perform a cesarean section to prevent damage to the fetus from the incompatibility problem

5. Failed to seek appropriate consultation

IX.

As a direct and proximate result of the negligence of the Defendant, the minor plaintiff, _____, has sustained serious and permanent bodily injury including, but not limited to, his maintaining a state of devastating brain damage, necessitating medical, surgical, and related care, and the reasonable expense thereof, and permanently impairing him from engaging in normal family, social, recreational and wage-earning activities for the rest of his entire life. He cannot walk, talk, crawl, stand, feed himself, or attend to any of his most private, personal needs, and he never will be able to do so. Great pain, distress, and anxiety have been suffered and always will be suffered by minor defendant _____ every day of his life. His capacity to enjoy life in the future is minimal or nonexistent. He has required hospital and medical care, aid, and attention, and will require the same in the future and for the rest of his life. His ability to earn a living in the future is nonexistent. Further, the parents of _____ must take complete care of their child and will have to continue doing so until the end of their lives or his life, whichever is sooner. He is virtually unable to do anything for himself. He is unable to respond to any verbal or tactile stimuli with the exception of crying many hours each day to verbalize his suffering. The parents of the minor plaintiff have not only been caused to become skilled in the nursing arts to care for their child, but have had to endure the agony and suffering of watching their child in a tremendously brain-damaged state. The parents have further been damaged by the loss of society, attention, comfort, and companionship of their son.

X.

By reason of all the foregoing, plaintiffs have been damaged in a sum in excess of the minimum jurisdictional limits of this court.

WHEREFORE, PREMISES CONSIDERED, plaintiffs pray that defendant be cited to appear and answer herein, and that upon final hearing and trial of this cause, plaintiffs have judgment against defendant in a sum in excess of the minimum jurisdictional limits of this court, prejudgment interest for their liquidated damages, together with interest thereon at the legal rate from the date of said judgment until paid, with all costs of this suit, and all such other and further relief, both general and special, at law and in equity, to which plaintiffs may justly be entitled.

§ 6.4 Sample Complaint: Fetal Injury from Failure to Test for Genetic Disorder

PLAINTIFFS' ORIGINAL COMPLAINT

I.

Plaintiffs are residents of the country of _____, and diversity jurisdiction exists between plaintiffs and defendant. The parent plaintiffs are Ashkenazi Jews.

II.

Defendant _____, M.D., is, and and was at all times relevant to this lawsuit, a physician duly licensed to practice his profession in the State of _____, specializing in genetics. Said defendant has his office in _____ county, state of _____ and service of process may be had upon him there.

III.

All the acts complained of herein occurred within the _____ jurisdiction. The matter in controversy exceeds, exclusive of interest and costs, the sum of $10,000.00.

IV.

Plaintiffs have fully satisfied the presuit requirements of § _____ of _____ code of the state of _____.

V.

In 1990, plaintiffs _____ gave birth to a stillborn child with multiple congenital problems. After the birth, plaintiffs consulted with defendant _____,

M.D., a local geneticist. Plaintiffs were extremely concerned about the possibility of giving birth to another child with congenital problems. Plaintiff _____ became pregnant again in early 1993 and once again consulted defendant _____, M.D. At all times, defendant _____, M.D., assured plaintiffs that the possibility of giving birth to another child with congenital problems was minimal, not higher than any normal pregnancy. On December 4, 1993, plaintiffs gave birth to their second child, _____. This child was subsequently diagnosed as having Tay-Sachs disease. Both parents have subsequently been diagnosed as carriers.

VI.

Defendant _____, M.D., was negligent in the following acts of commission or omission in that he:

1. Failed to do routine genetic testing to determine that plaintiffs were both carriers of Tay-Sachs disease.

2. Failed to take a careful genetic history.

3. Failed to diagnose both of the parent plaintiffs as carriers of Tay-Sachs disease.

4. Failed to advise the parent plaintiffs that because both parents were carriers, their risk of any child of theirs having Tay-Sachs was one in four.

5. Failed to counsel plaintiffs properly so that they could determine whether to terminate their second pregnancy.

6. Failed to perform or order an amniocentesis during the second pregnancy.

VII.

As a direct and proximate result of the negligence of the defendants, the parent plaintiffs were caused to give birth to a second child with Tay-Sachs disease.

§ 6.5 Sample Complaint: Mother's Death from Pregnancy-induced Hypertension

ORIGINAL COMPLAINT

Plaintiff, by and through attorney undersigned, and with leave of court, files his Original Complaint by alleging as follows:

I.

Plaintiff, _____ is the widower of _____, deceased, and the father of his deceased infant daughter, _____.

II.

The actions complained of herein occurred within _____ county, state of _____, and, at all material and relevant times, the plaintiff's decedents, and the defendant physicians were residents of _____ county, state of _____.

III.

On or about July 15, 1993, plaintiff's decedent _____ went to the defendant _____, M.D., as a patient, and was told by defendant that she was $11\frac{1}{2}$ weeks pregnant. Defendant agreed to become plaintiff's physician concerning that pregnancy and agreed to deliver her child at _____ Hospital. Throughout the second and third trimesters of the pregnancy, _____, the mother, had significantly elevated blood pressures, protein in her urine, and edema.

IV.

Thereafter, on January 14, 1994, _____ was admitted into _____ Hospital by defendant _____ with a diagnosis of pregnancy-induced hypertension. During this hospitalization, defendant _____, M.D., consulted with defendants _____, M.D., and _____, M.D., whose respective specialties are internal medicine and high-risk pregnancy.

V.

Thereafter, on January 18, 1994, plaintiff's decedent was discharged from the hospital and told to go home, even though her pregnancy-induced hypertension was not under control.

VI.

On January 29, 1994, plaintiff's decedent collapsed at home, began having seizures, and before she could be transported to the hospital, the mother and fetus died. The autopsy surgeon's opinion was that the cause of death of both mother and fetus was from the pregnancy-induced hypertension.

VII.

The deaths of _____ and _____ were directly and proximately caused by the negligence of the defendants, and each of them, by failing to:

1. Promptly and properly diagnose and treat both mother and child.

2. Keep both mother and child in the hospital during the first hospitalization in January with appropriate therapy.

3. Failed to terminate the pregnancy by cesarean section or assisted vaginal delivery.

4. Failed to adequately warn plaintiff of the risks and dangers to mother and child.

5. Failed to perform proper and necessary laboratory tests.

6. Failed to properly monitor the mother and child.

7. Abandoned the mother and child.

8. Failed to consult with each other.

9. Failed to consult with more qualified physicians.

10. Failed to properly evaluate mother and child.

11. Failed to institute proper therapy for both mother and child.

VIII.

As a direct and proximate result of the negligence of the defendants, and each of them, as aforesaid, and by reason of the wrongful death of mother and daughter, plaintiff _____, has been deprived of the aid, association, support, income, protection, services, comfort, care, love, devotion, and society of the decedents _____ and _____. Plaintiff _____ has further incurred funeral and burial expenses for the decedents, has suffered mental anguish and sorrow, and claims damages by reason of the wrongful deaths of his wife and child together with a sum to be determined by the court and a jury to be just and reasonable for exemplary damages.

IX.

The complained of conduct of the defendants, and each of them, was so outrageous as to make an award of exemplary damages appropriate to act as a deterrent to further outrageous behavior.

WHEREFORE, plaintiff prays for judgment against the defendants, and each of them, as follows:

1. For compensatory damages in such an amount as will reasonably, completely, and adequately compensate plaintiff for all of his injuries, damages, and losses as aforesaid.

2. For punitive damages in such an amount as will substantially deter the defendants from further outrageous conduct in the future.

3. For costs of suit necessarily and lawfully incurred herein.

4. For such other and further relief as the court deems just and proper in the circumstances.

§ 6.6   Goals of Interrogatories

Counsel must be extremely careful about giving away the anticipated plan with interrogatories. The office should have a standard set of interrogatories that are sent out to physicians in a prenatal injury case that consists of background information, requests for insurance, witnesses, and so forth. There are certain types of questions that must be asked that the defendant doctor should not know about beforehand. These should be reserved for depositions.

§ 6.7   Standard Interrogatories to Defendant Doctor

INTERROGATORIES PROPOUNDED TO DEFENDANT

TO: _____, M.D.

c/o _____, defense attorney

The following Interrogatories are propounded to you pursuant to the Rules of Civil Procedure, to be answered separately and fully in writing under oath within thirty-one (31) days after service, a copy of said answers to be served on plaintiff's attorney. You are under a duty seasonably to supplement and amend your answers.

1. Please list the name, address, and telephone number of each witness you intend to attempt to qualify as an expert witness and elicit any opinion as to any matter during the trial of this case.

ANSWER:

2. In connection with the answer to the preceding question, please state the following:

(a) State in detail the subject matter said expert witness is expected to testify to.

(b) Attach a copy of any and all reports received from such expert witness.

ANSWER:

3. Please state by name, address, and telephone number any potential witness that you may use in the trial of this case.

ANSWER:

4. Please state by name, address, and telephone number any individual whom you believe has personal knowledge of the relevant facts of your defense(s) in this lawsuit.

ANSWER:

5. Identify completely by company and insurance limits, all liability insurance in effect which would potentially cover defendant _____, M.D., for any acts of negligence during the time plaintiffs _____ and _____ were their patients. Please include primary insurance as well as any excess, group, corporate, or umbrella policies.

ANSWER:

6. Please state the name of all journals that you subscribed to at the time that plaintiff was a patient.

ANSWER:

7. Please state all obstetrical, gynecological, and neonatal textbooks that you own.

ANSWER:

8. Where did you attend medical school?

ANSWER:

9. Please state when and where you did your internship.

ANSWER:

10. If you did a residency, please state where you did it, the inclusive years, what the residency was, and whether or not you completed it.

ANSWER:

11. Are you board-certified? If so, in what specialty?

ANSWER:

12. Please name the professors you had for obstetrics and gynecology and pediatric care during medical school.

ANSWER:

13. Please name the professors you had for obstetrics and gynecology and pediatric care during your internship.

ANSWER:

14. Please name the professors you had for obstetrics and gynecology and pediatric care during your residency.

ANSWER:

15. Of what hospital staffs are you currently a member?

ANSWER:

16. Of what hospital staffs have you been a member of in the past that you are no longer a member?

ANSWER:

17. Have you ever had hospital privileges revoked, modified, or denied?

ANSWER:

18. Please list all seminars you have attended or other postgraduate education concerning obstetrics, gynecology, or neonatal care.

ANSWER:

19. Please name all claims made against you by any patient. A claim is any notice to you that a patient, or someone acting for a patient, alleges that you were negligent.

ANSWER:

20. Please name all malpractice cases that have been filed against you. Give the court, file number, county, and state in which the action was filed.

ANSWER:

21. Please state all other suits that you have been a part of, including family law and divorce suits.

ANSWER:

DATED this _____ day of _____, 19__ .

§ 6.8 Goals of Requests for Production

As with interrogatories, requests for production are used to set the stage for the defendant's deposition. If possible, answers should be received before any depositions are taken. Sometimes counsel cannot anticipate the subjects for production until after the depositions of the defendant physician have been taken. Material does not have to be admissible to be discoverable.

§ 6.9 Requests for Production: To Defendant Doctor in Fetal Injury Case

TO: _____, M.D.

c/o _____, defense attorney

Plaintiffs request defendant _____, M.D., to respond to plaintiffs' counsel pursuant to Rule 34, Federal Rules of Civil Procedure, by giving access to or making available and permitting the inspection and copying of:

1. Your curriculum vitae during the time that plaintiff _____ was your patient.

2. Your current curriculum vitae.

3. Any documents, correspondence, written memorandums, and the like concerning any denials, suspensions, or revoking of your hospital staff privileges at any time anywhere.

4. All liability insurance policies that would potentially cover you for any acts of negligence during the time plaintiffs were your patients. Please include primary insurance as well as any excess, group, corporate, or umbrella policies.

5. A copy of any and all articles, journals, pages from textbooks, and the like that will be relied upon to support your medical care in this case.

6. Any correspondence, memorandum, or other written documents concerning the care that you afforded your patient from any other physicians.

7. Copies of all charts in your possession of all patients you have treated with similar complications with identifying material deleted.

CHAPTER 7

NORMAL LABOR

Michael S. Cardwell, M.D.

Thomas G. Kirkhope, M.D.

§ 7.1 Mechanisms of Labor

The precise cause of the commencement of labor is still uncertain, although it is known that several factors play a part. The degree of distention of the uterus undoubtedly plays some role, since multiple pregnancies tend to go into labor earlier. The fetal brain plays some part, as is evidenced by the fact that when the fetus has certain brain anomalies, pregnancy is often prolonged. When it is considered desirable to terminate a pregnancy early, a synthetic maternal pituitary hormone, oxytocin, is used, demonstrating that the maternal pituitary gland has an important effect. Placental hormones are also involved as well. There is, however, no known individual signal that tells the uterus that the fetus is now mature and that labor should begin.

Labor is defined as rhythmic, coordinated, painful contractions of the uterine myometrium (muscle) that produce progressive dilatation and effacement of the cervix. The normal result of labor is expulsion of the fetus from the uterus, that is, delivery. Uterine contractions normally occur throughout the third trimester of pregnancy, but they are for the most part painless and are not accompanied by changes in the cervix. These are called Braxton Hicks contractions. They may occasionally cause some discomfort in the mother, and when they do it may be difficult for her to distinguish between these and real labor contractions. Observation in the labor and delivery suite at the hospital may be required to determine the difference.

§ 7.2   Fetal Position

The orientation of the fetus within the uterus is of crucial importance for the normal progress of labor. Several terms are used to describe this orientation. The normal fetal attitude with respect to itself is one of "universal flexion." That is, all joints, including the knees, hips, elbows, wrists, hands, and neck are in a position of flexion. If they are not, it may be related to a fetal anomaly or some malpresentation, and some investigation is required.

The fetal orientation with respect to the long axis of the mother is referred to as the fetal *lie* and may be vertical, transverse, or oblique.

Presentation refers to that part of the fetus presenting at the maternal pelvis, and likely to be the first part that comes out at delivery. In a vertical lie, the presentation may be "cephalic" or "breech." (In transverse and oblique lies, it is not really appropriate to discuss presentation, since no fetal part is presenting at the maternal pelvis for delivery.) Cephalic presentation is sub-divided into "vertex," "brow," and "face" presentation, referring to that part of the head which is leading and reflecting the position of the neck as flexed or extended.

Position is a subdivision of presentation and describes the orientation of the head or breech with respect to the maternal pelvis. Examples of presentation are: "right occiput posterior (ROP)," which describes a fetal head in a vertex presentation which is positioned obliquely in the maternal pelvis, with its posterior aspect in the right posterior quadrant of the pelvis; "left sacrum transverse" describes a fetus in a vertical lie, breech presentation, with the fetus facing the mother's right side.

The most common fetal orientation is vertical lie, vertex presentation, left occiput anterior (LOA) or right occiput anterior (ROA). These are most com-patible with normal labor and spontaneous vaginal delivery. If the orientation of the fetus is anything other than these, varying degrees of difficulty in labor and delivery can be anticipated.[1] It is therefore assumed in discussion of "normal" labor that this is the position of the fetus.

§ 7.3 Onset of Labor

Diagnosis of labor depends on the presence of regular, painful uterine contractions at gradually shortening intervals and gradually increasing intensity, accompanied by progressive dilatation and effacement of the cervix. If dilatation and effacement do not occur, the contractions are not considered labor, regardless of how strong or frequent they may be. The contractions are palpable by the observer through the abdominal wall as tightening and hardening of the uterus. The progressive cervical dilatation and effacement can be appreciated by vaginal digital examination.

The woman is usually instructed to call or to report to the labor and delivery area when the contractions are occurring at intervals of every five minutes. On admission, a number of procedures are routinely performed. The patient's general condition and that of the fetus are determined and an adequate physical examination performed. The maternal blood pressure, temperature, pulse, and respiratory rate are noted, and the prenatal record is reviewed. If any complications of pregnancy are present or anticipated, a plan of management is instituted.

Information is obtained regarding onset of regular contractions, interval between contractions, frequency, and duration. If there is a history or finding of significant bleeding from the vagina, cervical examination is avoided until placenta previa can be ruled out. If there is a history of watery discharge, spontaneous rupture of membranes may have occurred.

During abdominal examination, attention is focused on the uterine size, and the fetal weight is estimated by palpation. Fetal heart tones are counted and recorded. A fetal heart rate (FHR) that lies outside the usually accepted limits of 120 to 160 beats per minute requires further evaluation. "Leopold's maneuvers" are carried out to determine fetal position. Usually fetal lie and presentation, and often position, can be determined by clinical examination. If there is doubt, real-time ultrasound and occasionally an X-ray film may be needed.

The perineum and vagina are inspected for the presence of any lesions or growths that may obstruct fetal descent. The vulva is examined for the presence of lesions, such as herpes genitalis, which might contraindicate vaginal delivery.

The condition of the cervix is observed, including the percentage of effacement and the number of centimeters of dilatation. The position of the fetal head is determined, if possible, using the sutures and fontanels (spaces between the skull bones) as guidelines. The status of the amniotic membranes is important and if there is doubt, the examiner tests for the presence or absence of amniotic

---

[1] F. Cunningham, P. MacDonald, K. Leveno, N. Gant & L. Gilstrap III, Williams Obstetrics 493 (19th ed. 1993).

fluid by use of nitrazine paper or the presence of "ferning" of the vaginal fluid under the microscope. The station (level above or below the ischial spines) of the fetal head is observed and recorded.

Blood is drawn for hemoglobin and hematocrit. Many physicians find it prudent also to order blood type and screen (for antibodies), particularly if there has been some prenatal complication that may suggest a need for blood transfusion during the puerperium. Urinalysis may be ordered, and an intravenous solution is often started, especially if complications in labor are anticipated.[2]

§ 7.4   Fetal Surveillance in Labor

Continuous observation of the status of the fetus is of utmost importance during labor, but there is considerable difference of opinion among obstetricians as to how it should be accomplished. Since the advent of the electronic fetal monitor (EFM) in the late 1960s, the use of continuous observation by this method has become all but universal. Yet, most carefully controlled studies continue to show that intermittent auscultation (listening with a stethoscope) of the fetal heart is equivalent to continuous electronic monitoring in assessing fetal condition.[3]

Almost no study comparing continuous electronic FHR monitoring with intermittent auscultation in either high- or low-risk patients has shown a difference in intrapartum fetal death rates. Also, no study has shown that electronic FHR monitoring has been more effective in reducing the rates of low Apgar scores at birth or long-term neurologic morbidity.[4] (It should be noted that each of these studies on monitoring by intermittent auscultation has involved constant observation by nurses in a 1:1 nurse-to-patient ratio.) On the other hand, the use of EFM has been shown to be associated with a higher cesarean section rate.

Description of specific EFM patterns and their significance is beyond the scope of this chapter (see **Chapter 9**), but it should be noted that "reassuring"

---

[2] J. Scott, P. DiSaia, C. Hammond & W. Spellacy, Danforth's Obstetrics and Gynecology (7th ed. 1994).

[3] J. Garite & M. Nageotte, Fetal Heart Rate Patterns: Monitoring, Interpretation, and Management, ACOG Technical Bull. No. 207, American College of Obstetricians and Gynecologists (1995).

[4] R. Myers, E. Mueller-Huebach & K. Adamsons, *Predictability of the State of Fetal Oxygenation from Quantitative Analysis of the Components of Late Deceleration,* 115 Am. J. Obstet. Gynecol. 1083, 1094 (1973); R. Ball & J. Parer, *The Physiologic Mechanisms of Variable Decelerations,* 166 Am. J. Obstet. Gynecol. 1683, 1689 (1992); S. Davidson, J. Rankin, C. Martin Jr., & D. Reid, *Fetal Heart Rate Variability and Behavioral State: Analysis by Power Spectrum,* 167 Am. J. Obstet. Gynecol. 717, 722 (1992); S. Clark, M. Gimovsky & F. Miller, *Fetal Heart Rate Response to Scalp Blood Sampling,* 144 Am. J. Obstet. Gynecol. 706, 708 (1982); A. Haverkamp, M. Orleans, S. Langendoerfer, J. McFee, J. Murphy & H. Thompson, *A Controlled Trial of the Differential Effects of Intrapartum Fetal Monitoring,* 134 Am. J. Obstet. Gynecol. 399, 412 (1979).

and "non-reassuring" patterns are recognizable. When a non-reassuring pattern is seen, evaluation and management are approached as follows:

1. Determination of the etiology of the pattern, if possible.
2. An attempt to correct the pattern by correcting the primary problem, or by instituting general measures aimed at improving fetal oxygenation.
3. If attempts to correct are not successful, fetal scalp blood pH assessment may be considered.
4. Determination of whether operative intervention (cesarean section or operative vaginal delivery) is warranted and, if so, how urgently it is needed.

There are several steps that may be appropriate to try to relieve the non-reassuring pattern before considering operation. These include: oxygen to the mother by mask, change in maternal position, discontinuation or decrease in rate of oxytocin, amnioinfusion, tocolytic agents, fetal scalp stimulation, and vibro-acoustic stimulation.

§ 7.5   Progress and Management of the First Stage

The term *first stage* refers to that part of labor that begins with the onset of contractions and ends with complete dilatation of the cervix. Management of the first stage is directed toward careful observation and recording of fetal heart activity and uterine contractions. As noted in § 7.4, observation of fetal heart activity may be by EFM or by use of any one of a number of stethoscopes or Doppler ultrasound devices.

During the first stage of labor, the FHR is usually checked every 15 minutes by auscultation if high-risk factors are present and EFM is not used. There are no standards for frequency of auscultation in the absence of risk factors. Many individual hospitals, however, will specify a recommended frequency of auscultation in their nursing procedure manuals and provide a flow sheet on which the FHR is to be recorded.

The uterine contractions are observed for onset, duration, frequency, and intensity. If an electronic monitor is not being utilized, the palm of the hand can be used to gauge intensity, duration, and interval between contractions. The observations also are recorded in the nurses' notes.

The normal pregnant woman in labor need not be confined to lying supine in bed, especially early in labor and if analgesics have not been administered. She is often allowed to ambulate. If she prefers to remain in a labor room, a bedside chair may be used. If in bed, she is allowed to assume the position she finds most comfortable.

Administration of analgesic drugs to reduce pain and anxiety may be necessary, even in the early stages of labor. Experience with patients who have had special preparation for labor, (for example, Lamaze classes) indicates that their need for drugs is often reduced. Pain relief in labor may be indicated, however, whether or not there are any medical complications of the pregnancy or the labor. Maternal request is a sufficient justification for pain relief during labor.[5]

The maternal blood pressure and pulse rate are recorded every one to two hours in the first stage. It is usually recommended that these observations take place between contractions, since the blood pressure may be falsely elevated during a contraction. If the membranes are ruptured, the maternal temperature is recorded every hour.

In recent years, it has become common practice to allow the laboring patient to take fluids by mouth as desired, but to avoid solid foods during the first stage. This practice is to avoid vomiting with aspiration of stomach contents should it become necessary for some reason to administer general anesthesia. Intravenous fluids such as dilute electrolyte solutions or glucose are commonly, although not routinely, administered.

§ 7.6   Progress and Management of the Second Stage

The *second stage* of labor is defined as that portion from full dilatation of the cervix to delivery of the infant. The median duration of the second stage in multiparous patients is 20 minutes; in nulliparous patients, 50 minutes.[6] There is, however, wide variation. An old rule of obstetrics specified a maximum of two hours for nullipara, one hour for multipara. The intent was to avoid a prolonged second stage, which was commonly associated with fetal distress. Most obstetricians now feel that this rule is outdated. Equipment to monitor fetal well-being is sophisticated enough that such old "blanket rules" are no longer valid. If the fetus appears to be doing well and there is an obvious reason for the prolonged second stage, it may be allowed to continue.

Continued monitoring of fetal well-being in the second stage is essential. If continuous EFM is not being used, auscultation of the FHR every five minutes is recommended if the pregnancy is considered high-risk.[7] In the absence of high-risk factors, no firm recommendations have been made. Often, frequency of auscultation of the fetal heart in the second stage is dictated by individual

---

[5] American College of Obstetricians and Gynecologists, Committee on Obstetrics: Maternal and Fetal Medicine, Pain Relief During Labor, ACOG Committee Opinions No. 118, (1993); American Academy of Pediatrics and American College of Obstetricians and Gynecologists, Guidelines for Perinatal Care, 73 (3d ed. 1992).

[6] F. Cunningham, P. MacDonald, K. Leveno, N. Gant & L. Gilstrap III, Williams Obstetrics 379 (19th ed. 1993).

[7] J. Garite & M. Nageotte, Fetal Heart Rate Patterns: Monitoring, Interpretation, and Management, ACOG Technical Bull. No. 207, American College of Obstetricians and Gynecologists (1995).

hospital nursing procedure manuals. It is usually in the range of every 15 to 30 minutes.

As the second stage progresses, the mother usually has an urge to bear down, or to "push." This is encouraged by the labor and delivery attendants, because vigorous voluntary efforts are required to effect descent and delivery of the fetus. Transient slowing of the FHR during this expulsive phase is not uncommon. It is recognizable on the EFM tracing as the so-called early deceleration. These decelerations should promptly return to baseline levels when the contraction ends.

As the head descends, it begins to distend the perineum and separate the labia minora of the vulva. The fetal scalp becomes visible and preparations are made for delivery. At this point a decision must be made as to whether an episiotomy (incision of the posterior aspect of the vulva to allow more room for delivery) is needed.

In recent years more debate has taken place about the usefulness of routine episiotomy. The traditional teaching was that an episiotomy, by easing the stretching force, prevents tearing of the perineum. Tearing leads to poor healing with scar formation and distortion and dysfunction of the vulva. This traditional view is now being called into question, and fewer episiotomies are being performed. Cutting of an episiotomy is still recommended for appropriate indications, both fetal and maternal. Examples of fetal indications are: preterm delivery to protect the more malleable fetal head, shoulder dystocia, breech delivery, forceps or vacuum extractor application, and occiput posterior presentations. Episiotomy is also often used if frank rupture of the perineal floor appears imminent.

Following delivery of the fetal head, the nose and mouth are suctioned to minimize aspiration of amniotic fluid into the fetal lungs. This is particularly important if there is staining of the amniotic fluid by meconium (stool passed by the fetus in utero) since such aspiration can lead to a chemical pneumonia in the infant.

Various cord entanglements are looked for (for example, neck or shoulder) and, if found, an attempt is made to reduce these manually. If the cord cannot be untangled, it may have to be cut while the head is still on the perineum to avoid avulsion. Delivery of the shoulders is effected next. If there is no obstruction, the rest of the body of the fetus is usually delivered easily. The mouth and nose are again suctioned, and the cord is clamped and cut. If umbilical artery blood pH and acid-base analysis is to be performed, the blood is collected at this time.

There has been some discussion in recent years as to whether routine cord blood studies should be performed at all deliveries. Approximately 30 percent of university departments do so. Another 50 percent collect blood for analysis at all premature deliveries. The current recommendation of the American College of Obstetricians and Gynecologists (ACOG) states that cord blood gas and pH analysis should be performed in all cases in which the Apgar score is low, but that routine performance on all deliveries is not cost effective.[8]

---

[8] L. Gilstrap & S. Ramin, Umbilical Artery Blood Acid-Base Analysis, ACOG Technical Bull. No. 216, American College of Obstetricians and Gynecologists (1995).

§ 7.7 Progress and Management of the Third Stage

The third stage of labor begins with delivery of the infant and ends with delivery of the placenta. In ordinary circumstances, there is a short delay after delivery of the infant before the uterus begins to contract again. Subsequent contractions cause the placenta to separate from its attachment to the uterine wall, and to be expelled from the uterus. The dangers during this period include failure of the uterus to contract (atony), so that bleeding from the site of the partially separated placenta may occur, and conversely, that the uterus will contract too quickly, trapping the placenta inside.

If the uterus fails to contract and expel the placenta, it may be encouraged to do so by gentle massage of the fundus and traction on the umbilical cord. Vigorous massage and downward pressure is to be avoided because inversion of the uterus may result from excessive force. Uterine inversion is a very dangerous complication that could lead to severe hemorrhage and shock, and may require emergency hysterectomy.

If the placenta becomes trapped, manual removal be required. Insertion of the operator's hand up into the uterine fundus carries with it the dangers of post-partum endometritis (infection) and perforation of the uterus.

Normally, after delivery of the placenta, the uterus remains contracted firmly, shutting off the blood vessels leading to the raw placental bed. This is the physiologic mechanism for preventing postpartum bleeding. If contraction of the uterus is inadequate, massive hemorrhage can occur. Often the obstetrician will give a drug such as methergine or oxytocin to promote firm uterine contraction.

After delivery of the placenta, the vulva, vagina, and cervix are examined for evidence of bleeding, and any lacerations found may be repaired. The episiotomy, if any, is also repaired at this time.

§ 7.8 Elective Induction of Labor

Induction of labor is termed "elective" if performed for the convenience of the patient or the professional staff. When it is carried out because of medical, obstetric, or fetal complications of pregnancy it is termed "indicated" (see § 7.9).

Traditionally, elective induction of labor was considered unnecessarily hazardous and was disapproved by most conservative obstetricians. Some studies, however, have supported the safety and convenience of elective induction.[9]

---

[9] B. Black & W. McBride, *Children Born after Elective Induction of Labour,* 2 Med. J. Aust. 362 (1979); E. Friedman, M. Sachtleben & B. Wallace, *Infant Outcome Following Labor Induction,* 133 Am. J. Obstet. Gynecol. 718 (1979).

There is no doubt, however, that elective induction of labor is associated with an increased cesarean section rate.[10]

Probably the most compelling reason to favor waiting for spontaneous labor is that it tends to be associated with fetal maturity in the vast majority of cases. If labor is undertaken electively, there is no such assurance. It is reasonable, then, before undertaking an elective induction, to obtain corroborating evidence of fetal maturity. Fetal maturity may be assessed by amniocentesis for fetal pulmonary (lung) maturity studies. Fetal maturity may be assumed in the absence of amniocentesis if one of the following criteria is met:[11]

1. Fetal heart tones have been documented by nonelectronic fetoscope for 20 weeks, or for 30 weeks by Doppler ultrasound.
2. It has been 36 weeks since a positive serum or urine human chorionic gonadotropin pregnancy test was performed by a reliable method.
3. An ultrasound measurement of the crown-rump length, obtained at 6 to 11 weeks, supports a gestational age of 39 weeks or more.
4. An ultrasound scan, obtained at 12 to 20 weeks, confirms the gestational age of 39 weeks or more determined by clinical history and physical examination.

(If induction of labor is indicated by the medical condition of the mother or fetus, these criteria are of secondary importance.) Parents should be informed about the increased risks of both fetal immaturity and cesarean delivery if induction of labor is undertaken without medical indication.

If an obstetrics service permits elective induction, criteria and protocols should probably be established by the medical staff. In addition, periodic review of elective inductions should take place to assure that the criteria are being met, that the protocol is being followed, and that no untoward fetal or maternal morbidity is occurring.[12]

§ 7.9   Indicated Induction of Labor

The onset and progress of normal labor do not always occur under conditions that are optimal for the fetus. The normal duration of pregnancy, as mentioned in **Chapter 3,** is 40 weeks, plus or minus 2 weeks. It is well established that the

[10] P. Yudkin, A. Fumar, A. Anderson & A. Turnbill, *A Retrospective Study of Induction of Labour,* 135 Br. J. Obstet. Gynaecol. 239 (1979).

[11] W. Rayburn, *Induction of Labor,* ACOG Technical Bull. No. 217, American College of Obstetrics and Gynecology (1995).

[12] R. Creasy & R. Resnik, Maternal-Fetal Medicine Principles and Practice 535 (3d ed. 1994).

incidence of fetal problems, including intrauterine fetal death, rises rapidly after this time.[13] The aging placenta is no longer able to supply oxygen and nutrients as efficiently, and fetal well-being is affected.

There are also conditions for which delivery of the fetus prior to term would be beneficial. Examples of such conditions are diabetes mellitus, intrauterine growth restriction, premature rupture of membranes, and chorioamnionitis (intrauterine infection). These conditions may be evidenced by means such as serial ultrasound measurements during the prenatal course and amniocentesis for pulmonary maturity studies.

A number of methods of induction of labor have been developed. They are discussed in §§ **7.10** through **7.13.**

§ 7.10 Artificial Rupture of Membranes (Amniotomy)

Amniotomy is an effective method for induction of labor, particularly when the cervix is favorable.[14] (The "Bishop Score" (see **Appendix 7–1**) is used to determine the status of the cervix in the multiparous patient.) This method has the advantage of requiring no drugs. Labor usually begins within 12 hours when amniotomy is used as the only method of induction, but the technique is commonly used in conjunction with other methods of induction or augmentation.

Amniotomy also has several drawbacks. First, it is not always successful in inducing labor. If labor does not commence within a reasonable time period, bacteria may gain access to the endometrial cavity and cause chorioamnionitis. This problem can become severe enough to threaten the life of both mother and fetus. In addition, amniotomy can cause prolapse of the umbilical cord through the cervix, trapping it and causing acute oxygen deprivation to the fetus. This is particularly likely to occur if the presenting part is high and not well applied to the cervix.

In order to avoid these problems, some basic precautions are appropriate:

1. Amniotomy is performed only when the cervix is favorable for induction.
2. The procedure is performed only when the head is presenting, is engaged in the pelvis, and is well applied to the cervix. Cord presentation must be ruled out.
3. The fetal heart rate is assessed prior to and immediately after the procedure.

---

[13] R. Resnick, *Post-Term Pregnancy, in* R. Creasy & R. Resnik, Maternal-Fetal Medicine Principles and Practice 521 (3d ed. 1994).

[14] W. Rayburn, *Induction of Labor,* ACOG Technical Bull. No. 217, American College of Obstetrics and Gynecology (1995).

§ 7.11 Prostaglandins

Prostaglandin E_2 (PGE_2) is a drug which, when applied to the cervix, can produce cervical softening, effacement, and dilatation (cervical "ripening").[15] In 1992 it was given approval by the Food and Drug Administration for use in the induction of labor with a living fetus in the uterus. It is commercially available and is marketed under the names Prepidil and Cervidil. The drug may or may not cause contractions of the uterus. Most commonly it is given to a patient in order to prepare her cervix for induction of labor by the use of oxytocin (see § 7.12). On occasion, however, the uterus will go into labor after PGE_2 ripening with no further need for stimulation.

The most common side effects of prostaglandin are nausea, fever, and uterine contractions. Hyperstimulation (excessive uterine activity) of the uterus may occur in 1 to 5 percent of cases. If hyperstimulation does occur, removal of the gel from the vagina is usually effective in reversing this effect. If not, an agent such as terbutaline, given intravenously or subcutaneously, will result in rapid resolution in most cases.

Uterine rupture and intrauterine fetal deaths have been reported with the use of prostaglandin on a few occasions. Therefore it is considered prudent to monitor the FHR if PGE_2 is being used for preinduction cervical ripening.[16]

§ 7.12 Oxytocin

Oxytocin is a naturally occurring posterior pituitary hormone that has a role in the onset of normal labor. It has been synthesized and is available for use in induction and augmentation of labor. It is effective in inducing uterine contractions when administered by various routes, including intravenously, intramuscularly, and sublingually (under the tongue). The sensitivity of the uterus to the drug increases from about 30 weeks to term, and the sensitivity of an individual uterus at any given time is quite unpredictable. The usual mode of administration now used, therefore, in a patient with a living fetus in the uterus, is by intravenous infusion under carefully controlled conditions.

In most institutions, oxytocin is infused in a dilute intravenous solution using an electronically controlled infusion device. The induction solution is started "piggy-back" on another intravenous line so that it can be discontinued quickly, if complications are encountered, without losing the intravenous access line. The solution is started very slowly and gradually increased until a satisfactory

---

[15] R. Creasy & R. Resnik, Maternal-Fetal Medicine Principles and Practice 538 (3d ed. 1994).

[16] American College of Obstetricians and Gynecologists, Committee on Obstetrics: Maternal and Fetal Medicine, Prostaglandin E_2 Gel for Cervical Ripening, ACOG Committee Opinions, No. 123 (1993).

contraction pattern is attained. The rate of administration can then be titrated according to the uterine activity.

Appendix 7–2 shows four commonly used protocols for administration of oxytocin. The method selected depends on the clinician's training and experience and the clinical situation.

Another method of delivering oxytocin is pulsatile infusion. In this method the drug is given in pulses at 10-minute intervals. In some cases it is possible to use a smaller total amount of drug, which may be beneficial in patients in whom a lower fluid intake is desirable.[17]

Like prostaglandin (see § **7.11**), oxytocin can produce uterine hyperstimulation. This can take the form of tetanic (that is, unremitting) contraction. If the amount of drug administered is excessive at any moment for the particular uterus on which it is used, the uterus can contract tightly and fail to relax. A tetanic contraction shuts of the maternal blood supply to the placental bed, depriving the fetus of oxygen. If the contraction cannot be stopped, severe fetal distress and occasionally fetal death may ensue. In extreme cases, the uterus may contract so violently that there is danger of uterine rupture, leading to loss of the fetus, and sometimes the mother as well.

If stopping the intravenous infusion is not immediately effective in aborting a tetanic contraction, general anesthesia may be necessary, and, rarely, emergency cesarean section. Many institutions require the use of the EFM on all patients undergoing oxytocin induction or augmentation, so that fetal distress can be immediately recognized.

Other adverse effects of the use of oxytocin include antidiuresis (inhibition of urine formation) with consequent water intoxication, kidney failure, and ultimately heart failure. The amount of drug along with fluid intake and output must be carefully monitored to avoid this complication.

The Standards for Obstetric-Gynecologic Services published by the ACOG contains the following recommendations:

1. Induction or augmentation of labor with oxytocin may be initiated only after a responsible physician has evaluated the patient, determined that induction or augmentation is beneficial to the mother or fetus, recorded the indication, and established a prospective plan of management.

2. Only a physician who has privileges to perform cesarean deliveries should initiate the procedures.

3. A physician or qualified nurse should examine the patient vaginally immediately prior to the oxytocin infusion.

4. A written protocol for the preparation and administration of the oxytocin solution should be established by the obstetric department in each institution.

---

[17] K. Leveno, Induction and Augmentation of Labor, ACOG Technical Bull. No. 157, American College of Obstetricians and Gynecologists (1991).

5. Oxytocin should be administered only intravenously, with a device that permits precise control of the flow rate.

6. While oxytocin is being administered, an electronic fetal monitor should be used for continuous recording of fetal heart rate and uterine contractions.

7. Personnel who are familiar with the effects of oxytocin and are able to identify both maternal and fetal complications should be in attendance while oxytocin is being administered.

8. A qualified physician should be readily accessible to manage any complications that may arise during infusion.[18]

§ 7.13 Other Methods of Induction of Labor

There are other methods of induction of labor, of somewhat lesser importance. These include:

1. Stripping of membranes—On vaginal examination, the finger is introduced through the partially dilated cervix to the potential space between the amniotic membrane and the uterine wall. Although this method is commonly used, its safety and efficacy have never been thoroughly studied. The potential for infection, bleeding from undiagnosed placenta previa, and accidental rupture of the membranes are important considerations.

2. Laminaria—A form of dried kelp, which has been compressed and sterilized, can be placed into the undilated cervix. Over a period of several hours, the laminaria absorbs water and expands in size, forcing the cervix open. Other synthetic substances have also been used in a similar manner. These are usually used as preinduction cervical ripeners.

3. Foley Catheter—A rubber catheter is placed inside the cervix and held in place with a 30cc balloon filled with sterile water. The mechanism of action is not completely understood but is felt to be via stimulation of the release of endogenous prostaglandins.

§ 7.14 Augmentation of Labor

Augmentation of labor has been given considerably more attention in the last few years as the rate of cesarean section has risen in the United States. In the past, "previous cesarean section" was the most common reason given as an

---

[18] American College of Obstetricians and Gynecologists, Standards for Ob/Gyn Services 35 (6th ed. 1985).

indication for cesarean section. Previous caesarean section alone is no longer considered an acceptable indication in modern obstetrics. The next most common reason given for cesarean section today is failure of labor to progress. It is in these cases that augmentation of labor comes into play. *Augmentation* means, essentially, correcting ineffective uterine contractions.

The term "failure to progress" itself is very imprecise. Several attempts have been made to quantify the efficiency of labor contractions and the rate of progress in labor. But there are many confounding factors, such as whether the patient is primiparous (first pregnancy) or multiparous, the effect of anesthesia, type of equipment used in measuring intensity of contractions, the size of the fetus, and the size of the pelvis through which the fetus must pass. There is also undoubtedly an effect of social support and childbirth preparation, both of which have been shown to be associated with shorter durations of labor.

Labor can be augmented by amniotomy (artificial rupture of amniotic membranes) and by oxytocin infusion. The two are often used together. The goal of augmentation is to effect uterine activity sufficient to produce cervical dilatation and fetal descent. *Minimally effective uterine activity* is defined as three contractions in 10 minutes averaging greater than 25mm of mercury pressure, but there is wide variation.

The amount of oxytocin needed to achieve a normal labor pattern is usually less than that needed for induction of labor. The method of administration, however, is the same (see § **7.12**). The rates of infusion are currently matters of debate; there are both "low-dose" and "high-dose" regimens, both of which have their adherents. There are theoretical advantages and disadvantages to both. Risks of the use of oxytocin are described in § **7.12.**

Another technique of augmentation of labor, known as the "active management of labor," has been developed and practiced in Ireland.[19] One of its primary components is the use of much higher doses of oxytocin than are commonly used in the United States. However, this method is beginning to gain acceptance here, and must now be considered a "respectable minority" approach.

---

[19] K. O'Driscoll, M. Foley & D. MacDonald, *Active Management of Labor as an Alternative to Cesarean Section for Dystocia,* 63 Obstet. Gynecol. 485, 490 (1984).

§ 7.15 Appendix 7–1: Bishop Scoring System

As noted in **§ 7.10,** the Bishop Score[20] is important in evaluating the appropriateness of amniotomy.

Score	Dilatation (cm)	Effacement (%)	Consistency of Cervix	Station of Presenting Part	Position
0	Closed	0–30	Firm	Flat	Posterior
1	1–2	40–50	Medium	−2	Mid-position
2	3–4	60–70	Soft	−1, 0	Mid-position
3	≥5	≥80	Soft	+1,+2	Anterior

Factor (header spanning Dilatation...Position)

§ 7.16 Appendix 7–2: Examples of Protocols for Oxytocin Infusion

Reference	Initial Dose (mU/min)	Incremental Dose (mU/min)	Preferred Interval Between Doses (min)
Mercer et al. (1991)	0.5	Doubled	60
Chua et al. (1991)	2.5	2.5	30
Satin et al. (1994)	6	6	20–40
Muller et al. (1992)	1–2	1–2	30

Sources: Mercer, B., Pilgrim, P., Sibai, B. Labor induction with continuous low-dose oxytocin infusion: a randomized trial. Obstet. Gynecol. 1991; 77:659–663.

Chua, S., Arulkumaran, S., Kurup, A., Tay, D., Ratnam, S.S. Oxytocin titration for induction of labor: a prospective randomized study of 15 versus 30 minute dose increment schedules. Aust. N.Z. Obstet. Gynecol. 1991; 31:134–137.

Satin, A.J., Leveno, K.J., Sherman, M.L., McIntyre, D. High-dose oxytocin: 20- versus 40-minute dosage interval. Obstet. Gynecol. 1994; 83:234–238.

Muller, P.R., Stubbs, T.M., Laurent, S.L. A prospective randomized clinical trial comparing two oxytocin induction protocols. Am. J. Obstet. Gynecol. 1992; 167:373–381.

[20] E. Bishop, *Pelvic Scoring for Elective Induction,* 24 Obstet. Gynecol. 266 (1964).

CHAPTER 8

OBSTETRIC ANESTHESIA

Robert M. Knapp, D.O.

§ 8.1   Introduction

The practice of obstetric anesthesia includes the performance of invasive procedures and the administration of medications during labor and delivery. There are adjustments of technique and drug dosage that must be made in pregnancy, and the effects of each technique and drug on the fetus must be accounted for as well. These adjustments are widely disseminated in the anesthesia literature. All anesthesia practitioners are or should be aware of the elements of good obstetric anesthesia practice.

§ 8.2   Obstetric Anesthesia Texts

Obstetric Anesthesia: Principles and Practice (D.H. Chestnut, ed. 1994) is probably the most comprehensive and current text available.

Anesthesia for Obstetrics (3d ed) (S. Shnider & G. Levinson, eds. 1993) has been considered the reference text on the subject for many years. Compared with Chestnut, Shnider has the wider name recognition and far greater exposure to most clinicians.

In addition, numerous other texts, compilations, and handbooks are available. The number is sufficient that a large proportion of academic practitioners in obstetric anesthesia have written something about the field. It should be noted that obstetricians writing about anesthesia sometimes have significant biases that elicit strong opposition from anesthesiologists.

§ 8.3   The Medical Record

The anesthesia record is the document of greatest legal interest. It should hold the details of any procedures performed, the type and quantity of any medications administered, and the patient's vital signs as measured at appropriate intervals. There should also be a notation of the maneuvers that are specifically used to protect the fetus from the effects of the anesthetic procedure. These are brief and simple. The mother's right hip must be elevated during a spinal or epidural for cesarean section, the mother must have received an adequate amount of fluid (preload) prior to receiving an epidural or spinal, any drop in blood pressure must be rapidly and effectively treated following the administration of a spinal or epidural, and when general anesthesia is used the induction technique must provide safeguards against the mothers pulmonary aspiration of stomach contents. These maneuvers represent the fetus' primary defense against lack of oxygen during anesthesia.

The anesthesia record should indicate that specific monitoring devices were used during any surgical procedure. The American Society of Anesthesiologists (ASA) has approved and published the "Standards for Basic Anesthetic Monitoring." See **Appendix 8–1** in § **8.31.** These require the continuous use of a pulse oximeter and electrocardiogram, and the measurement of blood pressure every five minutes. In addition, the use of some form of carbon dioxide measurement during general anesthesia is strongly encouraged. It should be noted that these standards are somewhat involved, and that a specific disclaimer precludes their application to patients receiving pain relief for labor.

Two potential problems with the anesthesia record are unreliability, where information is recorded prospectively or retrospectively, and incompleteness, where information is either missing or illegible. Nursing records from the operating room and the recovery room can be used to verify the anesthesia record with regard to fluids given, blood loss, times, and some vital signs.

Before providing anesthesia, the anesthesiologist should interview the patient concerning facts that may affect the procedure. These include the time of the last meal, significant medical problems, a history of back problems, allergies, medications taken, previous anesthetics, and any family history of reactions to anesthesia. These should be written down and placed in the medical record. It is important to remember, however, that this interview is essentially a screen for significant contraindications to the contemplated anesthetic. The absence of information is not significant except where there is a failure to note an easily ascertainable fact that, if known, would have allowed avoidance of an injury-producing procedure.

§ 8.4   Anesthesia Provider

The person providing anesthesia should be either an anesthesiologist or a certified registered nurse anesthetist. This is important because an untrained person, such as an obstetrician, may not be aware of the precautionary measures needed to protect the mother or the fetus from the effects of the anesthetic. It is also possible that such a person may not recognize a problem if it occurs, or will be unable to properly compensate for it because of a lack of necessary skills or a preoccupation with other responsibilities.

In any case, no person should provide anesthesia services unless the hospital has granted the specific privilege to do so. As a matter of definition, the term *anesthetist* in this country usually refers to a nurse anesthetist. *Anesthesiologist* refers solely to a physician.

When a physician provides anesthesia, he is fully independently responsible for his own activities and the consequences that follow from them. A nurse anesthetist providing anesthesia may be supervised by an anesthesiologist who is immediately available for consultation and assistance. In some states the anesthetist may be supervised by the obstetrician. When there is no anesthesiologist available and when there is no legal provision for supervision by the obstetrician or surgeon, the nurse anesthetist acts independently for lack of anyone else equally qualified to make anesthesia-related judgments. The responsibility for the nurse anesthetist's activities may be shared, however, by the hospital as an employer or a credentialing entity, or by an anesthesiologist who should have been present to provide supervision but was not.

§ 8.5   Role of the Hospital

Hospitals generally arrange for anesthesia coverage either through direct employment of the anesthesiologist or through an exclusive arrangement with an individual or a restricted group. As a result, the hospital has several levels of responsibility for the provision of competent and timely anesthesia services.

The first responsibility occurs at the time each practitioner's privileges to practice anesthesia at the hospital are granted. Here, the hospital must verify that the anesthesiologist has had satisfactory training in her specialty, has maintained a satisfactory history of practice during her career, and is at least conversant with current practice.

Another level of responsibility exists when the hospital grants an exclusive privilege to practice anesthesia to an individual or a group. Under these circumstances, the hospital effectively controls its source of anesthesia services. Thus, it must be responsible for ensuring their day-to-day quality. This is particularly significant when the hospital fails to account for indicators of actual or potential substandard practice. Examples of this could include substantive complaints of irregular practices by the nursing staff or allegations of anesthetic malpractice brought by patients.

A final responsibility concerns the timely availability of anesthesia staff for obstetric procedures. Whether the anesthesia personnel are available from inside or from outside the hospital, they must be available to intervene within a reasonable amount of time when notified of an emergency situation. A reasonable amount of time, 30 minutes for example, should be specified somewhere within hospital or anesthesia department policies.

§ 8.6   Anesthesia Equipment

No matter how infrequently it may be used, anesthesia equipment in the delivery room must have the same life-support and patient safety capabilities as that used in the operating room. In particular, the ASA "Guidelines for Regional Anesthesia in Obstetrics" (see **Appendix 8–2** in § **8.32**) state that whenever regional anesthesia is sufficiently extensive to permit cesarean section or complex vaginal delivery, the "Standards for Basic Anesthetic Monitoring" shall be applied.

§ 8.7   Anesthesia Techniques

In general, the three anesthetic techniques used in obstetrics are epidural, spinal, and general anesthesia. Epidural and spinal share several similarities and are used somewhat interchangeably. General anesthesia involves a greater degree of risk of maternal death than does regional anesthesia. Its use is reserved for situations when its benefit can be shown to outweigh its risk. As a rule, the use of general anesthesia is justified by an unusual medical indication, a severe need for speed in the induction of anesthesia, or an absolute refusal by the mother to accept a regional anesthetic when a major anesthetic is needed.

§ 8.8   Epidural Anesthesia

The epidural takes its name from the covering around the spinal cord, known as the *dura*. There is a narrow space around the outside of this covering that can be filled with drugs such as local anesthetics and narcotics. There is no spinal fluid in this space. It is mostly empty except for veins and some connective tissue. The epidural anesthetic is performed by introducing a needle tip into this space and then either injecting medication directly or passing a plastic catheter into the space for later injection. The needle is then removed. If a catheter was passed through the needle, it is now taped to the patient's back to secure it in place.

There are two primary advantages to the epidural. The first is that the problem of a spinal headache is usually avoided. Spinal headaches result from spinal fluid leaking through a hole made in the dura. Since the epidural technique does not require such a hole to be made, the problem is usually avoided.

The other advantage comes from the catheter that is usually left in the epidural space. It allows for repeated dosing of the anesthetic. An epidural can thus be continued for hours or even days. With adjustment in medication, the same catheter can be used for both labor and cesarean section if need be.

The disadvantages to the epidural are inherent in the advantages. The tip of the epidural needle or the plastic catheter may find its way either into an epidural vein or under the dura and into the spinal fluid. A large amount of local anesthetic injected into a vein can result in seizures or cardiac arrest. A similar injection into the spinal fluid can produce a complete spinal block with respiratory arrest.

Despite these disadvantages, the incidence of harmful events is in reality quite small. The key to a reasonably safe epidural lies in the observance of certain key precautions.

§ 8.9 —Performance

Before an epidural is performed, approximately one liter of intravenous fluid should be given to the patient. This fluid should be lactated Ringer's solution or something substantially similar. It should not be 5 percent dextrose in water. This fluid preload is given to minimize the effects of lowered blood pressure, which sometimes accompanies epidural or spinal anesthesia.

Once the epidural space is located with the epidural needle, either medication is injected directly through the needle or else a catheter is placed through the needle and medication is injected through that. As the catheter enters the epidural space, it is common for the patient to feel a shock-like sensation, usually down one leg. This is a transient paresthesia thought to occur when the catheter brushes past a nerve root. It is not associated with harm to the patient.

Once the epidural catheter is in place, it should be aspirated with a syringe before medication is injected. Aspiration of any significant quantity of clear fluid or blood is a sign that the catheter is in the wrong place and must be replaced.

Even if no blood or clear fluid is aspirated, it is no guarantee that the catheter is correctly placed. Thus it is reasonable at this point to perform a test dose.

§ 8.10 —Epidural Test Dose

The *test dose* is a small dose of local anesthetic that contains epinephrine. It is the first dose of medication given through the epidural catheter, and it is accompanied by a close watch of the patient's heart rate for 30 to 60 seconds following the injection. The rationale behind the test dose is that if epinephrine is injected into a vein, it will produce a transient but noticeable rise in heart rate. Thus, the test dose plus heart rate observation serves to detect a catheter placed in an epidural vein even if no blood was aspirated.

The test dose is not a perfect screen for intravascular catheter placement, nor is there unanimous agreement over its effectiveness. Nonetheless, it is generally accepted that a test dose is a reasonable precaution to take against the possibility of intravascular injection of local anesthetic.

§ 8.11 —Intravascular Injection

There is a specific danger when a large amount of local anesthetic is injected directly into a blood vessel. Local anesthetics block the conduction of electrical impulses wherever they are generated in the body. This includes both the brain and the heart. A large amount of relatively undiluted drug placed in a blood vessel will go directly to the heart and from there to the brain. The heart can go into irregular rhythms and even full arrest. The brain can experience loss of consciousness and seizures.

These potential effects are serious enough to warrant the use of a test dose as the initial injection through an epidural catheter. They also suggest that it is prudent to limit any single injection of local anesthetic through an epidural catheter to an amount that is unlikely to cause serious effects. Examples of such limits would be 15 to 25 milligrams of bupivacaine and 100 milligrams of lidocaine.

§ 8.12 —Injection into Spinal Fluid

When the epidural needle or catheter pierces the covering around the spinal cord, there is the possibility that a large amount of local anesthetic will mix with the spinal fluid. This will result in a very high or even complete block of the spinal cord. The mother's blood pressure will drop and she will not be able to move her diaphragm or other muscles of breathing. Without immediate intervention by the anesthesiologist, the resulting lack of oxygen will cause brain damage and even death to both mother and fetus.

Aspirating the epidural catheter or needle with a syringe will often, but not always, produce clear fluid when the tip is in spinal fluid. On the other hand, clear fluid can sometimes be aspirated even when the tip is not in spinal fluid. The results of aspiration are thus no guarantee of proper position in the epidural space.

There is some opinion that any fluid aspirated from the epidural space should be tested for glucose using a reagent strip. The presence of glucose is then taken as presumptive evidence that spinal fluid is being aspirated. Unfortunately, this method only removes some of the ambiguity surrounding a fraction of the positive aspirations.Negative aspirations and even some positive ones do not benefit from this screen.

The definitive screen for spinal injections of epidural drugs must be close observation of each patient following each epidural injection. Both the labor nurses and the anesthesiologist must watch for signs of unexpectedly intense muscle weakness and numbness, low blood pressure, difficulty breathing, and unresponsiveness. If any of these occur, the anesthesiologist must be present to provide any treatment needed to ensure the safety of both the mother and the fetus.

The reason for insisting that the nurses share the burden of observation is that an unexpectedly extensive spinal blockade can occur as late as 20 to 30 minutes after an epidural injection. It is not reasonable to expect the anesthesiologist to personally remain with each patient for 30 minutes following each injection. However, it is reasonable to expect that the patient will be observed by someone who is trained and who has responsibility for the care of the patient. The labor nurse is the person in the best position to do this. In fact, in most hospitals the common obstetric practice following an epidural injection is to turn the observation of the patient over to the nurse after a brief interval. The nurse, in turn, is expected to notify the anesthesiologist if something unexpected or potentially harmful occurs.

§ 8.13 —Headaches and Backaches Afterward

Headaches and backaches are relatively frequent complaints after delivery. Back pain following delivery under an epidural may or may not be related to the epidural, and a causal link between the complaint and the anesthetic may be very difficult to establish in the particular case.

Studies on this subject have found a positive association when done in a retrospective manner, but no association when done in a prospective manner. The retrospective technique has inherent problems with bias that the prospective technique avoids.

When a patient complains of backache, the individual complaint needs to be evaluated on its merits. However, absent a strong and obvious link between epidural technique and symptoms, establishing causality is problematic at best.

Headaches, on the other hand, are usually more clear cut. A small percentage of epidural attempts result in puncture of the dura, the covering that holds the spinal fluid around the cord. A large percentage of these punctures result in spinal headaches, and they must be treated as such. Any patient who has had an epidural and complains of a headache, whether or not a dural puncture was evident at the time the epidural was done, should be referred to the anesthesiologist for evaluation of a potential spinal headache. Spinal headaches must be treated either before the patient's discharge or within some reasonable time after discharge if the headache persists.

§ 8.14 —Medications Used

Local anesthetics and narcotics are the primary anesthetics. Adjuvants such as epinephrine and bicarbonate may also be added to enhance certain characteristics of the primary agents.

The clinical use of these agents deviates significantly from the indications found in the *Physicians' Desk Reference* (*PDR*) and the various package inserts. With the local anesthetics, there is a large discrepancy between the maximum amounts of drug recommended by the manufacturers and the actual amounts used in clinical practice. This discrepancy is apparent from comparing past and current texts on anesthetic practice with their contemporary *PDR* entries. The significance of a these comparisons is that they highlight the fact that this discrepancy has existed for years, if not decades, without comment by the manufacturers. This would seem to call into question the significance of various claims made by the manufacturers with regard to local anesthetics.

Another common deviation between clinical practice and the package insert is the clinical use of a particular drug that finds no mention in the insert. This is true for the epidural use of most narcotics. Many of these are widely used as epidural analgesics, even though only morphine has its use documented in a package insert. This indicates the widespread appreciation by anesthesiologists that clinical acceptance, rather than FDA approval of a package insert, is the legal and ethical indicator of reasonable drug use.

Among the local anesthetics currently in use, two have had significant problems. Bupivacaine 0.75 percent has been contraindicated for obstetric use since 1983 due to an association with convulsions and heart arrhythmias in the mother. It should be noted that this prohibition extends only to the 0.75 percent concentration and only to use in epidurals. Spinal use of 0.75 percent bupivacaine is well accepted practice.

An older formulation of 2-chloroprocaine was associated with permanent damage to the lower portion of the spinal cord when a large volume was injected into the spinal fluid. In 1987, the present manufacturer removed the preservative suspected to be at fault. To date, there have been no published reports of similar damage associated with the new formulation.

§ 8.15   —Use in Labor

The "Guidelines for Regional Anesthesia in Obstetrics" provide a reasonable framework of safeguards for the performance of epidural analgesia in labor.

Just before the epidural is provided, 500 to 1000 milliliters (ml) of electrolyte solution should be given intravenously to minimize the incidence and effects of decreased blood pressure (hypotension) after the epidural is dosed. After the epidural is dosed, the anesthesiologist should remain with the patient for 10 to 15 minutes to observe for signs of intravascular injection, spinal injection, or hypotension. The patient's blood pressure should be taken every two to three minutes during this time. If the patient remains stable, the anesthesiologist may leave to attend other duties. The labor nurse should continue to check the blood pressure at reasonable intervals and to watch the patient for signs of unusually extensive block.

While an epidural is in progress, an anesthesiologist or a nurse anesthetist should be physically in the hospital. All dosing of the epidural should be done by anesthesia personnel.

§ 8.16 —Cesarean Section

Cesarean sections are frequently done under epidural anesthesia, particularly when the epidural has been previously placed for labor analgesia. The change from labor to surgery is accomplished by increasing the concentration of the local anesthetic.

The first responsibility of the anesthesiologist is to ensure that the block is sufficient to provide a reasonably pain-free surgery. The epidural will not always abolish all sensation, and this should be explained to the patient before-hand. However, any sensations the patient experiences under epidural should be no more than mildly to moderately uncomfortable and controlled by reasonable amounts of IV analgesics and sedatives. If the pain is severe, general anesthesia should be offered and provided unless there is a very strong reason not to do so.

Lower blood pressure should be anticipated during the 10 to 30 minutes after the surgical dose is injected. Prophylaxis consists of elevating the patient's right hip and quickly infusing IV fluid immediately before and after giving the anesthetic dose. Treatment consists of giving intravenous ephedrine in five to 15 milligram doses whenever a significant drop in blood pressure occurs.

Immediately after the infant and placenta are delivered, there is a period of acute blood loss while the uterus contracts and the incision made in the uterine wall is clamped and closed. Pitocin must be given intravenously during this time. The anesthesiologist must watch the surgery carefully to make certain that the blood loss is controlled in a reasonable time, and that any excessive loss is replaced with the appropriate fluid or blood.

§ 8.17 Spinal Anesthesia

A *spinal block,* also called a subarachnoid or a saddle block, is performed by injecting a small amount of local anesthetic directly into the spinal fluid. The quantity of anesthetic used is so much smaller than that used in the epidural that a toxic reaction is not seen if the injection should go into an inappropriate place.

The spinal has traditionally been a single-injection technique. Catheters that were small enough to pass through a spinal needle, and that could be used for repeated doses in the manner of an epidural catheter, appeared on the market briefly during the late 1980s. They have since had their marketing approval rescinded by the FDA for safety-related reasons. They should not be in clinical use at this time.

§ 8.18 —Performance

A spinal is performed in a similar manner and in the same place as an epidural. The major differences are the much finer needle used for the spinal and the further insertion of the spinal needle all the way through the dura and into the spinal fluid. In fact, the endpoint of spinal needle placement is the positive aspiration of clear fluid.

Once the spinal needle is placed and spinal fluid is obtained, the anesthetic agent is injected. The actual injection should go unnoticed by the patient. If the patient feels a distinct sensation as the agent is injected, and particularly a sharp or painful sensation, then a reasonable presumption may be made that the anesthetic is going into nerve tissue. Subsequent nerve damage may be the result of the injection.

On the other hand, a simple sensation as the needle is moved into place is a very common occurrence that is not associated with nerve damage. This sensation is most commonly describe as a sharp or electric shock sensation down one leg or at the insertion site. If the needle is positioned such that there is no sensation once it is at rest and there is no sensation as the anesthetic is injected, then previous sensations are of no real account.

§ 8.19 —Headache Afterward

A certain percentage of spinals are followed by spinal headaches. The percentage is dependent mostly on the diameter of the spinal needle and the age of the patient. Larger needles and younger patients are both associated with a higher incidence of spinal headaches. In fact, among patients in whom spinal anesthesia is relatively common, childbearing women have the highest incidence of spinal headaches.

Various symptoms are ascribed to the spinal headache, but the most common is a prominent postural quality. That is, when the patient sits up or stands, the headache becomes moderate to severe. When she lies down, it goes away. Other symptoms may be present, such as blurred vision, ringing in the ears, or nausea. Still, it is the postural nature that sets the spinal headache apart and ultimately makes the diagnosis.

A large percentage of spinal headaches occur the day after the day after the spinal anesthetic. This delay means that the anesthesiologist often depends on the obstetrician and the obstetric nursing staff to bring the patient with a potential spinal headache to his attention.

A large percentage of spinal headaches resolve on their own within a week. However, this leaves a significant percentage that persist for a longer time. Of these, a small number can go on for months. Fortunately, there is a definitive and relatively simple procedure that cures these headaches.

Spinal headaches can be extremely incapacitating to the patient. This means that an obstetrician who sees a patient with a spinal headache must not put her off with a promise that the headache will go away at some future time. Instead, that patient must be referred to an anesthesiologist for evaluation and treatment. Since an obstetrician is not, as a rule, privileged to perform the definitive procedure for treating a spinal headache, the patient must be sent back to the anesthesiologist or anesthesia group that performed the original spinal to receive treatment.

There a several treatments for spinal headaches. Most are temporizing measures that buy time for the headache to resolve on its own. This category includes simple waiting, the use of oral analgesics, and the use of oral and intravenous caffeine. These measures are both simple and noninvasive, but they are not necessarily curative.

There is a moderately invasive procedure that is curative in an extremely high percentage of cases. This is the epidural blood patch, wherein an epidural needle is introduced into the epidural space near the original dural puncture made by the spinal needle. A small quantity of the patient's own blood is injected into the space, where it seals the puncture site by clotting over it. Over 90 percent of patients are cured of their headaches following this procedure, with an extremely small percentage experiencing no more than transient discomfort afterward.

A spinal headache is an incapacitating complication of spinal anesthesia. Since there is a definitive cure available, it is reasonable to expect that any patient who has the problem should be treated in a systematic manner that leads to a timely cessation of the headache. This should begin with a referral of any patient with a suspected spinal headache to a responsible anesthesiologist for evaluation. Treatment options, from simple waiting to an epidural blood patch, should be explained to the patient in such a manner that she can make an informed decision about which course to pursue in her particular circumstance. If she elects to forgo the patch in favor of waiting, she should be told the patch can be done at any future time she elects, even on a outpatient basis. Furthermore, she should be told that a patch should be performed in any case if the headache does not resolve in some reasonable time.

§ 8.20 —Nerve Damage

When considering the possibility of nerve damage following delivery, it is important to know that a significant number of sensory and motor nerve deficits occur postpartum regardless of whether anesthesia was used. Weakness or numbness in either leg is generally related either to peripheral nerve entrapment in the lithotomy position or to nerve plexus trauma within the pelvis. These often resolve within several days, although a few continue much longer. The most helpful way to distinguish these from deficits clearly caused by anesthesia is to determine the number of spinal cord segments involved. The common postpartum deficits not related to anesthesia usually involve several such segments and often fall within the distribution of a peripheral nerve as well. In contrast, the circumstances surrounding anesthesia-related spinal cord trauma typically implicate a single segment of the cord. Because of the frequency of the common postpartum nerve deficits compared to the infrequency of spinal cord trauma, it is difficult to ascribe a given postpartum nerve deficit to anesthesia under most circumstances.

This said, it is also true that a very small incidence of actual nerve injury accompanies regional anesthesia in obstetrics. This incidence cannot be reduced to zero even with the most meticulous technique.

The majority of injuries are caused by needle- (or epidural catheter-) induced trauma. Most patients complain of severe pain or shock-like sensations called *paresthesias* at the time the traumatic block is done. This means that if severe pain occurs either as the needle is placed or as the spinal drug is injected, the anesthesiologist should cease the attempt, withdraw the needle, and begin again.

Note, however, that a great many spinals are accompanied by paresthesias of no consequence at all. To abandon every procedure in which any paresthesia occurs would raise the question of risking still more trauma. This is why the reasonable course is to remove and replace the needle whenever its placement causes a severe and persisting pain or if the injection of a drug causes pain.

Aside from direct trauma, the causes of nerve damage following spinal anesthesia are varied. There is little foreseeability among these varied causes, and usually a great deal of room for asserting that the anesthesiologist could not have expected the eventual outcome.

§ 8.21   —Medications Used

Local anesthetics are the primary spinal agents in obstetrics. However, narcotics are often combined with local anesthetics to enhance pain relief without interfering with the patient's blood pressure or her ability to control her legs. This use of narcotics as spinal agents has a well-documented clinical history, even though only morphine carries regulatory labeling documenting this use.

The dose of local anesthetic is more important than the actual drug selected. A dose in the high end of the generally accepted range will be more likely to lead to a very high or complete block. On the other hand, a low dose is no guarantee that a high block will not occur. Given this, it is not possible to establish an unreasonable risk to a patient solely by showing a deviation from some person's recommended dosing regimen. There is no substantial recognition for any particular method wherein the spinal dose varies incrementally according to incremental changes in the patient's body habitus or height.

On the other hand, it is reasonable to match an approximately sized dose with the extent of the procedure planned. For example, a vaginal delivery dose of a particular drug is clearly not as large as a cesarean section dose.

The unpredictable effect of a given dose is a known phenomena with spinal anesthetics, and particularly with spinals given during pregnancy. This means that a high or total spinal is not a complication in itself, but rather a rare but foreseeable outcome of any given spinal anesthetic. It is the manner in which the high spinal is managed that determines whether the appropriate standard of care is met.

When narcotics such as morphine, fentanyl, and sufentanil are used in spinals, the major concern is respiratory depression. There is a known potential for the patient to slow her breathing to the point where she receives insufficient oxygen. Given this, there must be some form of appropriate monitoring of the patient during the effective time of the particular narcotic used. Morphine causes the most concern in this regard because of a very long duration and a potentially very depressant effect on the brain's respiratory control center. It is not uncommon to institute 24 hours of hourly monitoring of the patient's breathing when spinal morphine is used.

§ 8.22 —High or Total

High or total spinal refers to a spinal that affects all or nearly all the patient's body. The dividing line between an acceptably high and a dangerously high spinal is found in the patient's ability to speak. As long as she can speak, the patient's breathing is adequate and the major concern is that her blood pressure remains satisfactory. When the patient can no longer speak, inadequate air is moving into her lungs. This causes dangerously low oxygen levels for her and for the fetus.

When the patient loses her ability to speak, the anesthesiologist must know almost immediately. This means that he must watch the patient closely for several minutes after the spinal is performed. Any speaking impairment requires immediate assistance with breathing, whether by face mask or by endotracheal tube. Furthermore, since this situation is by definition an extensive regional blockade, patient monitoring as defined by the "Standards for Basic Anesthetic Monitoring" should be instituted if it is not already in place. See **Appendix 8–1.**

Blood pressure tends to drop significantly during a high or total spinal. A significant drop should be noticed and treated immediately.

§ 8.23 —Drop in Blood Pressure (Hypotension)

A drop in blood pressure often follows the injection of a spinal or epidural dose of local anesthetic. This drop, also known as *hypotension,* is the most common side effect of spinal and epidural anesthesia. It is caused in part by the pregnant uterus as it compresses the inferior vena cava, the main blood vessel that brings blood up to the heart from the lower body. This compression occurs primarily when the mother lies flat on her back, thus the term "supine hypotension." Hypotension is also caused by a relaxing effect that a spinal or epidural block has on the body's blood vessels. As the vessels relax, they squeeze the flowing blood less tightly and the blood pressure goes down.

Hypotension may be harmful if it results in a significantly decreased blood flow to the placenta. This can damage the fetus by causing a deprivation of oxygen, particularly to the brain. In extreme cases, such as those associated with severe supine hypotension, the decrease in blood flow can be so great that the mother's brain loses consciousness.

It is not true that every drop in blood pressure causes harm. It is not even possible to predict that a given amount of drop sustained over a given time will result in permanent damage. Instead it is reasonable to say that when damage has occurred, a blood pressure that was allowed to languish at a level appreciably lower than normal for a significant time after an anesthetic was started could have contributed to the damage.

The correct response to spinal- or epidural-induced hypotension has been established. The response consists of rapid infusion of intravenous fluid, correct positioning of the uterus to push it off the vena cava, and immediate intravenous injection of a drug such a ephedrine that stimulates the heart to pump more forcefully. If this treatment is instituted immediately when a drop in blood pressure occurs, the result is the same fetal condition as if no drop in blood pressure occurred at all. On the other hand, delaying treatment until some particular level of blood pressure is reached will result in a significantly worse fetal condition than will providing immediate treatment.

Every patient receiving spinal or epidural anesthesia should have prospective treatment in anticipation of hypotension occurring. This includes (1) pre-anesthesia hydration with an intravenous electrolyte solution such as lactated Ringer's, one to two liters before a cesarean section and one-half to one liter before a labor anesthetic; (2) elevation of the right hip when supine. Additional measures taken in response to hypotension after the anesthetic include (1) further rapid infusion of electrolyte solution until the blood pressure is satisfactory; (2) 5 to 15 milligram injections of intravenous ephedrine.

Monitoring for hypotension consists of determining blood pressure every one to three minutes for 15 to 20 minutes after a spinal or epidural dose is given. Once the blood pressure reaches an acceptably stable level, it may be taken less frequently.

§ 8.24   —Use in Labor

Spinal anesthesia used for labor usually consists of a mixture of a small amount of local anesthetic, a narcotic, and possibly a third agent to enhance the duration of pain relief. It is a safe form of pain relief, provided that monitoring for hypotension and respiratory depression are carried out as they would be in any other setting in which spinal anesthesia is used. The anesthesiologist should be immediately available during this time to correct any problems that arise.

§ 8.25 —Vaginal or Cesarean Delivery

Spinal anesthesia used for delivery usually relies primarily on local anesthetic as the agent. There is always a potential for extensive blockade, and the patient monitoring and the actions of the anesthesiologist should reflect this. Again, the "Guidelines for Regional Anesthesia in Obstetrics" provide a reasonable framework for ensuring patient safety.

The considerations given for a cesarean section under epidural anesthesia apply equally to spinal anesthesia. Choosing between the two is almost invariably a matter of personal preference on the part of the anesthesiologist, except when the patient has a clearly expressed preference for one over the other. In that case, it should be possible to follow the wishes of the patient. However, the patient's choice of one particular kind of regional anesthesia is strictly a matter of preference and does not reflect a greater degree of safety. Even when an anesthesiologist expresses a preference for one kind of regional anesthetic due to a particular disease that may be present, such as preeclampsia, the preference is almost always based on anecdote or pure opinion.

§ 8.26 General Anesthesia

In obstetrics, general anesthesia carries a higher risk of severe injury and death for the mother than does spinal or epidural anesthesia. This suggests that the elective use of general anesthesia for delivery should be discouraged, and that any use requires some justification for the increased risk involved.

The most prominent risk is aspiration into the lungs of solid and acid material coming up from the stomach after the patient becomes unconscious. This risk increases significantly during pregnancy because the enlarging uterus pushes up on the stomach from below. It further increases during labor because the natural emptying actions of the stomach slow and even stop during this time. This leads to the clinical axiom that every pregnant woman undergoing anesthesia must be presumed to have a full stomach.

A secondary risk is the simple failure to maintain an open route for air to get into the lungs once the patient is unconscious. This is known as *difficulty maintaining an airway.* A number of causes can predispose a patient to having a difficult airway, including obesity. One of the serious problems with a difficult airway is that once the problem begins, when simply trying to get enough oxygen into the patient's lungs becomes a difficult task, the risk of stomach contents coming up into the throat and threatening the lungs becomes significantly higher.

The use of general anesthesia in obstetrics has declined as its risks have become clearly defined and the use of regional anesthesia more uniformly taught. Nonetheless, there are still situations when the balance of risk and benefit demand the use of general anesthesia, when regional anesthesia is simply impossible to establish, and when the patient steadfastly refuses a spinal or epidural anesthetic even when the risks of general have been explained to her.

§ 8.27   —Induction

In current practice, the use of general anesthesia in obstetrics requires endotracheal intubation. The endotracheal tube is considered the best protection for the lungs against the aspiration of stomach contents. Mask anesthesia is not used except in extraordinary circumstances, such as an inability to intubate the trachea.

Before general anesthesia is induced, the patient should breathe pure oxygen for a brief time. This oxygen replaces the nitrogen that takes up the majority of the air space in the lungs. This allows additional intubating time, a time when the patient gets no air into her lungs, before a critical lack of oxygen occurs.

Pharmacologic measures may also be taken to lessen the quantity and acidity of the stomach contents. The most consistently recommended measure is the ingestion of a nonparticulate antacid, such as sodium citrate, shortly before the induction of anesthesia.

From the time the patient loses consciousness until the endotracheal tube is in place, someone must depress the cricoid cartilage in the patient's neck so that it presses down into and occludes the esophagus. This provides a fairly effective barrier to rising stomach contents. It also means that the induction of general anesthesia properly requires two people, both of whom must be prepared to stay with the patient's airway until the endotracheal tube is in place.

Proper placement of the endotracheal tube is determined by the sounds of air going into and out of both lungs. More importantly, though, the placement is confirmed by the maintenance of satisfactory oxygen saturation as determined by the pulse oximeter and by the return of a satisfactory amount of carbon dioxide according to the end-tidal CO_2 monitor.

§ 8.28   —Failed Intubation

A small percentage of intubation attempts cannot be successfully completed. These are called *failed intubations*. Many of these can be at least suspected beforehand by a systematic examination of the patient's airway. The benefit to such an examination is that it allows alternative plans to be made, and necessary personnel or equipment to be assembled in all but the emergency situations.

Once an intubation attempt has failed, the anesthesiologist should have a sequence of steps in mind that leads to the establishment or maintenance of a reasonably safe airway for as long as is necessary to resolve both the anesthetic and the obstetric problem. At least one algorithm for the management of the difficult airway exists, and several texts offer commentary on how to deal with the problem. In dealing with this situation, the emphasis is always on anticipating that it can happen and planning the response beforehand.

§ 8.29 Care of the Infant

A great many, if not all, obstetric anesthesia texts devote a chapter to assessment and resuscitation of the neonate. The level of detail in these encourages a presumption of significant proficiency and participation in neonatal resuscitation by most anesthesiologists. Practical reasons intervene, however, to place limits on what most anesthesiologists are able to do in this regard.

Very few anesthesiologists are trained to perform neonatal resuscitation. The opportunity to gain actual training and experience is seldom available to anesthesia personnel at the various training institutions. Instead, these opportunities are usually taken by those in pediatric training.

At the same time, the anesthesia personnel have a particular responsibility to the patient on the operating table. They are seldom in a position to turn their complete attention away from her in order to provide intensive care to the neonate. This fact is reflected in the "Guidelines for Regional Anesthesia in Obstetrics," which call for a qualified person other than the anesthesiologist attending the mother to be available for resuscitating the newborn. See **Appendix 8–2.**

Despite the lack of training in full resuscitation and lack of continuous availability, the anesthesiologist does have expertise in securing and maintaining an infant's airway that may be called upon in an emergency situation. In this case, the anesthesiologist's actions may resemble those of a Good Samaritan or may resemble those of an expected provider. The result will depend heavily on the facts surrounding the individual situation, rather than on a presumption about what an anesthesiologist should do.

§ 8.30 Informed Consent

The issue of informed consent for anesthesia during labor has been addressed by a small number of appellate courts. The clear trend has been to find that informed consent was obtained even when the sole evidence was verbal assurance by the anesthesiologist that an exchange of information and consent took place. The stated elements that persuaded each court were remarkably similar: information given to each patient, the lack of objection by each patient, and the actual cooperation given by each patient during the procedure.

Another factor may have at least influenced the decisions of the courts. In most obstetric situations, there are remarkably few choices available with regard to anesthesia. For example, in cesarean section there is no real choice about needing the surgery, so it is a given fact that the patient must receive anesthesia. On the basis of risk, general anesthesia is least desirable. This leaves spinal and epidural anesthesia, and they are difficult to distinguish on the basis of risk. The patient is thus left with a choice based solely on personal preference, which in fact is usually settled by a difference in performance characteristics between the two techniques.

The practical fact of the obstetric setting is that sufficient consent can usually be found in the normal exchange of information that takes place between anesthesiologist and patient, and in the assent of the patient to the procedure performed.

In the obstetric case the anesthesiologist affects the greatest potential lifespan she is ever likely to encounter. Here, there are actually two lives affected that together may have over a century of functional life ahead of them. This is what makes it particularly important that the anesthesiologist exercise sound judgment and technique in every case. Also, it is equally important that all parties who influence the practice of obstetric anesthesia actively support a sound and reasonable anesthetic practice.

§ 8.31   Appendix 8–1: ASA Standards (Basic Monitoring)[1]

STANDARDS FOR BASIC ANESTHETIC MONITORING (APPROVED BY ASA HOUSE OF DELEGATES OCTOBER 21, 1986 AND LAST AMENDED OCTOBER 25, 1995)[1]

These standards apply to all anesthesia care although, in emergency circumstances, appropriate life support measures take precedence. These standards may be exceeded at any time based on the judgment of the responsible anesthesiologist. They are intended to encourage quality patient care, but observing them cannot guarantee any specific patient outcome. They are subject to revision from time to time, as warranted by the evolution of technology and practice. They apply to all general anesthetics, regional anesthetics and monitored anesthesia care. This set of standards addresses only the issue of basic anesthetic monitoring, which is one component of anesthesia care. In certain rare or unusual circumstances, 1) some of these methods of monitoring may be clinically impractical, and 2) appropriate use of the described monitoring methods may fail to detect untoward clinical developments. Brief interruptions of continual monitoring may be unavoidable. *Under extenuating circumstances, the*

---

[1] Standards for Basic Anesthetic Monitoring (approved 1986, last amended 1995) is reprinted with permission of the American Society of Anesthesiologists, 520 N. Northwest Highway, Park Ridge, Illinois 60068-2573.

responsible anesthesiologist may waive the requirements marked with an asterisk (*); it is recommended that when this is done, it should be so stated (including the reasons) in a note in the patient's medical record. These standards are not intended for application to the care of the obstetrical patient in labor or in the conduct of pain management.

§ Note that continual is defined as "repeated regularly and frequently in steady rapid succession" whereas continuous means prolonged without any interruption at any time."

STANDARD I

Qualified anesthesia personnel shall be present in the room throughout the conduct of all general anesthetics, regional anesthetics and monitored anesthesia care.

OBJECTIVE

Because of the rapid changes in patient status during anesthesia, qualified anesthesia personnel shall be continuously present to monitor the patient and provide anesthesia care. In the event there is a direct known hazard, e.g., radiation, to the anesthesia personnel which might require intermittent remote observation of the patient, some provision for monitoring the patient must be made. In the event that an emergency requires the temporary absence of the person primarily responsible for the anesthetic, the best judgment of the anesthesiologist will be exercised in comparing the emergency with the anesthetized patients condition and in the selection of the person left responsible for the anesthetic during the temporary absence.

STANDARD II

During all anesthetics the patient's oxygenation, ventilation, circulation, and temperature shall be continually evaluated.

OXYGENATION

OBJECTIVE

To ensure adequate oxygen concentration in the inspired gas and the blood during all anesthetics.

METHODS

1) Inspired gas: During every administration of general anesthesia using an anesthesia machine, the concentration of oxygen in the patient breathing system shall be measured by an oxygen analyzer with a low oxygen concentration limit alarm in use.*

2) Blood oxygenation: During all anesthetics, a quantitative method of assessing oxygenation such as pulse oximetry shall be employed.* Adequate illumination and exposure of the patient are necessary to assess color.*

VENTILATION

OBJECTIVE

To ensure adequate ventilation of the patient during all anesthetics.

METHODS

1) Every patient receiving general anesthesia shall have the adequacy of ventilation continually evaluated. While qualitative clinical signs such as chest excursion, observation of the reservoir breathing bag and auscultation of breath sounds may be useful, quantitative monitoring of the carbon dioxide content and/or volume of expired gas is strongly encouraged.

2) When an endotracheal tube is inserted, its presence in the trachea must be verified by clinical assessment and by identification of carbon dioxide in the expired gas. Continual end-tidal carbon dioxide analysis, in use from the time of endotracheal tube placement, until extubation or initiating transfer to a postoperative care location, shall be performed using a quantitative method such as capnography, capnometry or mass spectroscopy.*

3) When ventilation is controlled by a mechanical ventilator, there shall be in continuous use a device that is capable of detecting disconnection of components of the breathing system. The device must give an audible signal when its alarm threshold is exceeded.

4) During regional anesthesia and monitored anesthesia care, the adequacy of ventilation shall be evaluated, at least, by continual observation of qualitative clinical signs.

CIRCULATION

OBJECTIVE

To ensure the adequacy of the patient's circulatory function during all anesthetics.

METHODS

1) Every patient receiving anesthesia shall have the electrocardiogram continuously displayed from the beginning of anesthesia until preparing to leave the anesthetizing location.*

2) Every patient receiving anesthesia shall have arterial blood pressure and heart rate determined and evaluated at least every five minutes.*

3) Every patient receiving general anesthesia shall have, in addition to the above, circulatory function continually evaluated by at least one of the following: palpation of a pulse, auscultation of heart sounds, monitoring of a

tracing of intra-arterial pressure, ultrasound peripheral pulse monitoring, or pulse plethysmography or oximetry.

BODY TEMPERATURE

OBJECTIVE

To aid in the maintenance of appropriate body temperature during all anesthetics.

METHODS

There shall be readily available a means to continuously measure the patient's temperature. When changes in body temperature are intended, anticipated or suspected, the temperature shall be measured.[1]

---

[1] *To become effective January 1, 1996.*

§ 8.32   Appendix 8–2: ASA Guidelines (Obstetrics)[2]

GUIDELINES FOR REGIONAL ANESTHESIA IN OBSTETRICS
(APPROVED BY ASA HOUSE OF DELEGATES OCTOBER 12,1988
AND LAST AMENDED OCTOBER 30, 1991)

These guidelines apply to the use of regional anesthesia or analgesia in which local anesthetics are administered to the parturient during labor and delivery. They are intended to encourage quality patient care but cannot guarantee any specific patient outcome. Because the availability of anesthesia resources may vary, members are responsible for interpreting and establishing the guidelines for their own institutions and practices. These guidelines are subject to revision from time to time as warranted by the evolution of technology and practice.

GUIDELINE I

REGIONAL ANESTHESIA SHOULD BE INITIATED AND MAINTAINED ONLY IN LOCATIONS IN WHICH APPROPRIATE RESUSCITATION EQUIPMENT AND DRUGS ARE IMMEDIATELY AVAILABLE TO MANAGE PROCEDURALLY RELATED PROBLEMS.

Resuscitation equipment should include, but is not limited to: sources of oxygen and suction, equipment to maintain an airway and perform endotracheal intubation, a means to provide positive pressure ventilation, and drugs and equipment for cardiopulmonary resuscitation.

---

[2] Guidelines for Regional Anesthesia in Obstetrics (approved 1988, last amended 1991) is reprinted with permission of the American Society of Anesthesiologists, 520 N. Northwest Highway, Park Ridge, Illinois 60068-2573.

GUIDELINE II

REGIONAL ANESTHESIA SHOULD BE INITIATED BY A PHYSICIAN WITH APPRO-
PRIATE PRIVILEGES AND MAINTAINED BY OR UNDER THE MEDICAL DIRECTION[1]
OF SUCH ON INDIVIDUAL.

Physicians should be approved through the institutional credentialing process to
initiate and direct the maintenance of obstetric anesthesia and to manage procedurally related complications.

GUIDELINE III

REGIONAL ANESTHESIA SHOULD NOT BE ADMINISTERED UNTIL: 1) THE
PATIENT HAS BEEN EXAMINED BY A QUALIFIED INDIVIDUAL[2]; AND 2) THE
MATERNAL AND FETAL STATUS AND PROGRESS OF LABOR HAVE BEEN EVALU-
ATED BY A PHYSICIAN WITH PRIVILEGES IN OBSTETRICS WHO IS READILY
AVAILABLE TO SUPERVISE THE LABOR AND MANAGE ANY OBSTETRIC COM-
PLICATIONS THAT MAY ARISE.

Under circumstances defined by department protocol, qualified personnel may
perform the initial pelvic examination. The physician responsible for the patient's
obstetrical care should be informed of her status so that a decision can be made
regarding present risk and further management.[2]

GUIDELINE IV

AN INTRAVENOUS INFUSION SHOULD BE ESTABLISHED BEFORE THE INITIA-
TION OF REGIONAL ANESTHESIA AND MAINTAINED THROUGHOUT THE
DURATION OF THE REGIONAL ANESTHETIC.

GUIDELINE V

REGIONAL ANESTHESIA FOR LABOR AND/OR DELIVERY REQUIRES THAT THE
PARTURIENT'S VITAL SIGNS AND THE FETAL HEART RATE BE MONITORED
AND DOCUMENTED BY A QUALIFIED INDIVIDUAL. ADDITIONAL MONITOR-
ING APPROPRIATE TO THE CLINICAL CONDITION OF THE PARTURIENT AND
THE FETUS SHOULD BE EMPLOYED WHEN INDICATED. WHEN EXTENSIVE
REGIONAL BLOCKADE IS ADMINISTERED FOR COMPLICATED VAGINAL
DELIVERY, THE STANDARD FOR BASIC ANESTHETIC MONITORING[3] SHOULD BE
APPLIED.

---

[1] The Anesthesia Care Team (Approved by ASA House of Delegates 10/26/82 and last amended
10/25/95).

[2] Guidelines for Perinatal Care (American Academy of Pediatrics and American College of Obstetricians and Gynecologists, 1988).

[3] Standards for Basic Anesthetic Monitoring (Approved by ASA House of Delegates 10/21/86 and last
amended 10/25/95).

GUIDELINE VI

REGIONAL ANESTHESIA FOR CESAREAN DELIVERY REQUIRES THAT THE STAND-ARDS FOR BASIC ANESTHETIC MONITORING[3] BE APPLIED AND THAT A PHYSI-CIAN WITH PRIVILEGES IN OBSTETRICS BE IMMEDIATELY AVAILABLE.

GUIDELINE VII

QUALIFIED PERSONNEL, OTHER THAN THE ANESTHESIOLOGIST ATTENDING THE MOTHER, SHOULD BE IMMEDIATELY AVAILABLE TO ASSUME RESPON-SIBILITY FOR RESUSCITATION OF THE NEWBORN.[3]

The primary responsibility of the anesthesiologist is to provide care to the mother. If the anesthesiologist is also requested to provide brief assistance in the care of the newborn, the benefit to the child must be compared to the risk to the mother.

GUIDELINE VIII

A PHYSICIAN WITH APPROPRIATE PRIVILEGES SHOULD REMAIN READILY AVAIL-ABLE DURING THE REGIONAL ANESTHETIC TO MANAGE ANESTHETIC COMPLI-CATIONS UNTIL THE PATIENT'S POSTANESTHESIA CONDITION IS SATISFACTORY AND STABLE.

GUIDELINE IX

ALL PATIENTS RECOVERING FROM REGIONAL ANESTHESIA SHOULD RECEIVE APPROPRIATE POSTANESTHESIA CARE. FOLLOWING CESAREAN DELIVERY AND/OR EXTENSIVE REGIONAL BLOCKADE, THE STANDARDS FOR POST-ANESTHESIA CARE[4] SHOULD BE APPLIED.

1. A postanesthesia care unit (PACU) should be available to receive patients. The design, equipment and staffing should meet requirements of the facility's accrediting and licensing bodies.

2. When a site other than the PACU is used, equivalent postanesthesia care should be provided.

GUIDELINE X

THERE SHOULD BE A POLICY TO ASSURE THE AVAILABILITY IN THE FACILITY OF A PHYSICIAN TO MANAGE COMPLICATIONS AND TO PROVIDE CARDIO-PULMONARY RESUSCITATION FOR PATIENTS RECEIVING POSTANESTHESIA CARE.

---

[4] Standards for Postanesthesia Care (Approved by ASA House of Delegates 10/12/88 and last amended 10/19/94).

CHAPTER 9

PRIMARY COMPLICATIONS OF LABOR AND DELIVERY: CAUSES AND TREATMENT

Michael S. Cardwell, M.D.

Thomas G. Kirkhope, M.D.

ABNORMAL LABOR

§ 9.1   Abnormalities of the First Stage

The first stage of labor is divided into two phases, the latent and the active phase. Prolongation of the latent phase occurs if the duration is longer than 20 hours in nulliparas and 14 hours in multiparas. However, it is often difficult to ascertain the onset of true labor or if false labor was present initially. Prolonged latent phase is associated with excessive analgesia and sedation administered early, unfavorable or unripe cervix, and poor uterine contractile forces.[1] This abnormality is not related to cephalopelvic disproportion (CPD), nor is it associated with an increased risk for neonatal asphyxia. Unless complicated by fetal distress, is not associated with higher cesarean section rates. Management of prolonged latent phase involves sedating or resting the patient, or augmenting labor with oxytocin. Sedation may be accomplished by giving morphine or meperidine. After four to six hours, the patient may awaken in better labor or no labor. If oxytocin is chosen as the therapeutic modality, a standard for administration of oxytocin must be observed.

Protraction disorders are abnormalities of labor in which progress of cervical dilation and descent of the fetal head occur at a slower than normal in the active phase of labor. During this phase, the cervix normally dilates at least one centimeter per hour and toward the latter part of the first stage, the fetal head descends at least one centimeter per hour. Protraction disorders are frequently associated with CPD, use of conduction anesthesia, and malposition of the fetus.[2] Treatment is directed toward identification of a possible cause.

Arrest disorders are abnormalities during the active phase when the cervix has stopped dilating or the fetal head has not descended for more than two hours. These disorders are frequently associated with CPD. Management, as in protraction disorders, consists of careful maternal and fetal monitoring, physiologic and emotional support of the mother, and avoidance of difficult forceps delivery. If oxytocin is considered for augmentation of labor, it must be administered by protocol. If there is still no progress after two hours, cesarean section is performed unless forceps delivery can be accomplished with little or no difficulty.

---

[1] W.R. Cohen, E.A. Friedman, Management of Labor (1983).

[2] *Id.*

§ 9.2   Abnormalities of the Second Stage

Arrest of descent and rotation of the fetal head following complete cervical dilation may occur. If this is observed, reassessment of fetal size and position is made and consideration is given to further observation or termination of labor. It has generally been believed in the past that after two hours of the second stage, the infant must be delivered, often resulting in traumatic mid-forceps deliveries or unnecessary cesarean sections. It is now acceptable to allow the patient to go beyond the second stage for longer than two hours as long as both mother and fetus are well monitored, no signs of fetal distress are present, the mother is comfortable, not exhausted, and well-supported (physiologically and emotionally), there is reason to believe that further progress may be accomplished, and vaginal delivery is expected.

§ 9.3   Abnormalities of the Third Stage and Immediately Postpartum

Placental separation during the third stage of labor may be accompanied by massive bleeding or complicated by incomplete separation and expulsion, leaving placental fragments in the uterus and contributing to postpartum hemorrhage. The episiotomy or vaginal and vulvar lacerations that could occur during delivery also contribute to intrapartum and postpartum bleeding.

The most common cause of postpartum hemorrhage (over 500 milliters during first 24 hours postpartum) is uterine atony, or inadequate myometrial contraction following placental separation and expulsion. Associated or predisposing factors to uterine atony are high or excessive parity, uterine overdistention (as in twins), and prolonged labor, especially when stimulated or augmented by oxytocin.[3] Treatment of uterine atony includes vigorous bimanual uterine massage and administration of uterotonic drugs (oxytocin, ergot, prostaglandins). Blood transfusion and intravenous fluids should be administered when indicated. Hysterectomy is performed as a last resort if bleeding cannot be controlled.

§ 9.4   Maternal Complications

An abnormal labor pattern not only leads to added physical discomfort to the mother, but to her already existing anxiety and apprehension and that of her family. Prolongation of labor, especially if abnormal, can result in maternal exhaustion, emotional distress, and metabolic abnormalities, particularly if the patient has not been hydrated well. Maternal support, both physiologic (hydration,

---

[3] G. Cunningham et al., Williams Obstetrics (19th ed. 1993).

pain relief) and emotional (reassurance, physician or nurse presence), plays a very important role in the outcome of labor.

Prolongation of labor, especially if an abnormal pattern (arrest or protraction disorder) later manifests, is accompanied by an increased risk of operative intervention—either forceps delivery or cesarean section. The patient (and her family) must be continuously apprised of the progress (or nonprogress) of labor, options for management, and the present plan of treatment.

§ 9.5   Management of Abnormal Labor

When an abnormal labor pattern becomes apparent, careful and diligent maternal and fetal monitoring must be instituted. Accurate documentation of cervical dilation and fetal station are noted during each pelvic examination and written report of progress (or nonprogress) placed in the patient's chart. Discussions with the patient, her husband, or other family members, or with a consulting physician, as to options and plan of management should be recorded. Equally important to document are interpretations of the fetal monitor tracings and any change in plan of treatment.

If the abnormal labor pattern persists, identification of a possible cause is made. The use of x-ray pelvimetry in the United States has markedly decreased in the past decade. As long as careful and diligent maternal and fetal monitoring is used, further observation of labor in a patient with possible cephalopelvic disproportion is acceptable. In anticipation of a possible cesarean section, preparations for operative intervention are made, including availability of blood for cross-matching, or appropriately matched blood already available prior to surgery if the patient is anemic.

§ 9.6   Abnormal Fetal Presentation or Position

The normal fetal presentation is cephalic or vertex in about 96 percent of pregnancies at or near term. The fetus presents by the breech (buttocks or feet) in three to four percent of cases at or near term. Fetal and neonatal mortality and morbidity are higher in breech than vertex deliveries.[4] Problems associated with breech presentation and delivery include preterm delivery, preterm rupture of membranes, prolapse of the umbilical cord, congenital malformations, placenta previa, and abruptio placenta. Breech vaginal delivery may also be complicated by fetal injury or entrapment of the fetal head after the trunk and shoulders have been delivered.

---

[4] R. Creasy & R. Resnik, Maternal-Fetal Medicine: Principles and Practice (3d ed. 1994).

The current approach to management of breech presentation involves identification of patients who may be candidates for external version (to convert breech to vertex), patients who are at highest risk for complications of vaginal breech delivery (deliver by cesarean section), and patients who are carefully chosen (after thorough discussion with them of options and risks) as candidates for vaginal breech delivery.

Obviously, management of breech presentation, whether at term or not, requires the skills of a physician trained in obstetrics and management of labor and delivery at a facility in which intensive care nursery resources are available. Refer to textbooks with comprehensive discussion on approaches to management.[5]

Other more infrequent types of fetal malpresentation are shoulder (transverse lie), face, and brow presentations. Because of the frequency of other accompanying obstetric factors in these types of malpresentation, such as cephalopelvic disproportion, placenta previa, and premature rupture of membranes, delivery by cesarean section is often the management of choice. However, by themselves, these malpresentations (particularly shoulder presentations) are legitimate indications for abdominal delivery, although face presentations (chin anterior) are often delivered vaginally and the majority of brow presentations convert to either face or vertex presentation.

Management in general of abnormal fetal presentation involves confirmation of the type of presentation by ultrasound (or, in some cases, x-ray), identification of associated problems (inadequate pelvis, placenta previa, fetal anomaly), consultation with a neonatologist, and assessment of maternal and fetal risks for both vaginal delivery and operative intervention.

Maternal complications include increased possibility for operative intervention (with a longer and costlier hospital stay), increased emotional distress, and increased risks for postpartum complications (like hemorrhage and sepsis). Difficult forcep deliveries should be avoided and vacuum extraction, when available, should be used only by experienced operators after discussing options with the patient or her family.

In these situations the neonate is at higher risk for complications. Because of frequent association between fetal malpresentation and preterm infants, preterm rupture of membranes, placenta previa, and prolapse of the umbilical cord, the infant can be considered compromised even prior to delivery. This imposes additional stress, especially if difficult vaginal manipulations and forceps maneuvers are performed. Fetal and neonatal asphyxia and birth trauma are important potential complications.

---

[5] *Id. See also* G. Cunningham et al., Williams Obstetrics (19th ed. 1993).

§ 9.7   Preterm Labor

Preterm labor (PTL) is defined as labor occurring prior to the completion of 37 weeks' gestation.[6] PTL is responsible for at least 75 percent of neonatal mortality excluding congenital anomalies. The complications of prematurity include respiratory distress syndrome, hyperbilirubinemia, intraventricular hemorrhage, thermal instability, necrotizing enterocolitis, and a host of other problems.[7]

§ 9.8   Respiratory Distress Syndrome

Respiratory distress syndrome (RDS) accounts for about 30 percent of all neonatal deaths in the United States and 50 to 70 percent of premature deaths.[8] This usually occurs in preterm infants, although the susceptibility may depend more on the degree of lung maturity at the time of delivery than the age of gestation.

An infant with RDS presents with respiratory distress due to the inability of the lungs to adapt to extrauterine life resulting from anatomical and biochemical immaturity. There are two important prerequisites for a successful pulmonary adaptation to extrauterine life. First is the presence of surfactant, which is a surface-active substance. Second is the development of an adequate pulmonary capillary bed in close contact with air sacs covered by cells adapted for gas exchange of Type I alveolar cells. Surfactant is necessary in the maintenance of stability of the alveoli or air sacs at low pressures so that the lungs do not collapse at the end of expiration. This substance is produced by Type II alveolar cells that are found in smaller numbers in immature lungs, so that the surfactant that is produced may not be sufficient to maintain lung stability. The more immature the lung, the less developed are the capillary beds and the epithelial cells responsible for gas exchange of type II alveolar cells. It is not until about 34 weeks in appropriately grown infants that type II alveolar cells are capable of producing large amounts of surfactant to supply airways adequately perfused by blood from capillaries in close contact with well-differentiated type I alveolar cells for gas exchange. It is at this time that the lung is both anatomically and biochemically capable of carrying on the function of respiration.

Some infants with RDS may initially appear healthy, as normally grown premature infants with good Apgar scores, but many may have evidence of intrapartum asphyxia requiring resuscitation. Such infants will present with an abnormal pattern of respiration, either immediately or a few minutes after delivery.

---

[6] ACOG Technical Bull. 206, Preterm Labor (1995).

[7] A.A. Fanoroff & R.J. Martin, Neonatal-Perinatal Medicine: Diseases of the Fetus and Infant (5th ed. 1992).

[8] A.A. Fanoroff, R.J. Martin, Neonatal-Perinatal Medicine: Diseases of the Fetus and Infant (5th ed. 1992).

Large premature infants may present initially with tachypnea, and may remain pink for a while in room air. Asphyxiated infants, especially the small premature, may have ineffective respirations requiring early ventilatory support. As the disease progresses, infants have an increase in respiratory rate and increase in ventilatory effort. As the oxygen requirement increases, infants exert more effort to help the terminal airways open, becoming flaccid with marked peripheral vasoconstriction. Clinical findings in the lungs reveal poor air entry despite vigorous respiratory effort. Rales may not be heard initially, but as the disease progresses, coarse rales may be heard. A heart murmur is usually appreciated after 24 hours. In the presence of uncorrected acidosis and hypoxemia or hypovolemia, tachycardia is frequently present. The clinical course is one of increasing severity, characterized by an increase in respiratory effort and oxygen requirement, and worsening of the pulmonary function in about 48 to 72 hours, after which clinical improvement will be seen. This coincides with the evidence of regeneration of Type II alveolar cells and an increase in the production of surfactant. In severe cases, however, the clinical course may be different or modified by the initiation of ventilatory support. In some infants the course may be prolonged; chronic lung disease such as bronchopulmonary dysplasia may follow after long-term ventilatory assistance and exposure to high concentrations of oxygen.

§ 9.9   Patent Ductus Arteriosus

In utero, oxygenated blood from the placenta is brought to the fetus via the umbilical vein into the portal sinus where a variable portion of it profuses the liver. The remainder of the blood from the portal sinus is then shunted to the inferior vena cava via the ductus venosus where it mixes with blood coming from the kidney, skin, and gastrointestinal tract. About one-half of the blood in the inferior vena cava goes to the left atrium through the foramen ovale (a shunt present between the right and left atria) where it combines with small amounts of pulmonary venous blood. This relatively oxygenated blood then supplies the heart and the brain via the ascending aorta. The rest of the blood that enters the inferior vena cava goes to the right atrium to the right ventricle and then to the pulmonary artery. Since the pulmonary arterioles are constricted in utero, most of the blood that enters the descending aorta has less oxygen than that in the ascending aorta. After birth, with the expansion of the lungs and ligation of the umbilical cord, the blood flow to the lungs increases and systemic arterial and left atrial pressure increase. When the left atrial pressure rises above that of the right atrium, the foramen ovale closes. The increase in the systemic blood pressure and the fall in pulmonary arterial pressure causes the flow through the ductus arteriosus to go from left to right and the ductus arteriosus to constrict and close. The flow of blood becomes that of the adult pattern—with unoxygenated blood going to the right side of the heart, then to the lungs for oxygenation, and then to the left side of the heart to be distributed to the rest of the body via the aorta.

In fullterm infants, the ductus arteriosus undergoes rapid initial closure a few hours after birth, followed by a gradual final functional closure in one to eight days. In preterm infants the closure of the ductus arteriosus is delayed until full-term gestation, but most of the time may not present with clinical problems. However, in those who have severe respiratory distress, the ductus arteriosus may remain patent and cause serious heart failure leading to hypoventilation that aggravates the existing pulmonary problem. Premature infants of 30 weeks gestation and less frequently present with patent ductus arteriosus with congestive heart failure, whether they have respiratory distress syndrome or not. This usually presents with a systolic murmur at the left upper sternal border occurring at about the third to the fifth day of age, resulting from the decrease in pulmonary vascular resistance that allows a left to right flow through the patent ductus. If the shunt is larger, a murmur may not be heard. The peripheral pulses are bounding and the cardiac impulse is hyperdynamic. As the left to right shunting increases, congestive heart failure occurs and is manifested by tachypnea, tachycardia, chest retractions, diminished breath sounds on auscultation, and the presence of rales. Management is directed towards the control of heart failure, correction of hypoxemia and acidosis, and the closure of the ductus arteriosus.

§ 9.10   Hyperbilirubinemia

The rise in the concentration of bilirubin in preterm infants is higher than that of full-term infants and peak concentration reaches 10 to 15 milligram/deciliter by the fifth day of life. The impaired ability to conjugate bilirubin in the liver of premature infants accounts for the higher rise as well as the delay in the peak concentration of bilirubin. This hyperbilirubinemia effect of prematurity has been shown to be of the same degree from 28 to 36 weeks of gestation.[9]

Relative hypoproteinemia and acidemia in premature infants may make them susceptible to kernicterus, so that bilirubin levels in jaundiced premature infants should be closely followed and investigated.[10]

---

[9] Saigal et al., *Placental Transfusion and Hyperbilirubinemia in the Premature,* 49 Pediatrics 406 (1972).

[10] A. Fanoroff & R. Martin, Neonatal-Perinatal Medicine: Diseases of the Fetus and Infant (5th ed. 1992).

§ 9.11   Periventricular or
Intraventricular Hemorrhage

Periventricular or intraventricular hemorrhage is frequently seen in premature infants, occurring in about 40 to 60 percent of cases.[11] The risk of the lesion increases with decreasing gestational age.[12] This association with prematurity occurs because the human subependymal matrix does not dissipate until term. Periventricular or intraventricular hemorrhage originates in the germinal matrix of the subependymal area at the capillary level and capillary-venous junction.[13] The subependymal germinal matrix provides minimal support for the vessels that traverse it and at the same time there is impaired cerebral autoregulation in premature infants.[14] The usual site of the hemorrhages is at the level of the foramen of Monro. However, in premature infants of less than 28 weeks gestation, the hemorrhage is usually seen at the level of the caudate nucleus.[15] The hematoma that results from the bleeding of the capillaries around the periventricular area may be small initially but may enlarge, rupture through the ependyma, and spread into the ventricular system.[16] The cause of intraventricular hemorrhage is not definitely established, although several factors have been implicated, including arterial hypertension and hypotension, hypoxia, loss of autoregulation of the cerebral blood vessels, hypercarbia, alkali therapy, volume expansion, and alveolar rupture. It has been proposed that asphyxia impairs cerebral autoregulation leading to cerebral vasodilation. As a result, any changes in the systemic blood pressure can be transmitted easily to the poorly supported capillary beds of the germinal matrix resulting in hemorrhage.[17]

Two clinical syndromes have been associated with intraventricular hemorrhage: a saltatory deterioration and a rapid catastrophic deterioration.[18] The usual outcome of the rapidly deteriorating course is either death or hydrocephalus. The majority of infants who have a saltatory deterioration survive and a minority of them develop hydrocephalus.

---

[11] Papile et al., *Incidence and Evolution of Subependymal and Intraventricular Hemorrhage: A Study of Infants with Birth Weights Less than 1500 g.:*, 92 J. Pediatrics 529 (1978).

[12] J.J. Volpe, Neurology of the Newborn (3d ed. 1995).

[13] Hambleton & Wigglesworth, *Origin of Intraventricular Hemorrhage in the Preterm Infant,* 51 Archives Diseases Childhood 651 (1976).

[14] Lou et al., *Impaired Autoregulation of Cerebral Blood Flow in the Distressed Newborn,* 94 J. Pediatrics 118 (1979).

[15] P.I. Yakoulev & R.N. Rosales, *Distribution of the Terminal Hemorrhages in the Brain Wall in Stillborn Premature and Nonviable Neonates, in* Physical Trauma as an Etiologic Agent in Mental Retardation (1970).

[16] J.J. Volpe, Neurology of the Newborn (3d ed. 1995).

[17] Wigglesworth & Pape, *An Integrated Model for Haemorrhagic and Ischemic Lesions in the Newborn Brain,* 2 Early Hum. Dev. 179 (1978).

[18] J.J. Volpe, Neurology of the Newborn (3d ed. 1995).

§ 9.12   Apnea of Prematurity

Apnea is defined as cessation of respiration for 20 seconds and cessation accompanied by bradycardia and cyanosis. With long-term monitoring, apnea has been shown to occur in about 25 percent of premature infants.[19] Apneic episodes occur in association with periodic breathing.[20] It is proposed that periodic breathing results from the influence of a modulating system for respiration that is not fully developed in the premature. Apneic spells occur when there is an insult to the immature modulating system such as extreme prematurity, metabolic derangement, hypoxemia, pulmonary disease, and disease of the central nervous system.

Bradycardia occurs about 30 seconds following apnea and earlier in more severe and prolonged apneic spells. Hypotonia and unresponsiveness follow in about 45 seconds. Severe apneic episodes may cause brain injury to premature infants secondary to the accompanying hypoxemia and ischemia, although there is little data available regarding the neurologic status of these infants during severe apneic spells.[21]

Other problems associated with preterm birth are neonatal asphyxia, infection, temperature control, and metabolic disorders such as control of blood sugar, azotemia, hypoproteinemia, and hypocalcemia.

§ 9.13   Perinatal Asphyxia

Asphyxia is defined as hypoxia with metabolic acidosis.[22] Asphyxia occurs when there is a failure of gas exchange. Asphyxia is evaluated by measuring blood gases and is established by an elevated partial pressure of carbon dioxide, low partial pressure of oxygen, and acidosis. However, changes in the blood may vary, depending on the particular mechanism causing the asphyxia. In fetal asphyxia, the predominant change is hypoxemia or low partial pressure of oxygen with secondary metabolic acidosis. This is because there is still sufficient blood flow to the placenta to provide adequate carbon dioxide exchange except when there is complete cord occlusion. In neonatal asphyxia, there is an elevation of partial pressure of carbon dioxide as well as low partial pressure of oxygen and acidosis because of the failure of the lungs to inflate.

In early stages, asphyxia may be reversed if the cause is corrected or removed, but once it has advanced to the severe state, it is difficult to reverse because of

---

[19] Daily et al., *Apnea in Premature Infants: Monitoring Incidence, Heart Rate Changes and an Effect of Environmental Temperature,* 43 Pediatrics 510 (1969).

[20] Miller et al., *Severe Apnea and Irregular Respiratory Rhythms among Premature Infants,* 23 Pediatrics 676 (1959).

[21] Duel, *Polygraphic Monitoring of Apneic Spells,* 28 Archives Neurology 71 (1973).

[22] ACOG Technical Bull. 216, Umbilical Artery Blood Acid-Base Analysis (1995).

the neurologic and circulatory changes that have already set in. In early stages, the blood supply to the vital organs (such as the brain, heart, and the adrenal glands) is maintained or increased, while the blood supply to the less vital organs (such as skin, muscles, gut, and kidneys) is reduced by selective regional vasoconstriction. This redistribution of blood flow assures the maintenance of adequate oxygen supply to the vital organs in the presence of a low oxygen supply in the blood. In utero, the placenta is a vital organ, and its blood supply is maintained and even increased in the presence of asphyxia, except when there is complete obstruction of the umbilical cord. The lung in the fetus is a less vital organ and the reduction of its blood supply has no immediate consequence. In the newborn, however, it produces changes that can further compromise oxygenation.

Infants who are severely asphyxiated at birth present with coma, flaccidity, and unresponsiveness to noxious stimuli. Pupils are unresponsive to light and all complex reflexes and deep tendon reflexes are absent. There may be systemic hypothermia, apnea, and bradycardia. Multiple organ system involvement is common, and may include the brain, heart, kidney, liver, and gastrointestinal tract. Metabolic disturbances (such as hypoglycemia, hypocalcemia, and fluid and electrolyte imbalance) may occur as a result of acute renal failure. Ischemic-hypoxic encephalopathy results due to hypoxia to the brain and the presence of metabolic derangements can worsen the already compromised brain.[23]

§ 9.14 Neonatal Sepsis

Neonatal sepsis is a bacterial disease of newborns occurring during the first 28 days of the life, manifested by clinical illness and evidenced by a positive blood culture. The incidence is about 1 in 1,000 live births among fullterm infants and 1 in 250 premature live births.[24] The incidence varies among nurseries depending on the presence of conditions that predispose to infection. There are several obstetric complications present before and during delivery that could predispose the neonate to infection. Among these are prolonged rupture of membranes, premature labor, chorioamnionitis, and maternal fever.

Clinical manifestations of a neonate with sepsis are usually nonspecific in the child and may be described as not doing well, feeding poorly, and lethargy. It may present with multiple organ system involvement so that it should be considered in the differential diagnosis of a sick neonate with vague nonspecific signs and symptoms.

---

[23] A. Fanoroff & R. Martin, Neonatal-Perinatal Medicine: Diseases of the Fetus and Infant (5th ed. 1992).

[24] J.S. Remington & J.O. Klein, Infections Diseases of the Fetus and Newborn Infant (4th ed. 1995).

§ 9.15   Precipitate Labor and Delivery

Extremely rapid labor and delivery is termed *precipitate*. Precipitate labor is usually less than three hours and precipitate delivery is quite rapid, and uncontrolled, usually over an unprepared, unsterile field.[25] This may result from an abnormally low resistance of the soft tissues of the birth canal or from excessively strong uterine and abdominal contractions during the active phase and second stage of labor.

The extreme rapidity of labor and delivery often catches the attendants at birth unprepared—if the woman even makes it to the hospital. Lacerations of the genital tract may occur as a result of the rapid descent of the fetus accompanied by powerful uterine and abdominal forces. Amniotic fluid embolism, a rare obstetric complication, may result from vigorous labor forcing amniotic fluid into the maternal venous circulation. What follows may be varying degrees of respiratory distress and circulatory collapse. If the woman does not die immediately, profuse hemorrhage with severe coagulation defects ensues.

Because of rapid labor and delivery, the expulsion of the baby may not be controlled and injury may occur. Excessive and forceful uterine contractions could compromise fetal oxygenation and produce hypoxia. Delivery of the baby in an unprepared setting (taxicab, elevator) may also result in injury; resuscitation may not be available.

Management is directed towards removing the cause of the forceful uterine contractions if known, for example, during oxytocin stimulation or augmentation. Tocolytic agents, such as terbutaline (brethine) or magnesium sulfate, may help relax the uterus and slow down the labor.

§ 9.16   Forceps Delivery

Forceps are obstetric instruments used to shorten the second stage of labor, when an indication arises to assist the mother in delivering the baby. They are applied on the infant's head and used to rotate or pull the baby's head toward the vaginal introitus and out of the perineum.

Three types of forceps deliveries are recognized:

1. Outlet forceps. Criteria for use include:
    a. Scalp is visible at introitus without separating labia.
    b. Fetal skull has reached pelvic floor.
    c. Sagittal suture is in anteroposterior diameter or left or right occiput anterior or posterior position.

---

[25] W.R. Cohen & E.A. Friedman, Management of Labor (1983).

   d. Fetal head is at or on perineum.

   e. Rotation does not exceed 45 degrees.

  2. Low forceps. Criteria for use include:

   a. Leading point of fetal skull is 2+ station and not on pelvic floor.

   b. Rotation is permissible.

  3. Midforceps. Requires a station above 2+ cm, but head engaged.[26]

The termination of the second stage by use of forceps is indicated in any situation that requires immediate delivery as long as the criteria for forceps and delivery have been met. Whereas an outlet forceps delivery is generally uncomplicated in the hands of a skilled operator, low and midforceps deliveries are still accompanied by a higher maternal and fetal or neonatal morbidity and mortality rate even in the hands of experienced physicians. In current practice, difficult and potentially traumatic midforceps deliveries have been replaced by cesarean section, even though the latter is still accompanied by a higher maternal morbidity rate. However, because of the greater potential for damage to the fetus with midforceps deliveries, cesarean section is often preferred when an easy vaginal forceps delivery is not anticipated. Fetal injury in midforceps application can result in immediate death or long-term morbidity in the form of cerebral palsy or diminished intelligence.[27]

§ 9.17   Vacuum Extractor

The vacuum extractor, another obstetric tool applied on the fetal head for rotation and traction, is more widely accepted in Europe than in the United States. There are reports of fetal damage, such as lacerations and abrasions of the scalp, cephalhematomas, intracranial hemorrhage, and death. The indications are similar to those for forceps deliveries but the application requires a different kind of skill and experience.

§ 9.18   Birth Injuries

In breech presentation, the usual injuries involved are those to the soft tissues, injuries to the spine and the spinal cord, fracture of the extremities, and epiphyseal separations.

Soft tissue injuries are usually petechiae and ecchymoses. If the external genitalia is the presenting part, there may be hematoma, ecchymoses, and edema. In the male newborn, the pendulous urethra may be compressed against the

---

[26] ACOG Technical Bull. 196, Operative Vaginal Delivery (1994).

[27] G. Cunningham et al., Williams Obstetrics (19th ed. 1993).

maternal bony pelvis following protracted labor. Temporary hydronephrosis has been reported following such deliveries.

Injuries to the vertebrae, spine, and spinal cord may result from breech deliveries, especially those in which version and extraction have been used. The most common mechanism for the injury is probably a forceful longitudinal traction on the trunk while the head is still engaged on the pelvis. Clinical manifestations vary depending on the site of injury. Infants with a high cervical or brainstem lesion may be stillborn or delivered in poor clinical condition with respiratory depression and shock. Deterioration is rapid, and death occurs within several hours. In those infants in whom the lesion is in the upper or midcervical area, clinical manifestation may not be recognized for several days until paralysis of the legs is noted. If the lesion is high enough, intercostal muscles may be involved. Urinary retention and paralysis of the abdominal muscles may be present. The central respiratory depression may be complicated by pneumonia within hours or days. These infants die after several days. In those infants whose lesions are at the level of C_7 and T_1 or lower, the lesions may be mild and reversible or the condition could lead to permanent neurologic sequelae of the lower cord segment. If the injury to the spinal cord is partial, the infant may present with subtle neurologic signs of spasticity.

Phrenic nerve paralysis resulting in diaphragmatic paralysis can result from difficult breech delivery. *Avulsion* is overstretching of the third, fourth, and fifth cervical roots that supply the phrenic nerve, and results from enteral hyperextension of the neck. The initial manifestation may be episodes of cyanosis accompanied by irregular and labored respirations. There is absent excursion of the chest on the affected side with diminished breath sounds. In severe injury, there may be tachypnea, apneic spells, and weak cry. Early diagnosis is established by fluoroscopy that reveals abnormal elevation of the involved hemidiaphragm and seesaw movement of the two hemidiaphragms on respiration.

Brachial plexus palsy is paralysis involving the muscles of the upper extremity that results from mechanical trauma to the brachial plexus (C_5 to T_1). The injury usually follows a prolonged and difficult labor. Injury to the fifth and sixth cervical roots may follow a breech presentation with arms extended over the head. Brachial palsy presents in three forms:

1. duchenne-erb's or upper arm palsy resulting from injury to the fifth and sixth cervical roots
2. klumpke's or lower arm paralysis resulting from injury to the eighth cervical and the first thoracic roots
3. paralysis of the entire arm with the injury of nerve roots C_5 to T_1.

Unilateral paralysis of the vocal cord may result from excessive traction of the head during breech delivery. This is due to the injury to the recurrent laryngeal nerve. Rupture of the intra-abdominal organs (such as the liver and spleen) can result from difficult breech delivery. If undetected, deterioration may be rapid and diagnosis should be suspected in a neonate who presents with abdominal distention, shock, anemia, and irritability without any evidence of external bleeding.

§ 9.19   Cesarean Section

Cesarean section is defined as delivery of the fetus through incisions in the abdominal and uterine walls. The indication to perform a cesarean section arises when a situation demands that the pregnancy (or labor) be terminated because vaginal delivery is not safe for either the mother or infant, or vaginal delivery is not feasible.

The maternal complications of cesarean section include infection, hemorrhage, and damage to the urinary tract. These are found in higher rates—compared to maternal morbidity—from vaginal delivery. There is some circumstantial evidence implicating cesarean sections as a predisposing factor to transient tachypnea of the newborn.[28] Birth trauma in general is much less likely to occur with cesarean section than with vaginal delivery.

The timing of a repeat cesarean section on an elective basis is very important. There are distinct advantages to performing a repeat cesarean section, for whatever indication, on a predetermined day and time after certain criteria for ascertaining fetal maturity have been met. The operating room team, anesthesia personnel, resuscitation team, and nursery personnel can be better assembled to provide optimal care. Laboratory and blood-bank facilities are also better equipped to handle potential problems when well-staffed. Timing is of the essence since a premature infant may be delivered in an elective repeat cesarean section. Clinical evidence of fetal maturity should be present, such as:

Term gestational dates (more than 38 weeks) from the first day of the last known monthly period (LMP)

Audible fetal heartbeats by the fetoscope (not Doppler tone) for at least 20 weeks since the first time they were heard (about 18 to 20 weeks' gestation)

Uterine fundus growth consistent with menstrual dates

In case of any doubt, ultrasound study done between 20 and 30 weeks that correlates with fetal size (or uterine growth), if not menstrual dates.

Amniocentesis to detect mature lecithin-sphingomyelin ratio may be required in those instances that do not meet the other criteria.

---

[28] Sundell et al., *Studies on Infants with Type II Respiratory Distress Syndrome,* 78 J. Pediatrics 754 (1971); Avery et al., *Transient Tachypnea of the Newborn: Possible Delayed Resorption of Fluid at Birth,* 11 Am. J. Diseases Children 380 (1966).

Vaginal Birth after Cesarean Section

Because of better methods for maternal and fetal monitoring during labor, vaginal birth following cesarean section (VBAC) is now deemed safe as long as guidelines to determine candidates for VBAC and guidelines for labor are followed. The American College of Obstetricians and Gynecologists (ACOG) released its first ACOG Practice Patterns in August 1995. This pattern provides clinicians with clinical practice guidelines for managing a vaginal birth after a previous cesarean section.[29] The guidelines emphasize the following:

1. In the absence of contraindications, a woman with one prior low transverse cervical cesarean section should be encouraged to undergo a trial of labor.
2. A previous classical cesarean section is a contraindication.
3. Epidural anesthesia is not a contraindication for VBAC.
4. Oxytocin use is not contraindicated.
5. VBAC attempts should not be limited to tertiary care centers.
6. Appropriate monitoring, for example, electronic fetal monitoring, is necessary.

FETAL DISTRESS AND
ELECTRONIC MONITORING

§ 9.20   Signs of Intrapartum Fetal Distress

The presence of fetal hypoxia and acidosis during labor may manifest as intrapartum fetal distress and may be suggested by the following signs:

1. Presence of heavy meconium
2. Presence of one or more of the following patterns on electronic monitoring: persistent late decelerations, persistent severe variable decelerations, prolonged bradycardia, and markedly decreased or absent beat-to-beat variability
3. Presence of an abnormal fetal pH in fetal scalp sampling
4. Ultrasound evidence of disturbance in the biophysical profile.[30]

Heavy meconium.   The presence of heavy meconium in the amniotic fluid is not by itself pathognomonic of fetal distress, but the finding requires application

---

[29] ACOG Practice Pattern 1, Vaginal Delivery after Previous Cesarean Birth (1995).

[30] R.K. Freeman et al., Fetal Heart Rate Monitoring (3d ed. 1991).

of internal monitoring of the fetal heart rate and an internal uterine catheter for accurate pressure determination.

Electronic monitoring. The presence of one or more of the previously mentioned fetal heart rate patterns is suggestive of fetal distress and requires investigation as to possible etiology, such as hypotension in the supine parturient, hypotension induced by conduction anesthesia, drugs used for pain relief, such as heavy narcotics, and cord compression or prolapse. However, the diagnosis of fetal distress must be made within the context of all the circumstances at the time. If an abnormal heart rate pattern is persistent or worsens, preparations for cesarean section should be instituted. Fetal scalp sampling is still performed in some centers but its use is not widespread or standard.

Ultrasound. The biophysical profile, or observation of fetal breathing movement, fetal movement, fetal tone, and amniotic fluid volume by ultrasound during labor can help assess intrapartum fetal status.

§ 9.21 Intrapartum Electronic Monitoring

Monitoring of the fetal heart activity during and in between uterine contractions is indicated in high-risk pregnancies or labors with complications. The fetal heart rate (FHR) monitor has two components, one to detect uterine contractions and the other to detect fetal heart rate. Detection of both may be carried out by external leads strapped on the abdominal wall, or by direct application of the leads internally after rupture of the membranes—one lead inserted into the uterine cavity to gauge uterine pressure, and the other lead directly attached to the fetal scalp to detect heart rate. Readings are translated to an electrical signal and displayed on the monitor tracing or strip.

Terminology in Interpretation of Tracing

Basic FHR patterns include: (1) baseline features: heart rate and variability (between contractions); or (2) periodic changes: occurring during contractions. The baseline normal FHR is 120 to 160 beats per minute (BPM) between contractions. Tachycardia is FHR above 160 BPM and bradycardia is FHR below 120 BPM.

The FHR variability refers to the "jiggly" pattern observed in the FHR that represents a slight difference in interval from beat to beat. Normal variability occurs when the amplitude range of the variability is six BPM or greater. Decreased variability occurs when the amplitude range is less than six BPM. Absent variability occurs when the amplitude range is less than two BPM and the FHR line looks "flat." FHR variability of amplitude greater than 25 BPM is called *saltatory pattern*. Accurate assessment of variability can only be determined with internal fetal monitoring. The periodic changes are four: early decelerations, late decelerations, variable decelerations, and accelerations with contractions.

Early decelerations.   These are uniform decelerations that mirror contractions. They generally begin and end at the same time the uterine contractions begin and end. These decelerations are caused by fetal head compression; altered blood flow in the brain causes slowing of the heart rate through a vagal reflex. These decelerations are a reassuring fetal heart-rate pattern and are not associated with fetal acidosis, fetal hypoxia, or low Apgar scores.

Late decelerations.   These are similar to early decelerations in shape and uniformity, but the timing is delayed relative to the uterine contraction. The deceleration starts after the beginning of the uterine contraction and usually the return to baseline occurs after the contraction is over. The cause of late decelerations is usually uteroplacental insufficiency and may indicate fetal hypoxia.

Variable decelerations.   These are the most frequently seen fetal heart-rate deceleration pattern in labor. They are variable in duration, intensity, and timing in relation to the uterine contractions. Their probable cause is cord compression. The effect on fetal health depends on the duration and degree of cord compression, and other clinical events occurring at the time.

Accelerations with uterine contractions.   These constitute a reassuring pattern. They may occur with fetal movement or without apparent stimulus, or as a response to pelvic examination and stimulation of the fetal head. The risks and complications of internal fetal monitoring include:

1.   Fetal infection. Small scalp infections and, occasionally, scalp abscesses have been reported with the use of internal fetal scalp electrodes.
2.   Maternal infection. As an independent variable, fetal monitoring has little or no effect on infection.
3.   Uterine perforation from the catheter introducer guide.

   The effect of intrapartum electronic monitoring on morbidity and mortality rates relates to a decrease in the intrapartum stillbirth rate and a decrease in the neonatal mortality rate.[31]
   The effect of electronic fetal monitoring on cesarean section rates is the subject of debate. There is currently an increase in the cesarean delivery rate in the United States, and it is possible (although not likely) that contributing to the increase is the inappropriate use of the monitor and inadequate interpretation of

---

[31] R. Creasy & R. Resnik, Maternal-Fetal Medicine: Principles and Practice (3d ed. 1994).

FHR patterns. Also, there have been changes in philosophy as to management of certain situations, such as cesarean section for breech presentation. In addition, difficult forceps deliveries have been largely abandoned and more premature fetuses are given a chance of survival by the less traumatic approach of cesarean delivery because of better neonatal care and facilities. It is, therefore, difficult to conclude that electronic fetal monitoring has contributed to the increase in cesarean rate.

§ 9.22 Management of Fetal Distress

The management of fetal distress diagnosed during labor includes the following:

1. Identification of possible etiology for the deceleration (for example, hypertonus from Oxytocin stimulation) and removing the offending cause
2. Oxygen inhalation by mask or nasal catheter
3. Change in position, especially if patient is in supine position
4. Correct hypotension, if any
5. Correct any metabolic problem
6. Preparation for operative intervention.

CHAPTER 10

DRUG ADMINISTRATION DURING LABOR AND DELIVERY

William Banner, Jr., M.D., Ph.D.

§ 10.1   Introduction

The administration of medications during labor and delivery presents many challenges in a risk benefit analysis. In general, the emphasis has been on the use of these drugs to provide a maternal benefit with, it is hoped, minimal risks to the fetus. Few if any maternally administered drugs are intended directly to treat the baby. The use of digoxin to treat disorders of heart rhythm in the baby is one of the few examples of drug therapy targeted to treat the newborn. While it is recognized that a severely painful delivery may result in stress and compromise of the infant, the use of analgesics has never been construed to be useful to the newborn to avoid the pain of delivery. While this may seem to be a specious argument, unfortunately, it is representative of the type of logic that may be applied to perinatal drug therapy in the courtroom. Balancing the benefits of therapy with its attendant risks remains the challenge.

Since the focus of drug use in labor and delivery has been the benefit to the mother with acceptable risks to the infant, litigation often arises when an unacceptable outcome to the fetus outweighs the apparent benefits to the mother.

Since the infant's benefit from analgesia during delivery, particularly local analgesics, may arguably be minimal, from the fetal standpoint any risks associated with this therapy arguably may be considered unacceptable. The obvious balancing of the needs of the mother against the needs of the baby provides a difficult series of choices for the obstetrician, who, in general, views the mother as the patient rather than the infant. The pediatrician, on the other hand, may view pain as an acceptable risk to the mother in order to avoid possible side effects associated with the child's outcome. This chapter will not resolve this issue, but will attempt to provide a structure with examples for evaluating the role of drugs in adverse outcomes in the delivery process.

§ 10.2 Systematically Approaching the Problem

In reviewing a case involving a drug administered during the process of labor and delivery, the type of toxic reaction caused by the drug should be carefully evaluated. Obviously, since the child is the passive partner of the mother until the time of delivery, drugs that have direct adverse effects on the mother may have similar effects on the baby. For example, administration of a drug that causes profound decreases in maternal blood pressure, even if it does not cross the placenta, will decrease the amount of blood flow available to the placenta for oxygenation of the baby. To carry this to the absurd extreme, a drug that produces a fatal reaction in the mother is very likely to have the same effect on the baby.

   More importantly, some adverse effects are specific to the fetus and newborn. Thus, while the mother may not experience any side effects associated with the administration of the drug, a specific reaction occurs in the baby. For purposes of clarity, these issues are divided into three categories:

1.   Does the drug reach the fetus in a greater concentration than it does the mother?
2.   Is the baby experiencing a dose-related side effect?
3.   Is this an atypical response because of the specific anatomy and physiology of the newborn?

§ 10.3 Whether the Drug Reaches the Fetus in a
Greater Concentration Than It Reaches the Mother

Several mechanisms exist by which the baby may receive a higher concentration of drug than the mother. The largest amount of data available has been generated from the effects of local anesthetics.[1] First and foremost, direct injection of a

---

[1] Nau, *Clinical Pharmacokinetics in Pregnancy and Perinatology,* 8 Developmental Pharmacology Theraputics 149–81 (1985).

drug into the baby creates extremely high concentrations locally. Direct injections of local anesthetics into the fetal head or the intrauterine area while attempting local nerve blocks in the maternal pelvis can cause profound seizure activity and bradycardia from the high concentration of these drugs in the central nervous system.[2] While this sounds like an obvious error, it may be extremely difficult to document an accident of this type, which may be inapparent to the obstetrician. The initial concern of the pediatrician caring for such a baby is to control seizure activity and not to document the accident.

More subtle is the phenomenon of local blood flow producing relatively high fetal concentrations of local anesthetics. Injections into the maternal pelvis may cause locally high concentrations of the drug in the placenta and the infant as well as a high incidence of fetal bradycardia.[3] This phenomenon has been reviewed by Nau, who has pointed out the difficulty in study design taking into account free and total concentrations of drugs across the fetal-to-maternal barrier.[4] Since protein binding may be decreased in the newborn, seemingly lower concentrations of local anesthetics, as compared to concentrations in the mother, may actually represent higher free concentrations of these drugs.

The pH of the fetus may also affect the transfer of drugs. Lidocaine, a local anesthetic, is a weak base with a pH slightly above that of the physiologic. A weak base will tend to be trapped in a compartment that is relatively more acidic. By having an acidotic asphyxiated fetus, lidocaine may be trapped in the fetal compartment. While these effects are theoretically possible, there remain very little clinical data to associate true toxicity with the local administration of most anesthetic agents unless the drug is injected directly.

A third potential source of drug toxicity where drug concentrations in the fetus would exceed the concentration in the mother is related to transplacental drug transfer. Drugs are normally transported across the placenta in a relatively lipid soluble form. *Lipid solubility* is the ability of something to traverse fat-containing membranes. When compounds are transported to the fetus they may then be metabolized by the fetal liver. The result of that metabolic process may be a more water soluble and less lipid soluble compound. Since water soluble compounds are not readily transported out of the fetus, they may accumulate to higher concentrations than would normally be predicted based on the amount of drug transported into the fetus. Once again, while a theoretical possibility, and certainly a demonstrable phenomenon, the clinical impact of accumulation of active metabolites in the fetus is not a well documented phenomenon.

---

[2] Amato, Carasso & Ruckstuhl, *Neonatal Mepivacaine Poisoning Following Episiotomy,* 187(4) Zeitschriff Geburtshife Perinatologie 191 (1983); Van Dorsten & Miller, *Fetal Heart Rate Changes After Accidental Intrauterine Lidocaine,* 57(2) Obstetrics Gynecology 257 (1981).

[3] Ralston & Shnider, *The Fetal and Neonatal Effects of Regional Anesthesia in Obstetrics,* 48 Anesthesiology 34 (1978); Liston, Adjepon-Yamoah & Scott, *Foetal and Maternal Lignocaine Levels after Paracervical Block,* 45 Brit. J. Anaesthesiology 750 (1973).

[4] Nau, *Clinical Pharmacokinetics in Pregnancy and Perinatology,* 8 Developmental Pharmacology Therapeutics 149–81 (1985).

§ 10.4   Dose-Related Side Effects

A wide variety of pharmaceutical agents are used for maternal treatment of various disorders. Despite achieving safe concentrations of these drugs in the mother, and with no evidence of excessive accumulation of the drug in the fetus, drugs may still produce adverse reactions in the newborn of a type that are normally associated with higher drug concentrations and serum. These effects may be caused by an increased sensitivity on the part of the fetus to the effect of drugs, or unknown effects that cannot be well correlated with serum concentrations alone, such as accumulation in the central nervous system or the phenomenon of trapping as described in § 10.3. In particular, drugs used for narcotic analgesia of the mother and the treatment of maternal hypertension may be associated with a variety of side effects in the fetus.

The use of analgesic agents is a fact of life in the peripartum period. These may in fact facilitate fetal outcome in that a precipitous or poorly controlled delivery under severe pain and stress may be more hazardous to the infant than a smoothly controlled, less stressful event. At the same time, certain well recognized side effects of narcotic analgesics are important to consider. The major cause of concern for the fetus relating to narcotic effects is respiratory depression. Since no respiratory effort is needed until immediately postdelivery, a relatively long-term exposure in utero to narcotic agents is not necessarily a hazardous event until the first breath is desired. It does appear that the infant is more sensitive to the respiratory depressant effects of the narcotics, in particular, morphine. From a therapeutic standpoint, narcotic-induced respiratory depression can be reversed by a narcotic antagonist such as naloxone but not until the airway is preserved and artificially supported if necessary. A common error is to wait following the injection of an intramuscular dose of a narcotic antagonist instead of immediately proceeding with vigorous respiratory support, and then, reversal of the narcotic effect. An equally serious error in the management of any baby exposed to a narcotic analgesic is a failure to understand the pharmacokinetics of narcotic reversal. Naloxone (Narcan), the most readily available narcotic reversing agent, has a limited duration of action of about 30 to 45 minutes. Since many of the narcotics have a longer duration in the newborn, there can be a return to the depressed state as naloxone wears off. A physician who makes the judgment that a baby is sufficiently awake following naloxone to be sent to a nonmonitored situation, and then experiences the return of narcotic-induced respiratory depression under circumstances where an infant is not monitored, has clearly failed to recognize basic principles of narcotic reversal.

Another class of drugs that has a multitude of effects to which the fetus may be sensitive are the antihypertensive drugs. Life-threatening hypertension is part of the syndrome of eclampsia that worsens late in pregnancy. Continuing controversy surrounds the management of this hypertension in the period around the delivery. The overall question of whether there is an improved outcome with the treatment of hypertension has until relatively recently been an area of some controversy. A study by Berkowitz and others found that blood pressures in excess of 200/120 are associated with a high degree of perinatal mortality.[5] If one accepts the basic principle that maternal hypertension should be treated to improve outcome, the second critical question is whether a particular group of drugs is advantageous in improving the outcome of the fetus. For example, the results of a study by Arias suggest that hydralazine, a blood vessel dilator, is associated with a poor fetal outcome.[6] On the opposite side of the argument is a study by Redman.[7] Methyldopa, an antihypertensive agent that acts on the brain, was found to decrease dramatically fetal demise. Thus, the decision to treat maternal hypertension, as well as the choice of agents, is critical.

In general, the first drugs used in the treatment of hypertension in pregnancy are the diuretics, drugs that decrease the sodium in the body. The thiazide diuretics were thought in the past to be associated with depression of fetal platelet counts. This has not been supported in better controlled studies.[8] The major concern in the use of thiazide diuretics in the perinatal period is the effect of these drugs on bilirubin binding to the protein, albumin. By occupying binding sites on albumin, these drugs cause displacement of the bilirubin that would normally be bound, and a greater tendency for bilirubin to be free to cause central nervous system toxicity. While this kind of argument is valid in theory, in practice it would appear that the amount of drug retained in the infant following maternal treatment with thiazide diuretics would not mandate that a very useful category of drugs be discontinued from perinatal clinical use. Recent references, however, have still argued against the use of these compounds.[9] This effect of drugs to displace bilirubin should serve as a caution, however, that in the first few days of life, the neonate with hyperbilirubinemia should not be directly treated with highly protein-bound drugs in the presence of an elevated serum bilirubin.

The next major category of antihypertensive drugs that may have effects on the fetus is also an area of great controversy. The vasodilator drugs lower blood pressure by increasing the caliber of the blood vessel and lowering the resistance to flow. Nitroprusside is a rapid and potent vasodilator that is used in perinatal hypertension based on some data showing favorable effects of this compound on fetal outcome.[10] Animal data on nitroprusside have suggested the potential for

---

[5] Berkowitz, *Antihypertensive Drugs in the Pregnant Patient,* 35 Obstet. Gynecol. Surv. 191 (1980).

[6] Arias & Zamora, *Antihypertensive Treatment and Pregnancy Outcome in Patients with Mild Hypertension,* 53 Obstetrics Gynecology 489 (1979).

[7] Redman, Beilin, Bonnar & Ounsted, *Fetal Outcome in Trial of Antihypertensive Treatment in Pregnancy,* 2 Lancet 753 (1976).

[8] Jerkner, Kutti & Victorin, *Platelet Counts in Mothers and Their Newborn Infants with Respect to Antepartum Administration of Oral Diuretics,* 194 Acta Med. Scand. 473 (1973).

[9] Lindheimer, Marshall & Katz, *Medical Intelligence: Current Concepts: Hypertension in Pregnancy,* 313(11) New Eng. J. Med. 675 (1985).

[10] Stempel, O'Grady, Morton & Johnson, *Use of Sodium Nitroprusside in Complications of Gestational Hypertension,* 60(4) Obstetrics Gynecology 533 (1982).

severe toxicity in the infant, because nitroprusside is broken down into cyanide and thiocyanate.[11] It does not appear that these metabolites accumulate to a degree sufficient to cause significant toxicity providing the mother has normal renal function and the dose used is low.[12] In the presence of maternal renal failure or at high doses, infusion of nitroprusside may be relatively contra-indicated unless careful monitoring of thiocyanate can be performed.

Diazoxide, another direct acting vasodilator drug, was shown in several early studies to depress uterine activity and lower fetal blood pressure.[13] One study in particular found that the rapid injection of diazoxide had profound effects on maternal circulation, causing evidence of fetal distress.[14] It is a well-recognized fact that sudden drops in blood pressure cause a decrease in blood flow to certain critical areas such as the brain and heart. In the pregnant patient, the uterus is probably also at risk for having critical blood flow cut off if a sudden and dramatic drop in blood pressure occurs. The rapid injection of diazoxide there-fore appears to be a hazard to the pregnant female and should be discouraged. No data exist on relatively slow infusions of diazoxide in terms of fetal outcome. However, the slow infusion of diazoxide has been used in large numbers of adult patients with relatively few side effects and the same principles may apply to the pregnant female. A third drug that is relatively commonly used as a vasodilator during pregnancy is hydralazine. The same basic arguments on sudden reduc-tions in blood pressure have been applied to hydralazine and indeed, some studies have suggested that hydralazine may be relatively hazardous.[15]

It would appear that all vasodilators should be used with close monitoring and maintenance of adequate blood pressures at all times in the mother during the peripartum period. Rapid lowering of blood pressure as may be experienced with the bolus injection of vasodilator drugs appears to be hazardous to the fetus by decreasing uterine blood flow.[16]

[11] Naulty, Cefalo & Lewis, *Fetal Toxicity of Nitroprusside in the Pregnant Ewe,* 139(6) Am. J. Obstetrics Gynecology 708 (1981).

[12] Shoemaker & Meyers, *Sodium Nitroprusside for Control of Severe Hypertensive Disease of Pregnancy: A Case Report and Discussion of Potential Toxicity,* 149(2) Am. J. Obstetrics Gynecology 171 (1984).

[13] Morishima, Caritis, Yeh & James, *Prolonged Infusion of Diazoxide in the Management of Premature Labor in the Baboon,* 48 Obstetrics Gynecology 203 (1976); Morishima, Cohen, Brown, Daniel, Neimann & James, *The Inhibitory Action of Diazoxide on Uterine Activity in the Subhuman Primate: Placental Transfer and Effect of the Fetus,* 1 J. Perinatal Med. 13 (1973); Milner & Chouksey, *Effects of Fetal Exposure to Diazoxide in Man,* 47 Archives Diseases Children 537 (1972); Newayhid, Brinkman III, Katchen, Sympchowiez, Martinek & Assali, *Maternal and Fetal Hemodynamic Effects of Diazoxide,* 46 Obstetrics Gynecology 197 (1975).

[14] Neuman, Weiss, Rabello, Cabal & Freeman, *Diazoxide for the Acute Control of Severe Hyper-tension Complicating Pregnancy: A Pilot Study,* 53 Obstetrics Gynecology 50 (1979).

[15] Redman, Beilin, Bonnar & Ounsted, *Fetal Outcome in Trial of Antihypertensive Treatment in Pregnancy,* 2 Lancet 753 (1976).

[16] Stempel, O'Grady, Morton & Johnson, *Use of Sodium Nitroprusside in Complications of Gestational Hypertension,* 60(4) Obstetrics Gynecology 533 (1982).

Another category of drugs is the sympatholytic drugs. These drugs act to block the fight or flight response and are generally used for the more chronic management of hypertension in pregnancy. Clonidine, one commonly used antihypertensive in adult patients, has been associated in a single case report with Robert's Syndrome including facial and limb abnormalities.[17] As is discussed in **Chapter 6,** it is difficult to interpret a single case report. However, in the absence of data on safety, use of this drug would appear to be relatively contraindicated early in pregnancy. Reserpine has been demonstrated to cause newborn nasal obstruction and hypothermia. This drug is not recommended for use in the management of maternal hypertension. Methyldopa has been extensively studied in the perinatal period. While it does appear that methyldopa readily crosses the placenta and appears in therapeutic concentrations in the human fetus, it still appears that it is relatively safe and is associated with an improvement in outcome when compared with untreated control hypertensive patients.[18] Some of the newer drugs for the management of hypertension such as captopril have been found to coincide with an alarming increase in malformations in animals, and thus have not been recommended for use during pregnancy.[19]

One major area of controversy in the use of sympatholytic drugs involves the use of the drug propranolol. Several large series have demonstrated that propranolol and other beta blockers are well tolerated and effective for the management of hypertension in pregnancy.[20] It is also well recognized, however, that propranolol may cause a prolongation of the labor process and a decrease in blood sugar and heart rate at the time of delivery.[21] In addition, these drugs may delay the onset of breathing. Animal studies have also demonstrated that propranolol is capable of decreasing intrauterine fetal growth in a dose-related fashion.[22] Despite these findings, these drugs have been strongly advocated for use in pregnancy.[23]

Thus, the treatment of maternal hypertension producing rapid changes in blood pressure may be associated with unacceptable fetal side effects. With judicious antihypertensive treatment, the overall improvement outcome of the mother and fetus outweighs the risks. In this respect, failure to control blood pressure may be a more appropriate reason for litigation than the use of drug

---

[17] Stoll, Levy & Beshara, *Robert's Syndrome and Clonidine,* 16 J. Med. Genetics 486 (1979).

[18] Mutch, Moar, Ounsted & Redman, *Hypertension During Pregnancy, With and Without Specific Hypotensive Treatment,* 1 Early Human Dev. 47 (1977).

[19] Pipkin & O'Brien, *The Effect of a Specific Angiotensin Antagonist on Blood Pressure in the Conscious Pregnant Ewe and Her Foetus,* 269(1) Physiolog. Soc. 63 (1977).

[20] Rubin, *Beta-Blockers in Pregnancy,* 303 New Eng. J. Med. 1323 (1981).

[21] Cottrill, McAllister, Gettes & Noonan, *Propranolol Therapy During Pregnancy, Labor and Delivery: Evidence for Transplacental Drug Transfer and Impaired Neonatal Drug Disposition,* 91(5) J. Pediatr. 812 (1977).

[22] Schoenfeld, Epstein, Nemesh, Rosen & Atsmon, *Effects of Propranolol during Pregnancy and Development of Rats. I. Adverse Effects during Pregnancy,* 12 Pediatric Res. 747 (1978).

[23] Rubin, *Beta-Blockers in Pregnancy,* 303 New Eng. J. Med. 1323 (1981).

therapy, particularly when a variety of agents have been demonstrated safe and effective.

In summary, the baby is exposed at the time of delivery to a variety of drugs intended primarily to treat disorders such as pain or hypertension due to eclampsia in the mother. Since the placenta does not act as a barrier to prevent drug access to the fetus, the fetus is exposed to many of the same drug influences that the mother is receiving. In many respects, however, the fetus is more responsive to the effects of these drugs. Thus, a dose-related adverse reaction may occur despite the demonstration that concentrations of a drug in the baby may be lower than in the mother. For example, all patients may have a dose-related respiratory depression from narcotics; however, the extreme sensitivity of the baby to narcotic-induced respiratory depression needs to be considered in the risk benefit analysis. Any time a drug is used in the time surrounding the delivery of a child, the possibility that an exaggerated response to that drug may be observed is a reasonable assumption. Fortunately, many of these adverse reactions can be readily reversed, as can be seen with the use of a narcotic antagonist such as naloxone. Since data have been accumulated on exaggerated responses to the same agents in older patients, often the therapy is simply an extension of the same therapy that would be used in an adult who had an adverse reaction to the same medication. This is in contrast to reactions that are based on some specific anatomic or physiologic peculiarity of the newborn.

§ 10.5   Atypical Responses Because of the Specific Anatomy and Physiology of the Newborn

One peculiar aspect of drug use during labor and delivery is that if one searches only for the responses observed in the mother, one may miss some peculiar idiosyncratic response of the newborn because of the newborn's anatomy and physiology. One dramatic example of this is in the use of drugs to stop the labor process once it is under way. Indeed, the whole area of stopping the process of labor (tocolysis) when a premature birth is the likely outcome has been controversial.[24] In the past, decisions on tocolytic therapy have been based upon how effective a drug was at stopping the labor process, rather than on the outcome of the baby. Hemminki and Starfield have reviewed 18 clinical trials of tocolytic therapy.[25] Strikingly, it appeared that when inappropriate methodologies were eliminated, less than one-half of the studies were actually able to demonstrate that these drugs were able to halt the labor process. Further, it was almost impossible to draw the conclusion that the newborn's outcome was

---

[24] Caritis, *Treatment of Preterm Labour: A Review of the Therapeutic Options,* 26(3) Drugs 243 (1983); Souney, Kaul & Osathanondh, *Pharmacotherapy of Preterm Labor,* 2(1) Clinical Pharmacology 29 (1983).

[25] Hemminki & Starfield, *Prevention and Treatment of Premature Labour by Drugs: Review of Controlled Clinical Trials,* 85 Brit. J. Obstetrics Gynaecology 411 (1978).

improved. Despite the lack of hard objective data, the clinical experience of many neonatologists would suggest that if begun early, some methods of decreasing the labor process may be useful to delay the delivery of the premature baby.

There are, however, exceptions. The drug indomethacin is a good example of a tocolytic drug in which a very unusual adverse response was observed in the newborn. Indomethacin is an inhibitor of the synthesis of prostaglandins. It was found to be extremely effective at stopping premature labor. On the basis of clinical and animal trials, however, it appears that this drug is capable of closing the ductus arteriosus in the fetus.[26] The ductus arteriosus is a muscular blood vessel connecting the pulmonary artery and the aorta. Since blood does not need to pass through the lungs in utero, this vessel allows oxygenated blood from the placenta to reach the fetal circulation. At birth, this structure closes and eventually disappears. By causing closure of the ductus arteriosus in utero, indomethacin causes the development of pulmonary hypertension and a high degree of fetal morbidity. Even in the face of this evidence, several authors have concluded, based on relatively small series of patients, that these drugs were effective and safe.[27] A similar drug, naproxen, has been reported to have similar toxic properties and, thus, all drugs in this category may be suspect.[28]

Another drug that has continued to be used as a tocolytic is alcohol. Ethyl alcohol, taken either orally or intravenously, has now been shown in large series to be a severe depressant of metabolism and glucose, as well as the central nervous system, in the newborn period and is associated with a high degree of mortality.[29]

Another major category of drugs useful in the delay of labor are the sympathomimetic drugs. These drugs appear to act by stimulating blood flow to the uterus and causing it to relax. One drug, isoxsuprine, was initially the standard of care until a study appeared in 1981 that associated the use of isoxsuprine with hypocalcemia and poor gastrointestinal motility in the newborn following

[26] Csaba, Sulyok & Ertl, *Relationship of Maternal Treatment with Indomethacin to Persistence of Fetal Circulation Syndrome,* 92 J. Pediatrics 484 (1978); Levin, Mills & Parkey, *Constriction of the Fetal Ductus Arteriosus After Administration of Indomethacin to the Pregnant Ewe,* 94 J. Pediatrics 647 (1979); Manchester, Margolis & Sheldon, *Possible Association Between Maternal Indomethacin Therapy and Primary Pulmonary Hypertension of the Newborn,* 126 Am. J. Obstetrics Gynecology 467 (1975).

[27] Atad, Moise & Abramovici, *Classification of Threatened Premature Labor Related to Treatment with Prostaglandin Inhibitor: Indomethacin,* 37 Biology Neonate 291 (1980); Van Kets, Thiery, Deron, van Egmond & Baele, *Perinatal Hazards of Chronic Tocolysis with Indomethacin,* 18 Prostaglandins 893 (1979).

[28] Wilkinson, Aynsley-Green & Mitchell, *Persistent Pulmonary Hypertension and Abnormal Prostaglandin E Levels in Preterm Infants After Maternal Treatment with Naproxen,* 54 Archives Diseases Children 942 (1979).

[29] Lopez & Montoya, *Abnormal Bone Marrow Morphology in the Premature Infant Associated with Maternal Alcohol Infusion,* 79 J. Pediatr. 1008 (1971); Fuchs, Fuchs, Lauersen & Zervoudakis, *Treatment of Pre-Term Labour with Ethanol,* 26 Danish Med. Bull. 123 (1979).

maternal treatment.[30] In addition, for unknown reasons, it was found that there was an increased incidence of neonatal mortality associated with this drug. It is part of the paradox of obstetrical and neonatal care that a drug could be in use as the standard of care without having demonstrated an improvement in outcome. In contrast to this rather poor outcome, ritodrine, terbutaline, and salbutamol have all been used to treat premature labor, and have been felt to be relatively safe. However, subtle effects such as neonatal hypoglycemia and fetal cardiac hypertrophy have been associated with the use of these drugs and some studies have even suggested unacceptable outcomes.[31]

Another rather unusual area of responses of the newborn is the development of intraventricular hemorrhage (IVH) in the premature infant. Very little is known about the administration of maternal drugs and the production of IVH. Some studies, however, have suggested that drugs that cause a sudden surge in blood flow to the central nervous system of babies born prematurely may predispose an area called the germinal matrix layer to hemorrhage. The germinal matrix layer is a tissue of growth for the central nervous system that disappears after about 36 weeks of gestation. This has led to the suggestion that premature newborns be sedated and not subjected to drugs that may cause a dramatic increase in blood flow or blood pressure to the central nervous system in order to decrease the incidence of IVH. The inappropriate resuscitation of premature infants in the delivery room with large doses of caffeine as a respiratory stimulant is an example of a drug-induced side effect peculiar to the premature newborn. By injecting large doses of caffeine, an increase in fetal heart rate and blood pressure is observed that may contribute to development of IVH.[32] In addition, this practice is associated with a high incidence of seizures in the newborn. The use of caffeine appears to be inappropriate given its lack of effectiveness in the delivery room as a primary respiratory stimulant and these possibly severe side effects.

As demonstrated in this chapter, the side effects of medications during the process of labor and delivery can be categorized as to their origin. An important first screening for categorizing these reactions is determining whether the infant achieved a higher serum concentration than the mother, was merely more sensitive to a typical side effect, or had a side effect peculiar to the newborn physiology and anatomy. In reviewing the literature in this area, it is often surprising to find out how little is actually known about the effects of these medications on fetal outcome in any systematic way. Considering the unusual

---

[30] Braxy, Little & Grim, *Isoxsuprine in the Perinatal Period. II. Relationships Between Neonatal Symptoms, Drug Exposure and Drug Concentration at the Time of Birth,* 98 J. Pediatr. 146 (1981).

[31] Caritis, *Treatment of Preterm Labour: A Review of the Therapeutic Options,* Kristoffersen & Hansen, *The Condition of the Foetus and Infant in Cases Treated with Ritrodrine,* 26 Dan. Med. Bull. 121 (1979).

[32] Banner & Czajka, *Acute Caffeine Overdosage in the Neonate,* 134 Am. J. Diseases of Children 495 (1980).

and diverse disorders of intraventricular hemorrhage and premature closure of the ductus arteriosus, it should be apparent that the introduction of a new pharmaceutical agent into therapy during labor and delivery would require much more extensive investigation than occurs in the case of drugs introduced into use in the adult.

Despite this greater need for knowledge, the willingness of investigators to pursue the effects of these drugs on the fetus and the willingness of pharmaceutical manufacturers to support research of this type is limited. For many investigators, the primary consideration is efficacy in the disorder under treatment and not improvement in fetal outcome. In addition, the liability assumed by the pharmaceutical manufacturer in investigating peripartum drug use discourages close investigation into drug use. Thus, as with drug use during pregnancy in general, the number of medications that may be used in the peripartum period is relatively limited. Even more surprising is the fact that despite some rather spectacular examples of drug misuse in the peripartum period, the number of actual events directly attributable to drug-induced reactions in the newborn period are extremely few in standard obstetrical practice.

CHAPTER 11

THE NURSE'S ROLE IN LABOR AND DELIVERY

Karen Carter Lyon, Ph.D., R.N.

§ 11.1 Introduction

The role of the nurse during labor and delivery may differ by practitioner and clinical setting. For example, a licensed vocational nurse in a small, rural hospital may have total nursing responsibility for laboring patients, with only intermittent supervision from a registered nurse. The same nurse, caring for a high-risk population in a tertiary center, may have a supportive or technical role if allowed to work in an obstetrical unit at all.

Registered nurses working at hospitals staffed entirely by private physicians ordinarily assume a great deal of responsibility for assessment of patient status and decision making. In a teaching facility with house-officers, interns, or residents in constant attendance, registered nurses generally have less opportunity to engage in the technical aspects of medical care for laboring mothers. However, in both settings, registered nurses are responsible for assessment, nursing diagnosis, nursing interventions, and evaluation of care. While important to consider classification of nursing personnel and the particular facility in order to determine scope of responsibility, it is imperative that any registered nurse who practices in the obstetrical arena have the requisite knowledge, skills, and experience. Guidelines for practice should be set out in individual job descriptions, policy and procedure manuals, or the standard operating procedures of the unit. This chapter addresses the responsibility of labor and delivery nurses when it is the greatest; that is, when the physician is not in constant attendance in the hospital.

§ 11.2   Allied Health Personnel

As indicated, education and subsequent classification of nursing attendants to a large extent determines their role. Note, however, that experience and on-the-job training often increase responsibilities and tasks assumed by staff members. In jurisdictions that have permissive nursing statutes, role distinctions may become quite blurred.

Nurse's Aide or Technician

In most areas of the United States, nurse's aides are trained in formal, certification programs offered by community colleges or vocational schools. Courses range from six weeks to three months. Depending on the state or jurisdiction, certification may be required. In addition to certification, many hospitals require that potential employees pass an in-house examination.

Obstetrical technicians are trained beyond the basic level of an aide. Programs may be conducted in a formal, post–high school setting or in a hospital. Obstetrical technicians act under the supervision of licensed personnel. In general, their function is to carry out specified, delegated tasks. Although these tasks (for example, setup of delivery equipment, paperwork, or instrument care) often do not include direct patient care, certain patient care responsibilities may be delegated to the technician. Examples of commonly delegated tasks include taking vital signs (temperature, pulse, respiration, fetal heart rate, and blood pressure), timing uterine contractions, applying external electronic fetal monitors, doing perineal shaves and enemas, and identification procedures for newborns.

Many acts, however, are specifically reserved to licensed personnel and are not delegable. These include, but are not limited to, vaginal examination, venipuncture, administration of medications, assessment of fetal heart rate patterns, and resuscitation procedures beyond basic CPR.

In general, the responsibilities of unlicensed personnel are task-oriented and require no interpretation of data or independent judgment. However, aides and technicians must be knowledgeable about the normal limits of the assessments performed. It would not be sufficient for an aide to take and chart a dangerously elevated blood pressure without any further action; the aide must be aware of its abnormality and promptly notify the nurse. Responsibility for the actions of assistant personnel resides with the supervising nurse.

Licensed Vocational or Practical Nurses

Licensed vocational or practical nurses (LVN, LPN) usually train beyond high school for one year. Training programs are state-accredited and located in a community college or vocational school. Students are taught basic anatomy, physiology, and pharmacology as well as the technical aspects of patient care. Clinical experience and didactic courses are provided. After completion of the educational program, a student is required to pass a state licensing examination.

As discussed in § 11.1, roles of LVNs vary widely in accordance with the facility in which they work; however, actions must always be limited to the scope outlined by the nurse practice act of any state. For example, the administration of intravenous medication is often statutorily beyond the scope of the LVN's license to practice. The employing facility may further restrict the responsibilities of LVNs via job descriptions and procedure manuals.

An LVN acting as the primary nurse for women in labor assumes the responsibilities of a registered nurse. However, the LVN's practice must always be supervised by a registered nurse who is in charge of the individual unit or is supervising several units.

Registered Nurses

A registered nurse (RN) is the typical provider of nursing care to laboring women. While the level of education required for basic entry into practice as an RN is controversial, there are three types of programs. The most traditional program for training RNs is conducted by hospitals over a three-year period. These programs are state accredited and include a large component of clinical bedside experience. Hospital-based programs are currently being phased out; however, most nurses trainees prior to 1950 were educated in these so-called diploma programs.

An associate degree nurse (AON) has graduated from a two-year program, often administered by a community college. Emphasis in these programs is fairly evenly divided between didactic classroom training and bedside clinical experience. Nurses receive very little preparation in nursing management or community health issues. Their training prepares them for basic hospital practice. AONs often require prolonged employment orientation in order to function in alternative health settings and managed care environments.

Many nursing graduates attended baccalaureate programs and hold bachelor's degrees from a university or college. BSN programs usually extend over four academic years and attempt to balance clinical care with didactic experience. In addition, leadership and management skills and nursing theory are integral parts of the program. BSN graduates are well versed in community-based practice and managed care.

Upon completion of a basic nursing program, all graduates must pass the NCLEX licensing examination, a national test administered by the state. Because the NCLEX is a national examination, once a nurse is licensed in one state, licensure in others is usually by reciprocity. An RN working on a labor and delivery unit is the nurse most often responsible for continual assessment of a mother and fetus in labor. This nurse is also a primary source of support and information for patients and families during the childbearing process. In the absence of an obstetrician, certified nurse, or midwife, the laboring family turn to an RN for guidance through this mystifying and exciting life experience. The science of being a nurse rests in accurate assessments and appropriate actions that aid a mother and her baby in emerging from parturition safely. The art of nursing facilitates a family's comfort, ease, dignity, and satisfaction.

Certain aspects of care described in later sections may be carried out by other members of the health care team, but the registered nurse is most likely to be the responsible person at the bedside.

Nurse Practitioners and Clinical Specialists

The advanced nurse practitioner has attended a post-RN course and received a certificate or graduate degree in a field of specialization such as obstetrics and gynecology. States vary in their recognition and requirement for advanced specialty training. Although most OB/GYN nurse practitioner work in prenatal ambulatory care settings, they may be found in the labor and delivery suite. Nurse practitioners usually continue in a role similar to the registered nurse, but their duties and responsibilities are expanded and may include teaching other health care providers. Clinically, the nurse practitioner may be trained and given authority to perform some procedures most often reserved to the physician. For example, amniotomy (artificial rupture of the membranes) and placement of an internal uterine pressure catheter are often assumed by nurse practitioners.

The clinical nurse specialist functions in much the same way as the nurse practitioner. The clinical specialist, however, always holds a master's degree and is often involved in clinical research and education.

Primary Care Nurses

The primary care nurse is typically an RN. The role of the primary care nurse is to coordinate the nursing care being given to a particular patient, including the development of a nursing care plan. The primary care nurse is completely responsible for the clinical management of one or more patients, depending on the distribution of case load on the unit. While this type of distribution is most effective in a unit where a patient's stay will extend over several days or weeks, it can also work in the short-stay environment. In the fast-moving world of labor and delivery, the primary care nurse becomes the nurse who is responsible for a particular patient's total care.

Charge Nurses

The charge nurse is usually an RN who has the responsibility of coordinating nursing care for all the patients on the unit during a particular shift. The charge nurse usually assigns patients and tasks to individual personnel and evaluates the care being provided. The charge nurse must make it his or her business to know the basic status of each patient at all times. Most importantly, he or she must be aware of the levels of knowledge and skill of the nursing personnel supervised. It is the charge nurse's ability to appropriately match nursing skills to patient needs that will often avert problems.

When lapses in nursing care occur, it is the charge nurse's responsibility to recognize and rectify them. Organization of new nursing personnel often is the responsibility of the charge nurse. Ascertaining the ability of a new nurse to appropriately assess and intervene before releasing that nurse to full staff status is of primary importance.

Certified Nurse-Midwives

A certified nurse-midwife (CNM) is an individual who is educated in the two disciplines of nursing and midwifery and possesses evidence of certification according to the requirements of the American College of Nurse-Midwives (ACNM).[1] A CNM is trained in midwifery after completion of training as a registered nurse. Programs are accredited by the ACNM at the certificate, master's degree, or doctoral level. Graduates must satisfactorily complete a national examination administered by the ACNM to become certified. The practice of a *nurse-midwife* is defined by the ACNM as:

> The independent management of care of essentially normal newborns and women, antepartally, intrapartally, post-partally and/or gynecologically. This

---

[1] S. M. Cohen et al., Maternal Neonatal, and Women's Health Nursing 19 (1991) [hereinafter Cohen].

occurs within a health care system which provides for medical consultation, collaborative management, and referral and is in accord with the "functions, standards and qualifications for Nurse-Midwifery Practice" as defined by the ACNM.[2]

Authorization to practice midwifery varies among states. Some states have specific legislation concerning the practice of midwifery. In others, midwives practice in the absence of any statutory authority. CNMs practicing in hospital settings must meet the standards of the particular facility. CNMs are often employed by physicians and hospitals. They may be in independent practice, with an arrangement with a physician for backup in case complications develop. In all cases, written protocols must be agreed upon between the CNM and the backup physician. Protocols delineate medical tasks and procedures, and set guidelines for referral and consultation. Within these protocols, a CNM assumes the actual decision making responsibilities and management of care. Some states grant CNMs the authority to prescribe certain medications to patients. In most hospital settings, staff nurses carry out the orders of a CNM just as they would for an obstetrician.[3] The CNM assumes some duties that are typically the physician's, but may retain many nursing care responsibilities.

§ 11.3   Initial Assessment of Patients

A woman presenting to a labor and delivery unit requires an initial assessment, usually performed by a nurse, prior to notifying the physician that the patient has arrived. Elements of a typical nursing admission assessment are listed in **Appendix 11–1.** The history, with special emphasis on previous childbearing, can alert the nurse to risk factors. Accurate estimation of gestational age of the fetus is required because a medical decision to facilitate or arrest the labor hinges in large part on this information. Careful questioning concerning the onset of true labor and the time of rupture of membranes is indispensable for continued evaluation of labor progress. Notation of the color of the amniotic fluid is made if membranes have ruptured. A green to greenish-brown color is indicative of meconium in the fluid and may signal the possibility of fetal distress. Allergies, current medication, and time of last meal are data needed if analgesia and anesthesia are later considered.

Physical assessment includes vital signs of mother and fetus. An abdominal palpation yields valuable data to an experienced examiner. Palpation provides information concerning labor mechanism (frequency and quality of uterine

---

[2] *Id.*

[3] For basic information concerning the status of CNMs in various states, see generally 29 J. Nurse-Midwifery (Mar./Apr. 1984).

contractions) and fetal presentation. Certain abnormalities may be appreciated on abdominal palpation. For example, the nurse may note that the height of the uterine fundus is unusually large or that fetal small parts (arms and legs) are palpable in many quadrants of the uterus, indicating the possibility of a multi-fetal pregnancy. Conversely, an exceptionally small uterus alerts the nurse to the possibility of a premature or growth-retarded fetus.

Finally, a sterile vaginal examination is performed by an experienced examiner. The status determined during the initial assessment forms the basis for subsequent evaluation and must be accurate. The nurse notes:

Dilation. This measures the degree of opening of the cervix, in centimeters, from 0 to 10.

Effacement. This measurement is of the degree of thinning of the cervix, in percentiles. The normal pregnant cervix is roughly one inch thick. During the weeks prior to and at the onset of labor, the cervix thins, or *effaces,* to facilitate dilation. A thick cervix would be indicated as long, or 0 percent. A completely effaced cervix is said to be 100 percent.

Station. These measurements are of the level of the presenting part (usually the fetal skull) in relation to the bony prominence at the center of the maternal pelvis (the ischial spines). This is measured or stated in increments of one centimeter above or below the spines: 0 is the level of the spines; −1, −2, and so forth equals 1 centimeter and 2 centimeters above, respectively; and +1,+2 equal 1 centimeter and 2 centimeters below.

Membranes. The presence or absence of palpable amniotic membranes must be noted. See § **11.2.**

Fetal presentation or position. The nurse confirms the presentation of the fetus by noting the hard, regular surface of the fetal skull versus the softer angularity of the breech, foot, or shoulder. Determining position is often difficult, even for the skilled and experienced nurse, especially if the cervix is not greatly dilated and the presenting part is high. The examiner locates the *occiput* (the spot in the rear of the fetal head where the skull bones meet) and ascertains its relationship to maternal pelvis. See **Chapter 7.**

Once the complete assessment is finished, the nurse is able to identify the patient's needs and priorities. A nursing plan is developed incorporating the patient's and the infant's status, the policies of the facility and the physician, and the birth plans of the patient and her family.

§ 11.4 Responsibility to Inform Physicians

Following initial assessment, the nurse informs the physician of the patient's arrival in the unit and the results of the assessment. It is always wise to reacquaint the physician with significant history because the patient's name may trigger no recall for someone in a large and busy obstetrical practice. The physician then gives orders for admission and care of the patient. Orders are given in conversational shorthand (especially in the middle of the night), like "OK, thanks," which translates into, "Admit her and use my standing orders." The nurse points out and pursues any questionable aspects of the mother or fetus's condition. It is the responsibility of the nurse to confirm that the medical practitioner has a clear understanding of the patient's condition and that medical orders are consistent with the nursing assessment.

It is basic policy for any nurse to inform the physician when the status of the mother or fetus deviates significantly from the norm in a manner that jeopardizes the health or well-being of either. If physicians were called from their office, surgical suite, or bed for every deviation, they would be forced to hover at the bedside of laboring patients. Although commendable, this practice would necessitate a very small practice for the obstetrician, and most assuredly raise the cost of maternity care.

It is critical, therefore, for the nurse to identify deviations and their severity, initiate appropriate nursing interventions, reassess, and inform the physician as necessary. Guidelines for exactly when a physician should be summoned are not listed in any textbook. Making this decision is a skill developed through experience. Two factors are weighed in the decision of whether to notify the physician immediately: (1) the degree of threat to the well-being of the mother and infant; and (2) the probability that nursing measures will alleviate the problem. For example, a nurse noting variable decelerations of the fetal heart with rapid recovery (see § 11.6 for a discussion of decelerations) might reason that rapid recovery limits compromise to the fetus and that a change in the maternal position often eliminates decelerations altogether. Awaiting the results of this intervention over a reasonable period of time is proper. On the other hand, a deceleration that plunges below 60 beats per minute, persists for more than a minute, then climbs slowly back to baseline, with the pattern repeating during the next contraction, warrants an immediate call to the physician. The danger (in this instance, oxygen supply) is severe and nursing actions may not suffice to eliminate the threat of hypoxic brain injury.

Differences of opinion over which deviations constitute threats to the mother or her fetus are as plentiful as practitioners. It is, therefore, incumbent upon the individual nurse to assess, diagnose, act, and document. Of special note is the need (or attempt) to document reports to the physician. The precise nature of the report, its time, and the physician's response must be distinctly spelled out in the nursing notes.

§ 11.5 Monitoring the Mother

A primary function of labor and delivery nurses is to monitor the signs of the progress and status of the mother and fetus. Although highly technological devices have come to the aid of the nurse for these purposes, it is almost continuous nurse-patient interaction that provides the basis for assessment.

Vital Signs

Maternal vital signs—temperature, pulse, respiration, and blood pressure—are checked frequently throughout labor. They are often early warning signs of impending complications. Pulse, respiration, and blood pressure are usually evaluated every hour, and the temperature every four hours. Deviations from the norm or significant medical history would, or course, require more frequent readings.[4] Ruptured membranes of greater than 12 hours duration is an indication for a temperature reading every two hours. **Appendix 11-2** sets out the norms for maternal vital signs, significance of deviations, and nursing actions.

Blood pressure is given special attention because of the possibility of pre-eclampsia, a form of pregnancy-induced hypertension. The nurse should note a blood pressure greater than 140/90 or a diastolic (lower numeral) pressure that is elevated more than 15 points above early pregnancy readings. The nurse should check for the presence of protein in the urine by means of a dipstick test, for the presence of edema not confined to the maternal ankle, and for hyperactivity of the deep-tendon reflexes (usually the knee jerk). The mother should also be questioned concerning persistent frontal headache and epigastric pain. The presence of one or more of these symptoms, coupled with a second elevated blood pressure, should be reported to the physician. See **Chapter 4.**

Contraction Patterns

Uterine contractions may be monitored externally, either manually or electronically, and internally by means of an electronic pressure gauge. The contraction pattern consists of three elements: frequency, duration, and intensity.

To manually assess contractions, the nurse places the fingertips on the maternal abdomen over the fundal (top) portion of the uterus. The nurse will be able to palpate the gathering or tightening of the uterine muscle under the fingers, the strength or firmness at its peak, and the return to a relaxed state. Noting the time between the onset of one contraction to the onset of another gives the *frequency.* *Duration* is calculated as the average time from beginning to end of each

---

[4] Cohen at 666–67; G.F. Butnarescu & D.M. Tillotson, Maternity Nursing: Theory to Practice 328–29 (1983).

contraction. *Intensity* is tested by attempting to indent the muscle with the fingers. A strong contraction is unindentable, much like the bicep of a body-builder in full flex. Palpation of four to six contractions at least hourly is required for a meaningful estimation of the contraction pattern.[5]

Electronically, the external tocodynamometer (toco) on the direct intrauterine pressure catheter may be utilized to monitor contractions. The external toco is usually applied by the nurse, who must take care to place it appropriately on the uterine fundus. Checking that the toco is accurately recording contractions is done by intermittent manual palpation and comparison of these findings with those displayed on the monitor strip. An improperly placed toco may exaggerate or underestimate the intensity and duration of a contraction, thus presenting inaccurate data for management evaluation.

The intrauterine pressure catheter consists of a small, water-filled tube placed in the uterus, alongside the fetus, and attached to the pressure gauge of the fetal monitor. Pressure exerted on the column of water in the tube by the force of a uterine contraction is measured by the pressure gauge in millimeters of mercury and recorded on the graph. The nurse is typically responsible for:

1. Setting up and attaching the pressure gauge
2. Maintaining an air-free and patent column of water next to the baby
3. Testing the graphing device to ascertain whether the recorded pressures are accurate (the resting tone, or completely relaxed stage of the uterine muscle is indicated as the baseline of the graph).

The critical responsibility is to recognize deviant patterns. Normal uterine pattern is a regular rhythm of contractions, gradually increasing in force and frequency, but with adequate resting time between contractions to allow resumption of uteroplacental perfusion, hence fetal oxygenation. During normal labor, the frequency ranges from about every 10 minutes in early labor to every two minutes during peak activity. Likewise, duration increases from 30 to 90 seconds. Intensity, characterized as mild to strong on palpation, is measured from 20 to 60 mm Hg with the internal device.[6]

The normal pattern of contractions every two to four minutes is the most efficient for progress in labor. Infrequent mild contractions increase the length of labor. Abnormal patterns reduce the efficiency of labor and fetal oxygen supply.

Nursing measures for infrequent contractions might include encouraging the patient to ambulate or to increase the rate of oxytocin infusion, if used, within

---

[5] R.A. Knuppel & J.E. Drukker, High-Risk Pregnancy: A Team Approach 478–79 (1993); H.A. Pritchard & P.C. MacDonald, Williams Obstetrics 664–67 (16th ed. 1980).

[6] Cohen at 610–15; G.F. Butnarescu & D.M. Tillotson, Maternity Nursing; Theory to Practice 325 (1983).

the guidelines of the medical orders. A poor contraction pattern, coupled with failure to progress in labor, should be reported to the physician.

Interventions for abnormal patterns consist of measures to increase the resting time of the uterus, such as discontinuing or decreasing any infusion rate of oxytocin, if used, or repositioning the mother onto her side. Persistent abnormal patterns, especially coupled with failure to progress or abnormalities of the fetal heart rate, should be reported.

Friedman Labor Curve

Assessment of what constitutes normal progress in labor has been the object of much research and controversy. Disagreement is widespread as to when the progress (usually the lack of progress) is such that intervention is required. Whether the facilitation of a more rapid labor is for the well-being of the mother and her fetus or for convenience of the health care provider can be at issue. The basis of the problem is that human labor seems to be as individual as the mother herself, and one mother may experience entirely different labor patterns with each of her pregnancies.

Perhaps the most widely accepted guideline for the "normal" progression of labor is that developed by Dr. Emanuel Friedman.[7] The Friedman Labor Curve is a graphic depiction of the average changes in cervical dilation and fetal descent (station) over time. Important differences in labor patterns between nulliparas (no prior births) and multiparas (at least one prior birth) are addressed by assigning different time expectations for these categories.

The nurse should be aware of expected progress and report deviations. Guidelines are not absolute, but it is critical to advise the physician of deviations.

§ 11.6   Monitoring The Fetus

Due to the location of the fetus within the maternal uterus, the most frequently utilized methods of medical monitoring cannot be used. Direct palpation, visualization, and listening are modes of data collection denied to those caring for the intrauterine life. Although such signs as excessive or decreased fetal movement and the presence of meconium in the amniotic fluid give clues to fetal well-being, currently the only valuable indicator is the pattern of the fetal heart rate. The ability of an individual fetus to cope with the stresses of labor, the pressure variants, and the fluctuations in oxygen supply have all been found to be reflected in these identifiable patterns.

---

[7] E.A. Friedman, Labor Clinical Evaluation and Management (2d ed. 1978).

Methods

Like monitoring uterine contractions, the health care provider has several methods available to monitor the fetal heart rate: manual or electronic, external or internal. Controversy rages over the pros and cons of each.

Manual auscultation of the fetal heart rate (FHR) with a fetal stethoscope placed on the maternal abdomen by trained personnel has been shown to produce perinatal outcomes equivalent to electronic fetal monitoring.[8] Manual, or clinical auscultation should be performed through an entire contraction, including 10 seconds into the relaxation period. The fetal heart rate should be counted every 30 minutes in early labor and every 15 minutes during the active phase. Unusual patterns, with the exception of short-term variability, can be accurately identified by a trained listener. It is usual, however, to confirm a suspected abnormal pattern by using an electronic monitoring device. Although application of the electronic monitor is generally covered by the physician's specific order or hospital policy, most facilities encourage labor nurses to apply the monitor when in doubt as to what they are hearing with the stethoscope or whenever there is a concern about fetal well-being.

Electronic fetal monitoring is accomplished by means of an ultrasonic transducer externally or an electrode placed internally (transvaginally) on the fetal presenting part. Nurses are now commonly being trained in the application of the fetal electrode. Often, internal application requires a specific order; however, many institutions allow discretionary application by the nurse, especially when noninvasive techniques have failed to elicit adequate information. Note that, with the exception of nurse-midwives and nurse practitioners, nurses generally do not perform artificial rupture of the membranes, and ruptured membranes are a prerequisite to application of the electrode. Care must be taken to avoid placing the electrode over a fontanelle or suture in the fetal head.

Placement of the external ultrasonic transducer so that a clear, uninterrupted tracing of the FHR is obtained is often easier said than done. Fetal position and movement as well as contours of the maternal abdomen and movement of the mother conspire to move the fetal heart away from a direct line to the transducer. The nurse sometimes needs to readjust the placement to obtain a meaningful tracing of the FHR.

Variability

Variability, or normal irregularities in the fetal heart rate, is an important indicator of fetal well-being. *Long-term variability* is the degree of waviness of

---

[8] R.K. Freeman & T.J. Garite, Fetal Heart Rate Monitoring 56–59 (1981); J.A. Pritchard & P.C. MacDonald, Williams Obstetrics 376–77 (16th ed. 1980).

the tracing line and runs three to five cycles per minute. *Short-term variability* involves the time elapsed between each beat of the fetal heart (thus, beat-to-beat variability).

A decrease, or flattening, of the variability pattern is often associated with a decrease in fetal oxygenation (hypoxia). Factors such as fetal sleep, certain drugs, and fetal immaturity will also affect variability.[9] On recognizing a decreased variability pattern, without other abnormal changes, that persists for greater than 15 to 20 minutes, the nurse should encourage changes in maternal position, external manual stimulation of the fetus, and, if allowed, a drink of a fluid high in glucose (for example, orange juice). Decreased variability that persists or is associated with decelerations should be reported to the physician.

Accelerations

Accelerations are transient changes above the baseline heart rate and are associated with fetal well-being. Accelerations are most commonly found in association with movement of the healthy fetus and are reassuring.[10]

Tachycardia

The normal baseline fetal heart rate (FHR) ranges between 120 and 160 beats per minute (BPM). A baseline greater than 160 BPM is considered to be tachycardia.[11] As maternal fever and infection are the cause of much fetal tachycardia, the nurse should assess the maternal temperature, pulse, hydration, duration of ruptured membranes, and presence of other infectious processes. Tachycardia between 160 and 180 BPM persisting longer than 30 minutes or a baseline greater than 180 BPM should be reported.

Bradycardia

The opposite of tachycardia is *bradycardia*. This is defined as a baseline fetal heart rate below 120 beats per minute (BPM). Bradycardia without a decrease in variability is not usually considered ominous. During the second stage, as the mother begins to push, mild bradycardia may be present.[12] Changes in maternal position, especially to the left side, may relieve the bradycardia. Persistent low baseline or any baseline less than 80 to 90 BPM should be reported.

---

[9] R.A. Knuppel & J.E. Drukker, High-Risk Pregnancy: A Team Approach 323 (2d ed. 1993).

[10] R.K. Freeman & T.J. Garite, Fetal Heart Rate Monitoring 64–65 (1981).

[11] *Id.* at 79.

[12] *Id.* at 63.

§ 11.7 —Decelerations

Decelerations are periodic changes in the fetal heart rate below the baseline. The type of deceleration, and thus its indication of fetal status, is defined according to its relation to uterine contractions.

Early Decelerations

Early decelerations are considered mirror images of the contraction: beginning, peaking, and ending with the contraction. Early decelerations are usually mild (rarely extending below 100 beats per minute) and are associated with compression of the fetal head. The pattern is benign and no intervention is indicated.[13]

Variable Decelerations

This frequent pattern varies in shape, timing, and degree. The shape of variable decelerations is a steep, rapid drop in fetal heart rate and a rapid return to baseline, a *V* shape. Because the causative factor in variable decelerations is most likely pressure on the umbilical cord, change of maternal position may alleviate the problem.[14] Severe variable decelerations consistently last longer than 45 seconds, with slow, gradual return to baseline. There may be a concomitant increase in the baseline or decrease in variability. Nursing measures for severe variables include:

1. Change maternal position
2. Discontinue oxytocin
3. Perform vaginal examination (check for cord prolapse or imminent birth)
4. Administer oxygen[15]
5. Notify physician.

Late Decelerations

A late deceleration has a late relationship with all elements of the contraction. The deceleration begins late in relation to the onset of the contraction; its lowest point is after the peak, and it returns to baseline after the completion of the contraction. The shape of the deceleration is a shallow *U*. The deceleration usually falls no more than 40 beats per minute below baseline. The cause of late decelerations is *uteroplacental insufficiency*—an inability of the placenta to

---

[13] R.K. Freeman & T.J. Garite, Fetal Heart Rate Monitoring 64 (1981).

[14] *Id* at 67.

[15] *Id.* at 69–70.

furnish adequate oxygen from its reserve to last through the impaired perfusion of blood created by a contraction.[16] The following nursing measures are aimed at increasing placental perfusion:

1. Turn mother to her left side
2. Discontinue oxytocin
3. Administer oxygen
4. Check blood pressure—increase IV flow rate if hypotensive
5. Notify physician.

The physician should be notified concerning even mild late decelerations. Late decelerations, combined with decreased variability, are usually considered ominous.

§ 11.8 Analgesic Administration

As with the administration of any medication, the nurse must be aware of correct indications and dosage, as well as any possible side or toxic effects. In labor, it is also necessary to be aware of effects on the fetus. Most narcotic analgesics have a depressive effect on the fetus, which is problematic when the infant is born at a time when the action of the drug is in force. Because many physicians order pain relief on an *as necessary* (prn) basis, the nurse's judgment in giving these medications becomes paramount. The decision may include not only the timing of administration but also selecting from a variety of prn medications and dosages. Factors such as current status in labor, parity, rapidity of progress, and any fetal problems that put the infant at higher risk (for example, prematurity or growth retardation) must be considered before administration of analgesia.

§ 11.9 Oxytocic Administration

Oxytocin is a potent natural hormone that causes the uterine muscle to contract. Synthetic oxytocics have also been developed. Oxytocin has been used to stimulate labor in its intravenous, intramuscular, or buccal (placed under the tongue) forms. Due to the unpredictable nature of the uterine response, current administration is commonly limited to the intravenous route antipartally in order to retain optimal control. In addition, an infusion pump is invariably used to guard against inadvertent overdosage.

The nurse is usually given an order to dilute the drug in an intravenous solution and begin administration at a specified low infusion rate. The rate is

---

[16] *Id.* at 95.

increased every 15 to 20 minutes by a specified increment until an adequate contraction pattern is established.

The nurse must keep special vigilance on the patient being stimulated because the uterus may react with a hyperstimulated (too frequent) pattern or a tetanic (prolonged) contraction, both of which reduce fetal oxygenation and can ultimately rupture the uterus, causing death to both mother and fetus. Electronic monitoring is indicated. Placement of an intrauterine pressure catheter is highly recommended. Upon recognition of hyperstimulation, the nurse should discontinue the oxytocin, turn the patient to her side, and notify the physician.

§ 11.10 Emergency Measures

Labor nurses must be prepared to identify emergencies and intervene appropriately until medical help arrives. Measures taken by labor nurses in more common intrapartum emergencies follow.

Antepartum Hemorrhage

The two most prevalent causes of antepartum hemorrhage are abruptio placenta and placenta previa. The nurse should gather sufficient data so that a diagnosis can be made and appropriate actions taken in preparation for the physician's arrival.

The signs of *abruptio placenta* (premature detachment of the placenta) to be noted by the nurse are vaginal bleeding (although it is possible to have no apparent bleeding), a hard, boardlike uterus, and pain. The latter are caused by entrapment of blood between the placenta and the uterine wall. Fetal heart tones should be ausculated because a true abruption is frequently quickly fatal to the infant. Blood pressure should be taken since hypertension is often an underlying cause of abruptio.

The patient's physician must be notified immediately. The nurse should consider eliciting the aid of the nearest obstetrician as well. In cases of severe abruptio, due to the rapid progression and risk of fetal death, a prompt Cesarean section performed by any available obstetrician may well be of life-saving value.

Placenta previa is caused by the abnormal implantation of the placenta over the cervix, with subsequent peeling away as the cervix begins to change. The patient usually presents with mild to severe, painless, vaginal bleeding. For severe bleeding, preparations for a Cesarean should be initiated. For all significant antepartum hemorrhage, the nurse should:

1. Replace blood volume by initiating intravenous infusions
2. Draw blood studies as ordered

3. Initiate continuous fetal monitoring
4. Not perform a vaginal examination (due to the risk of exacerbating a bleeding previa)
5. Immediately notify the physician.

Seizures and Eclampsia

Seizures of a laboring patient are generally caused by an underlying seizure disorder (for example, epilepsy) or eclampsia. *Eclampsia* is the progression of the preeclamptic triad of hypertension, proteinuria, and edema to the point of convulsion. When a patient begins a seizure, the nurse should:

1. Place a tongue blade or airway in the patient's mouth to maintain the airway and prevent tongue-biting
2. Suction the mouth to remove secretions
3. Administer oxygen
4. Protect the patient from injury (for example, falling from bed to floor)
5. Ask another person to summon a physician
6. Be prepared to administer drugs as ordered (for example, valium or magnesium sulphate)
7. Note type and duration of seizure.

Cardiopulmonary Resuscitation

Every nurse should be well versed in the steps of cardiopulmonary resuscitation (CPR). Recognizing a cardiac arrest, the nurse should immediately:

1. Have the facility's CPR team summoned
2. Clear the airway
3. Begin mouth-to-mouth resuscitation
4. Begin external cardiac massage.

Once the team has arrived, the nurse should assist as directed and notify the attending physician. The arrest of the mother results in anoxia of the fetus. Once the maternal condition is stabilized, attention should be turned to evaluation of the fetal status.

Infant Resuscitation

In the absence of the physician, or when the physician is involved with another maternal emergency, the responsibility of neonatal resuscitation can fall on the nurse. In larger facilities with level 2 and or level 3 nurseries, neonatal intensive care nurses can be called upon to assist with resuscitative measures.

The infant should be dried well and initially placed in a warm area (ideally beneath a radiant heater) in a head down position. The airway should be cleared by means of a bulb syringe, de Lee mucus trap, or wall suction. Stimulation by means of rubbing the back or genitalia or flicking the soles of the feet may be effective.

If the infant fails to respond, face-mask oxygen is given. In cases of little or no respiratory effort, positive pressure is initiated by means of a bag and mask with the infant's neck in a neutral position. Insertion of a feeding tube into the stomach is encouraged to prevent gastric distention. The nurse should recall the time and nature of medication prior to birth. The order to administer a narcotic antagonist (for example, Narcan) is appropriate only when narcotic analgesia is very likely to be present in the fetal circulation.

Notation of bradycardia in the infant (less than 60 heart beats per minute) once respirations are established requires external cardiac massage. Two fingers and a ratio of three compressions to each ventilation with the bag and mask is appropriate.

After the physician has arrived, the nurse should be prepared to assist with endotracheal intubation if previous measures have failed. Once the tube has been placed, the nurse assists with attachment of the positive pressure oxygen bag, maintaining appropriate ventilatory and cardiac massage efforts, ausculation for proper placement of tube, monitoring of heart rate, and securing the position of the tube with tape. Administration of emergency medications may be ordered.[17]

After the infant has been stabilized, careful documentation of all resuscitative efforts is important. Appropriate preparations for transfer of the infant, to include continuous ventilation, should be made.

§ 11.11   —Postpartum Hemorrhage

Postpartum hemorrhage is usually caused by failure of the uterus to adequately contract to close off blood vessels left open after birth of the placenta (atony) or by unrepaired lacerations of the birth canal. Upon noting heavier than normal postpartum bleeding, the nurse should first suspect uterine atony. Measures to correct uterine relaxation include:

1. Massage the uterus and extrude any clots
2. Increase infusion rate of any intravenous oxytocin
3. Empty maternal bladder

---

[17] R.K. Freeman & T.J. Garite, Fetal Heart Rate Monitoring 68–69 (1981).

4. Obtain blood pressure and pulse readings
5. Inform physician if measures are unsuccessful or blood loss is extreme.

The existence of a firm, well-contracted uterus points to a vaginal or cervical laceration as the causative factor of continued bleeding. The physician should be summoned to reexamine the birth canal and suture any lacerations as needed.

§ 11.12 —Delivery by the Nurse

When labor progresses with such rapidity that it is apparent that no physician will be in attendance, the nurse must be prepared to provide for a safe birth. Every labor suite should have an emergency pack of necessary equipment. The nurse gathers the equipment, instructs another person to contact the physician, and remains with the patient. Instilling the mother with confidence and a sense of control are perhaps the most important elements of conducting a birth, since it is the mother who, in fact, delivers her child.

The nurse should be aware of the mechanisms of normal birth and facilitate the maternal efforts only when necessary, applying gentle pressure to the emerging head to control a gradual birth and prevent trauma associated with rapid delivery. The performance of an episiotomy is usually not indicated; however, the preparation of the nurse and hospital policy will guide the decision.

Once the head is born, the mouth and nose are suctioned for secretions and the neck area checked for presence of the cord around the neck. Gentle downward pressure on the infant's head facilitates the birth of the shoulders, and with a lift upward the rest of the body will be born. The unskilled birth attendant should be aware that the danger of dropping a slippery infant is absent if the mother is kept in bed or the obstetrical delivery table is not broken (that is, the table is not removed from under the mother's buttocks and legs).

After birth, the cord may be doubly clamped and cut between the clamps if sterile equipment is available. The nurse should keep a watchful eye for maternal bleeding. Unless there is bleeding or the nurse is certain concerning placental separation, there is no need to manipulate or hurry delivery of the placenta.

§ 11.13 High-Risk Patients

The patient at high risk for maternal or fetal complications often requires additional nursing care during labor. Care should be taken by the person making patient assignments that the nurse assigned to a high-risk patient possesses the requisite skill to recognize and deal with the complications inherent in various high-risk conditions.

Previous Cesarean Section

Not long ago, once a patient delivered via Cesarean section, subsequent deliveries had to be Cesareans too. However, with widespread utilization of lower-segment uterine incisions for Cesareans, mothers may choose a vaginal birth after Cesarean (VBAC) for subsequent deliveries. The danger of allowing vaginal birth has been the risk of uterine rupture of the old uterine scar, causing massive hemorrhage with maternal and fetal deaths.

Historically, Cesarean sections were performed through a vertical incision high in the uterine fundus, the so-called classical incision. This method remains common in undeveloped countries. In the United States, Europe, and most other developed nations, uterine incisions are routinely done in the less vascular, noncontractile tissues of the lower segment. The incision can be vertical or horizontal. Because of an increased chance that a vertical incision will extend into the upper segment and also because it heals less optimally, many physicians restrict VBAC to patients with horizontal, lower segment scars. Note that the position of the external abdominal scar is not an indication of the placement of the uterine incision.

The nurse's responsibility includes eliciting information concerning the patient's uterine scar and plans for VBAC or repeat Cesarean. The physician should be notified immediately of the arrival of a previous Cesarean patient in active labor. If VBAC is an option, the nurse monitors the contraction pattern especially closely. Hyperstimulation in the previously scarred uterus may be a direct cause of dehiscence (separation) and rupture (extrusion of the uterine contents into the abdominal cavity). A hyperstimulated pattern or the patient's complaint of a burning or searing abdominal pain should be reported.

Multiple Gestation

Multifetal pregnancies, typically twins, may not have been identified prior to the patient's admission in labor. During initial assessment, the nurse may note a fundal height greater in proportion to gestational age, fetal movement in all quadrants, palpation of two fetal heads, and auscultation of two distinct heart beats. A suspicion of multifetal pregnancy should be reported to the physician for definitive diagnosis.

Once labor has begun, it is important to ascertain the presentation of both infants. Often an ultrasound or X ray is indicated. Abnormal presentations and irregular contours of multiple infants should alert the nurse to the greater risk of cord prolapse when membranes rupture. An immediate vaginal exam should be performed by the nurse on membrane rupture. If the cord is palpated, the nurse should keep a hand in the vagina, instruct the patient to turn to a knee-chest position, and attempt to elevate the fetal head off the cord. At no time should the nurse remove the hand from the vagina. The assistance of a physician should be called for immediately. Often it is required that the nurse continue elevating the fetal head as a Cesarean section is begun until such time as the surgeon reaches for the infant.

During labor the nurse must monitor both fetuses—often using two fetal monitors—and be alert for signs of dysfunctional labor and hypertension, both of which have an increased incidence in multiple gestations.

In the delivery room, extra nursing responsibilities are created by an additional infant. Auscultation of fetal heart rates is important, especially for the second twin born. Following the first twin's delivery, the obstetrician may ask the nurse to assist by gently guiding the second twin toward the pelvis externally. Preparations to receive two infants must be made. Of special importance is the accurate identification of each twin and cord bloods. If twins are not discovered until the time of birth, there is a need to summon additional help.

Preeclampsia

Preeclampsia is defined as the presence of hypertension during pregnancy, accompanied by proteinuria, edema, or both. Although the disease has no known etiology, it has been well documented since the mid-1700s. The dangers of preeclampsia are the inherent complications of seizure, coma, and death for mother and fetus. Less drastic but severe complications include detachment of the retina and kidney damage.

The only cure[18] for preeclampsia is delivery. At best, treatment is aimed at the symptoms and prevention of convulsions. Various drugs and drug combinations have been used over the years with varying success.

Because preeclampsia often initially presents during labor, the nurse must be aware of its signs and symptoms. Two blood pressure readings of greater than 140 over 90 should be reported. A systolic (upper number) reading 30 points above, or a dyastolic (lower number) reading 15 points above the early pregnancy readings should be reported. Upon a finding of hypertension, the nurse should look for other signs of preeclampsia by checking for edema, checking the knee-jerk for hyperflexia, and checking the urine for more than a trace of proteinuria. The patient should be questioned concerning the presence of frontal headache, epigastric pain, and visual disturbance. Any positive finding should be reported.

A patient with moderate to severe preeclampsia should receive constant nursing care if possible. Frequent taking of vital signs, including blood pressure every 15 minutes, is often needed. In addition, monitoring the potent drugs administered is essential. The antihypertensive of choice is hydralazine hydrochloride, a potent vasodilator administered as IV boluses, or continuous IV infusion. Magnesium sulfate is the agent of choice of prevention. When given intravenously, it should be infused by means of a pump for control of eclamptic seizures. Before administration of the magnesium sulfate or at regular intervals

---

[18] S.B. Olds et al., Obstetric Nursing 782–87 (1980).

during IV infusion, reflexes are checked and respiration monitored every 15 minutes. Absence of reflexes are noted and reported. Magnesium levels are monitored every 6 to 8 hours, the therapeutic range being 4 to 7 meg/l. Calcium gluconate should be available at all times as an antidote to magnesium toxicity.

As decreased urine output can be a side effect of magnesium sulfate, a strict record of output is maintained. A Foley catheter with uremeter is indicated for accuracy. Fluid intake record is equally important. Typically, several IV infusions may be running simultaneously. The risk of fluid overload is increased and the effects on hypertensive patients are greater.

Additional responsibilities include close scrutiny of fetal well-being because of the higher risk of fetal distress. Laboratory tests are ordered with frequency and need to be followed promptly. Finally, the nurse should work to maintain a quiet, calm atmosphere, preferably in a darkened room to prevent overstimulation. Precautions and equipment should be available in the event of eclamptic seizure. See § **11.10.**

Diabetes

Depending on the classification of diabetes, pregnancy and birth may become life-threatening to both mother and infant. The nurse's role in the care of the laboring diabetic is to ensure strict adherence to ordered intravenous fluid and insulin dosages. Frequent monitoring of blood glucose levels is necessary. The nurse should be alert for signs of diabetic or insulin coma. Tachycardia, hunger, weakness, pallor, and sweating should be reported.

Because the infant of an uncontrolled diabetic pregnancy is often unusually large, the nurse should carefully monitor labor progress, especially fetal descent, for indications of cephalopelvic disproportion. There is a greater risk for shoulder dystocia (see **Chapter 13**) and other birth trauma more common in large for gestational age infants. Hypoglycemia should also be anticipated and intravenous glucose therapy for the infant should be readily available.

§ 11.14   Patient Advocacy

The issue of patient advocacy may not be addressed in hospital policy manuals or even in nursing schools. It is, however, a responsibility of the nurse to attempt to protect a woman and her fetus from harm. Such harm may not be caused by the intrinsic factors of the individual patient, but rather by iatrogenesis.

It is incumbent upon the nurse to advise patients of their right to refuse treatment. The nurse should be prepared to recognize and question potentially harmful or incorrect orders. If a physician persists in the order of an action the nurse is convinced will be harmful, the nurse should refuse to perform the action, immediately inform the supervisor, and document all conversations. There are many gray areas in obstetrical care; however, nurses are obligated to follow the standard of professional conduct as outlined in state nurse practice acts and the dictates of their consciences and knowledge in order to protect patients.

Similarly, protection of patients from inappropriate behaviors of physicians, and other hospital personnel is important. If incapacitation of any health care provider from alcohol, drugs, or other causes is suspected, the nurse should notify a supervisor. In the case of a physician, especially in an emergency, the physician's partner or the chief of the department may need to be summoned. The nurse faces a serious dilemma under such circumstances. Fear of job loss or repercussions may be an issue. However, more is required of nurses than simply to do no harm. As patient advocates, it is a nurse's responsibility to protect patients and their children from harm by others. Quality nursing care includes appropriate assessment and nursing interventions, communication and collaboration with other care providers, and constant vigilance to maintain a safe environment. Nurses provide a vital link between patients and doctors—a link so precious in maternal-fetal health care that the well-being of future generations literally depends on it. While risks are inherent in obstetrical nursing practice, the rewards of association with the gift of life are great.

§ 11.15 Appendix 11–1: Nurse's Sample Admission Form

Physician/Nurse Midwife _____

Admission Date _____ Time _____ via: stretcher/ambulatory/W.C.

Age _____ Last Menstrual _____ Period   Estimated Date of _____ Confinement   Gestational _____ Age

Gravida _____ Term _____ Premature _____ Abortions _____ Living _____

Onset of Labor _____ Rupture of Membranes: Time _____ Color _____

Bleeding _____ Temp. _____ Pulse _____ Resp _____ BP _____ FHR _____

Last meal: Time _____ light _____ heavy _____

Allergies: Medications _____ Food/Substances _____

Current Medications _____

Past Medical/Obstetrical History: _____

Past Surgical History: _____

Present Pregnancy Complications _____

Abdominal Palpation: Fundal Height _____ Presentation _____

Uterine Contractions: Frequency _____ Duration _____ Quality _____

Vaginal Examination:

Dilitation _____ Effacement _____ Station _____ Position _____

Birth Plans: _____

Prenatal classes: Yes _____ No _____ Anesthesia Planned _____

Breast feeding: Yes _____ No _____

Pediatrician: _____

Comments: _____

Patient's Name _____

Hospital Number _____ Signature of Admitting Nurse _____

§ 11.16 Appendix 11–2: Intrapartal Physical Assessment Guide: First Stage of Labor

Intrapartal Physical Assessment Guide: First Stage of Labor

Assess	Normal Findings	Deviations and Possible Causes	Nursing Interventions
Vital signs Blood pressure	90–140/60–90	High blood pressure (essential hypertension, preeclampsia, renal disease, apprehension or anxiety)	Evaluate history of preexisting disorders and check for presence of other signs of preeclampsia
Pulse	60–90 beats/min	Increased pulse rate (excitement or anxiety, cardiac disorders)	Evaluate cause. Report to physician.

Assess	Normal Findings	Deviations and Possible Causes	Nursing Interventions
Respirations	16–24/min (or pulse rate divided by 4)	Marked tachypnea (respiratory disease)	Report to physician (Note: Do not assess respirations during a uterine contraction.)
Temperature	36.2–37.6C (98–99.6F)	Elevated temperature (infection, dehydration)	Assess for other signs of infection or dehydration.

Source: Adapted from *Obstetrical Nursing* by Olds, et al. Copyright © 1980 by Addison-Wesley Publishing Company. Reprinted by permission.

CHAPTER 12

NURSE-MIDWIFERY PRACTICE

Diane Hodgman, C.N.M., M.S.N.

Christine Whelan Knapp, C.N.M., M.S.

§ 12.1 History in the United States

In the early 1900s in response to a high incidence of infant mortality, Congress legislated the Sheppard-Towner Act, which provided monies for midwifery training. Nurse-midwifery practice began in the United States in 1925 with British midwives brought to Kentucky to care for the rural population. The Lobestine Midwifery School in New York, started in 1932, was the first educational program for nurse-midwives in the United States. The American College of Nurse-Midwives (ACNM), the professional organization for nurse-midwives, was incorporated in 1955. Located in Washington, D.C., the ACNM defines, sets standards for and certifies nurse-midwives in this country.[1] A joint statement written in 1971 and reaffirmed in 1994 by both the

---

[1] H. Varney, Nurse-Midwifery, 8–21, (2d. ed., 1987).

ACNM and the American College of Obstetricians and Gynecologists (ACOG) defined practice relations between the two organizations and solidified the practice of nurse-midwifery in the United States. (See **Appendix 12–1** in **§ 12.5.**)

Today there are over 5,000 nurse-midwives in the United States and its territories. In 1992 certified nurse-midwives (CNMs) attended 185,000 births. Nearly ten percent of births in this country will be attended by a nurse-midwife by the year 2000. Currently there are 43 nurse-midwifery educational programs in this country.[2]

A definition of CNM is as follows: "A Certified Nurse-Midwife is an individual educated in the two disciplines of nursing and midwifery, who possesses evidence of certification according to the requirements of the American College of Nurse-Midwives.[3]

§ 12.2   Credentialing

In the United States, nurse-midwifery programs have to be affiliated with institutions of higher learning. A program can offer a certificate in midwifery or a master's or doctoral degree.

In addition, there are three precertificate programs for registered nurses to gain the education necessary to perform the core competencies for basic nurse-midwifery practice as defined by the ACNM. This route allows for the education of registered nurses (RNs) who practice as professional midwives and the credentialing of foreign trained nurse-midwives. Students in this type of program must be RNs in the United States or its territories and show that they are recognized as midwives in their country or state. There are also accelerated programs that enable nonnurses with bachelor's degrees in other fields to obtain an RN and a master's degree in nurse-midwifery. After graduation, the student is eligible to take the National Certification Examination given by the ACNM. Successful passage enables the student to use the professional initials CNM.[4] The CNM then applies to a state licensing agency to obtain a license to practice nurse-midwifery. This process can take a myriad of avenues.

Depending on the state, nurse-midwives are regulated by the board of nursing, the board of medicine, the department of public health, or some similar body. Each state has specific laws and regulations regarding CNM practice. These can

---

[2] 26 Quickening 2 (Mar./Apr. 1995).

[3] American College of Nurse-Midwives, 818 Connecticut Ave. NW, Ste. 900, Washington, DC 20006 (Position Statement 1978, 1992).

[4] L.E. Slattery & H.V. Burst, *ACNM Accredited and Preaccredited Nurse-midwifery Education Programs, Program Information,* 40 J. Nurse Midwifery 349–365 (July/Aug. 1995).

be found in general statutes, such as public health laws, or in specific legislation, such as a nurse practice act.

Thirty-six states currently allow nurse-midwives to have prescriptive drug privileges.[5] CNMs usually apply to various institutions for privileges and are subject to their bylaws. Written practice protocols serve as guidelines for care provided by CNMs.[6]

§ 12.3 Practice

The ACNM defines nurse-midwifery practice, consultation, collaboration, and referral. (See **Appendix 12–2** in **§ 12.6.**)

CNMs provide comprehensive care including histories, physical examinations, appropriate testing, counseling, and teaching. In labor and delivery, nurse-midwives manage labor and birth. They detect deviations from normal and provide interventions. Nurse-midwifery care and management may continue in situations where some degree of abnormality exists. Practice protocols must outline what the nurse-midwifery functions can be. Nurse-midwives conduct spontaneous vaginal deliveries, perform and repair episiotomies, repair lacerations, administer local and pudendal anesthesia, and provide immediate evaluation and care of newborns. CNMs are skilled in emergency management of many situations, such as shoulder dystocia, postpartum hemorrhage, and immediate care of unstable newborns while awaiting arrival of the backup or collaborating physicians.

In some locales CNMs have expanded their role into areas such as ultrasonagraphy, circumcision, colposcopy, use of vacuum extraction, low forceps delivery, and external version.[7] Practice in these and other areas continues to evolve. The ACNM has guidelines for incorporation of new procedures into nurse-midwifery practice. See **Appendix 12-3** in **§ 12.7.** The ACNM also encourages peer review of practices and has a continuing competency assessment program. The continuing competency assessment program is mandated by the ACNM for "all CNM's in clinical practice or whose employment is based on knowledge of nurse-midwifery practice. It is designed to demonstrate CNM competency in practice to colleagues, consumers, and other professionals."[8]

---

[5] V. Lops, L. Dixon & L. Hunter, *The Evolving Practice of Nurse Midwifery* 1 Adv. Prac. Nurs. Q. 29–36 (1995).

[6] D. Williams, *Credentialing Certified Nurse-Midwives,* 39 J. Nurse Midwifery, 261 (July/Aug. 1994).

[7] M. Avery & G. DelGiudive, *High-Tech Skills in Low-Tech Hands,* 38 J. Nurse Midwifery 9S–17S (Mar./Apr. 1993).

[8] ACNM Member Information Continuing Competency Assessment Program (Apr. 1992).

§ 12.4   Current Issues

As previously noted, nurse-midwifery practice varies widely according to locale. Issues that continue to be at the forefront are Medicaid reimbursement and restraint of trade. In some states, Medicaid reimbursement is at a much lower rate for CNMs than for physicians. Also, many hospitals have obstructed CNMs from obtaining independent privileges. The ACNM has been very active in addressing these issues.

In Washington state, according to the Board of Registered Nursing, as of January 1, 1995, nurse-midwives must have a master's degree in nursing or a related health care field in order to become licensed as an Advanced Registered Nurse Practitioner (ARNP). The ACNM is proceeding with a judicial review of the board's action.[9]

The ACNM has recently published *Nurse-Midwifery Today: A Handbook of State Legislation*. This publication notes statutory and regulatory provisions pertaining to the practice of nurse-midwifery in the United States.

§ 12.5   Appendix 12–1: Joint Statement of Practice Relations Between Obstetrician/Gynecologists and Certified Nurse-Midwives (Reaffirmed 1994)

It is critical that obstetrician/gynecologists and Certified Nurse-Midwives have a clear understanding of their individual collaborative and interdependent responsibilities. As agreed upon in previous Joint Statements by the American College of Nurse-Midwives, the American College of Obstetricians and Gynecologists, the maternity care team should be directed by a qualified obstetrician/gynecologist. The American College of Obstetricians and Gynecologists and the American College of Nurse-Midwives believe that the appropriate practice of the Certified Nurse-Midwife includes the participation and involvement of the obstetrician/gynecologist as mutually agreed upon in written medical guidelines/protocols. The American College of Obstetricians and Gynecologists and the American College of Nurse-Midwives also believe that the obstetrician/gynecologist should be responsive to the desire of Certified Nurse-Midwives for the participation and involvement of the obstetrician/gynecologist. The following principles represent a joint statement of the American College of Obstetricians and Gynecologists and the American College of Nurse-Midwives and are recommended for consideration in all practice relationships and agreements.

1. Clinical practice relationship between the obstetrician/gynecologist and the Certified Nurse-Midwife should provide for:
    a. Mutually agreed upon written medical guidelines/protocols for clinical practice which define the individual and shared responsibilities of

---

[9] 26 Quickening 1, 15 (May/June 1995).

the Certified Nurse-Midwife and the obstetrician/gynecologist in the delivery of health care services.

   b. Mutually agreed upon written medical guideline/protocols for on-going communication which provide for and define appropriate consultation between the obstetrician/gynecologist and the Certified Nurse-Midwife.

   c. Informed consent about the involvement of the obstetrician/gynecologist, Certified Nurse-Midwife, and other health care providers in the services offered.

   d. Periodic and joint evaluation of the services rendered, *e.g.,* chart review, case review, patient evaluation, review of outcome statistics.

   e. Periodic and joint review and updating of the written medical guidelines/protocols.

2. Quality of care is enhanced by the interdependent practice of the obstetrician/gynecologist and Certified Nurse-Midwife working in a relationship of mutual respect, trust and professional responsibility. This does not necessarily imply the physical presence of the physician when care is being given by the Certified Nurse-Midwife.

3. Administrative relationships, including employment agreements, reimbursement mechanisms, and corporate structures, should be mutually agreed upon by the participating parties.

4. Access to practice within the hospital setting for the obstetrician/gynecologist and Certified Nurse-Midwife who have a practice relationship in concurrence with these principles is strongly urged by the respective professional organizations.

The American College of Obstetricians and Gynecologists and the American College of Nurse-Midwives strongly urge the implementation of these principles in all practice relationships between obstetrician/gynecologists and Certified Nurse-Midwives, and consider the preceding an ideal model of practice.[10]

§ 12.6 Appendix 12–2: Collaborative Management in Nurse-Midwifery Practice for Medical, Gynecological, and Obstetrical Conditions

Clinical Practice Statement

Nurse-midwifery practice is the independent management of women's health care, focusing on pregnancy, childbirth, the postpartum period, care of the

---

[10] American College of Obstetricians and Gynecologists: Joint Statement of Practice Relations Between Obstetrician/Gynocologists and Certified Nurse-Midwives. Washington, DC, ACOG (reaffirmed 1994). Reprinted with permission.

newborn, and the family planning and gynecological needs of women. The certified nurse-midwife practices within a health care system that provides for consultation, collaborative management or referral as indicated by the health status of the client. Certified nurse-midwives practice in accord with the current *Standards for the Practice of Nurse-Midwifery,* as defined by the American College of Nurse-Midwives.

Nurse-midwifery care is primarily intended for healthy women. However, when women experience medical, gynecological and/or obstetrical complications, the certified nurse-midwife can continue to be instrumental in their care.

This collaboration (co-management) provides for the following patterns of care for the high-risk client:

1. *Consultation* is the process whereby a certified nurse-midwife, who maintains primary management responsibility for the woman's care, seeks the advice or opinion of a physician or another member of the health care team.

2. *Collaboration* is the process whereby a certified nurse-midwife and physician jointly manage the care of a woman or newborn who has become medically, gynecologically or obstetrically complicated. The scope of collaboration may encompass the physical care of the client, including delivery, by the certified nurse-midwife, according to a mutually agreed-upon plan of care. When the physician must assume a dominant role in the care of the client due to increased risk status, the certified nurse-midwife may continue to participate in physical care, counseling guidance, teaching and support. Effective communication between the certified nurse-midwife and physician is essential for ongoing collaborative management.

3. *Referral* is the process by which the certified nurse-midwife directs the client to a physician or another health care professional for management of a particular problem or aspect of the client's care.[11]

§ 12.7   Appendix 12–3: Guidelines for the Incorporation of New Procedures into Nurse-Midwifery Practice

Nurse-Midwifery practice will continue to evolve, depending on the needs of the client, the need of the site, the expectations of the institution, and the nurse-midwife's desire to improve care to women and their families. Procedures incorporated into the practice of nurse-midwifery should be in concert with the **Philosophy of the American College of Nurse-Midwives** and the *Standards*

---

[11] Approved by the American College of Nurse-Midwives' Board of Directors, July 17, 1992. Reprinted with permission of ACNM.

for the Practice of Nurse-Midwifery of the American College of Nurse-Midwives (ACNM) and should not conflict with any current clinical practice statements of the ACNM.

While the ACNM does not approve or disapprove the incorporation of new clinical procedures into nurse-midwifery practice, the following guidelines were developed by the Clinical Practice Committee and approved by the Board of Directors to assist the nurse-midwife in expanding clinical practice:

1. Identify need for the procedure, taking into consideration:
   a) consumer demand
   b) safety considerations
   c) institutional request
   d) availability of qualified personnel
   e) interest of nurse-midwives
2. Cite relevant statutes/documents that would constrain or support incorporation of the procedure, including:
   a) statutes and regulations
   b) institutional bylaws
   c) legal opinions
3. Evaluate procedure as a nurse-midwifery function, including:
   a) relevant literature
   b) use by other nurse-midwives
   c) risks/benefits
   d) management of complications
4. Develop process for educating nurse-midwives to perform this procedure, using:
   a) bibliography
   b) formal study
   c) supervised practice
   d) protocols
   e) evaluation of learning
5. Evaluate use of procedure, documenting:
   a) outcome statistics
   b) satisfaction with procedure
      —consumer
      —institution
      —nurse-midwifery practice
   c) maintenance of competency

6.   Any new procedure incorporated into nurse-midwifery practice will be done according to the "Guidelines for the Incorporation of New Procedures into Nurse-Midwifery Practice" as outlined in the *Standards for the Practice of Nurse-Midwifery* and reported on the form provided by the American College of Nurse-Midwives. The completed form shall be mailed to the ACNM for reporting purposes. Supporting documents, as outlined in the "Guidelines," should be placed with the written policies of the nurse-midwifery practice/service.[12]

---

[12] 1987; amended Nov. 1992. Reprinted with permission of ACNM.

CHAPTER 13

TWO SPECIAL MEDICOLEGAL ISSUES: PLACENTAL PATHOLOGY AND SHOULDER DYSTOCIA

Michael D. Volk

§ 13.1   Introduction

This chapter discusses two special medicolegal problems that are important today. The first is the discipline of placental pathology. The second is the problem of shoulder dystocia when it is encountered during delivery with a resulting permanent brachial plexus palsy to the newborn. The material is not meant to be all-inclusive, but an introduction to these two special medicolegal problems.

PLACENTAL PATHOLOGY

§ 13.2   Introduction to Placental Pathology

A diseased foetus without its placenta is an imperfect specimen, and a description of a foetal malady, unless accompanied by a notice of the placental condition, is incomplete. Deductions drawn from such a case cannot be considered as conclusive, for in the missing placenta or cord may have existed the cause of the disease or death. During intrauterine life the foetus, the membranes, the cord and the placenta form an organic whole, and disease of any part must react upon and affect the others.[1]

The discipline of *placental pathology* is the pathological study of the placenta, after delivery of the fetus, in the laboratory.

The fetus cannot live without the placenta—it allows the fetus to survive by serving the metabolic needs of the fetus, including respiration, nourishment, and excretion.[2] Damage or compromise to the fetus depends on the following factors:

1.   Severity of the insult to the placenta

2.   Adequacy of residual placental function

3.   Time remaining in utero.[3]

---

[1] J.E. Ballantyne, Manual of Antenatal Pathology and Hygiene: The Embryo (1904).

[2] J.M. Lage, M.D., *The Placenta, in* Pathology in Gynecology and Obstetrics 448 (1994).

[3] *Id.*

Placental pathologists generally believe that the placenta has recorded in its tissues a "diary" of certain intrauterine events that can sometimes be known by pathological inspection and evaluation. However, we must remember that the placental pathologist does not have the opportunity to see the happenings in vivo, but must attempt to draw conclusions sometimes weeks or months after the event. Some placental pathologists believe it is their calling to attempt to protect their obstetrical brothers and sisters from claims against them and have a bias in favor of the health care professional. This bias can cause them to attempt to stretch the science of placental pathology to assist a health care provider. The important debate for the medicolegal discipline is to what extent there is a recording of intrauterine events, whether the diary can be opened and translated in a given case, and how valid the medical translation is.

§ 13.3 A Brief History of Placental Pathology

The knowledge of the placenta, or afterbirth, in early times was obviously very imperfect. One of the earliest attempts to learn more about this organ came from drawings by illustrators, among them Andreas Vesalius (1514–1564).[4] In Vesalius' first edition to his work that was published in 1543, he depicted the annular carnine placenta as an attachment to the human fetus. He later corrected this in his second edition, published in 1555.[5] The Greeks labeled the afterbirth the chorion, which means "little gut." The afterbirth was probably named placenta by Gabriele de Falloppio (1523–1562), whose name is also the origin of the term fallopian tubes.[6]

The first scientific, thorough description of the placenta was recorded in 1669 by a Dutchman, Nicolas Hoboken (1632–1678), especially with regards to the vascular properties of the placenta.[7]

Reinier de Graaf (1641–1673), also Dutch, probably drew the most concise and up-to-date medical illustrations of his time, including those of the placenta.[8]

A physician from Estonia, Karl Ernst von Baer (1792–1876), further advanced the knowledge and study of placental pathology. His placental pathology book was dedicated to an East Prussian physician who believed that the causes of many fetal abnormalities resulted from the custom at that time of women wearing tight corsets! Von Baer investigated the possible connection between maternal and fetal bloodstreams and proved, at least in dog studies, that the two are separate. He was not able to obtain sufficient numbers of placentas

---

[4] K. Benirschke, *The Placenta in the Context of History and Modern Medical Practice,* 115 Arch. Pathol. Lab. Med. 663 (July 1991).

[5] *Id.*

[6] *Id.*

[7] *Id.* at 664.

[8] *Id.*

to study, ran out of funds, and for the rest of his life studied physical geography in Russia.[9]

An anatomy professor from Vienna, Austria published an atlas of the human placenta that included 160 color injection studies.[10]

The science of placental pathology progressed fairly rapidly after these trail-blazers. A professor of anatomy, Otto Grosser (1873–1951), produced a seminal work that included the "Grosser Classification," which deals with the comparative depth of placental invasion. Starting in the 1940s, the pathology and obstetrics team of Hertig and Rock further advanced the study.[11]

§ 13.4   Textbooks

Several placental pathology textbooks are available at this time. Some of these textbooks are set out below:

1. *Pathology in Gynecology and Obstetrics,* by Claude Gompel, M.D. & Steven G. Silverberg, M.D. (1994)
2. *Textbook of Fetal and Perinatal Pathology,* by Jonathan S. Wigglesworth, M.D. & Don B. Singer, M.D. (1991)
3. *Fetal and Neonatal Pathology,* edited by Jean W. Keeling, M.D. (1993)
4. *Disorders of the Placenta, Fetus, and Neonate: Diagnosis and Clinical Significance,* by Richard L. Naeye, M.D. (1992)
5. *Pathology of the Placenta,* by EVDK Perrin, M.D. (1984).

§ 13.5   Journals

Some journals that have placental pathology articles are set out below:

1. *Placenta*
2. *Archives of Pathological and Laboratory Medicine*
3. *Journal of the American Medical Association*
4. *Obstetrics and Gynecology*
5. *American Journal of Obstetrics and Gynecology*
6. *Journal of Perinatology*
7. *Journal of Reproductive Medicine*

---

[9] *Id.* at 665.

[10] K. Benirschke, *The Placenta in the Context of History and Modern Medical Practice,* 115 Arch. Pathol. Lab. Med. 663, 665 (July 1991).

[11] *Id.*

8. *Archives of Pathological and Laboratory Medicine*

9. *Journal of Child Neurology.*

§ 13.6   Indications for Examination

Placental pathologists believe that all placentas should be examined by a competent examiner.[12] However, not all placentas are examined because of lack of training in placental pathology in residency, disinterest in pathological evaluation from the attending physicians, the cost of placental evaluation, and the problems of paying the pathologist for the examination.[13] Further, the overwhelming number of general pathologists have little training in the interpretation of pathological changes in the placenta.

The recommendation has been made for the placenta to be examined by the attendant at delivery, and a written report made in the medical record, in an attempt to identify those placentas that have some characteristics that require a detailed inspection and examination by a pathologist.[14]

If there are indications, such as those set out below, the placenta would automatically be sent to pathology for inspection and evaluation.

Maternal indications would include an abnormal pregnancy such as poor fetal growth, hyperemesis, alpha-fetoprotein abnormalities, preterm labor, premature rupture of membranes, abruptio placenta or vaginal bleeding that is unexplained, maternal fever, chorioamnionitis or septicemia, pre-eclampsia, eclampsia, hypertension, diabetes, blood dyscrasias, or malignancy.[15]

Fetal indications would include stillbirth, neonatal death, multiple gestation, prematurity, intrauterine growth retardation, congenital anomalies, erythroblastosis fetalis, admission to the neonatal intensive care unit, ominous fetal heart monitor tracing, and an Apgar score of less than five at one minute and less than seven at five minutes.[16]

Placental or umbilical indications would include placental infarcts, placental abruption, vasa previa, placenta previa, abnormal calcifications, and abnormal appearance of the placenta or cord.[17]

---

[12] C.M. Salafia & A.M. Vintzileos, *Why All Placentas Should Be Examined by a Pathologist in 1990*, 163 Am. J. Obstet. Gynecol., 1282–93 (No. 4, 1990).

[13] *College of American Pathologists Conference XIX on the Examination of the Placenta: Report of the Working Group on the Role of the Pathologist in Malpractice Litigation Involving the Placenta*, 115 Arch. Path. Lab. Med., 717 (July 1991).

[14] *College of American Pathologists Conference XIX on the Examination of the Placenta: Report of the Working Group On Indications for Placental Examination*, 115 Arch. Path. Lab. Med. 701 (July 1991).

[15] *Id.* at 449.

[16] *Id.*

[17] *Id.*

Further indications include:

1. Fetal—untoward obstetric outcome, small or large for gestational age, and oligohydramnios
2. Placental—cloudy, foul-smelling membranes, excessively large or small placenta for gestational age, hematomas, and thrombi
3. Umbilical—cysts, knots, single umbilical artery, webs, and bands
4. Abnormalities of chorionic membranes—white spots on fetal surface, yellow streaking, extrachorial gestation, and cysts.[18]

Still another author includes the history of drug use, poor previous obstetrical history, and meconium as further indications for placental examination.[19]

§ 13.7   The Exam of the Placenta

The placental examination is obviously divided into the gross or macroscopic exam and the microscopic. In the gross exam, which may be done in the delivery area or in the pathology department, the following should be looked for:

1. In the extraplacental membranes:
    a. Adherent blood clot
    b. Color
    c. Transparency
    d. Site of rupture relative to placental margin
    e. Amnion nodosum
    f. Velementous vessas
    g. Chorionicity if multiple gestations.
2. With regard to the umbilical cord:
    a. Length
    b. Diameter
    c. Color
    d. Vessel number especially if there is a single artery
    e. Angioma, allantoic and omphalomesenteric remnants
    f. True knots
    g. Insertion—whether it be central, marginal, or velamentous.

---

[18] J.M. Lage, M.D., *The Placenta, in* Pathology in Gynecology and Obstetrics 449 (1994).

[19] N.R. Schindler, *Importance of the Placenta and Cord in the Defense of Neurologically Impaired Infant Claims,* 115 Arch. Pathol. Lab. Med. 685 (July 1991).

3. In the chorionic plate:
   a. Color and transparency
   b. Dimensions and shape
   c. Vascular pattern
   d. Subchorionic thrombi.
4. On the maternal surface:
   a. Completeness
   b. Adherent blood clot, placental indentation
   c. Calcifications.
5. In the villous parenchyma:
   a. Infarction, intervillous thrombosis
   b. Color
   c. Location and dimensions.
6. If a chorioangioma is present:
   a. Color
   b. Dimensions
   c. Solitary or multiple.
7. Whether or not there is maternal floor infarction
8. Whether or not there is perivillous fibrin deposition
9. Whether or not there is pallor to the placenta.[20]

The Working Group of the College of American Pathologists has the following recommendations:

1. All placentas must be examined by gross inspection promptly after delivery.
2. The examination should include:
   a. Inspection for immediate clinical relevance including incomplete membranes, incomplete maternal surface, retroplacental hematoma, cord hematoma, and ruptured membranous vessels;
   b. Umbilical cord length should be measured. The most accurate measurement is in the delivery room prior to division of the cord;
   c. Some studies are best performed in the delivery area, such as cultures for microorganisms.[21]

The information that should be transmitted with the placenta if it is sent to pathology for inspection and analysis by the pathologist is the following:

---

[20] C.M. Salafia & A.M. Vintzileos, *Why All Placentas Should Be Examined by a Pathologist in 1990,* 163 Am. J. Obstet. Gynecol. 1282–93 (No. 4, 1990).

[21] 115 Arch. Pathol. Lab. Med. 701, 704–05 (1990).

1. The infant's gestational age
2. The reason the placenta is being submitted to pathology
3. The infant's weight
4. The infant's Apgar scores
5. An estimation of amniotic fluid
6. Any questions the delivering doctor would like the pathologist to answer
7. The name of the delivering doctor and the name of the infant's pediatrician.[22]

If the placenta is sent to pathology, the gross exam should include the following steps:

1. The placental dimensions are measured
2. The disc shape is recorded
3. The fetal surface, membranes, and cord are examined
4. The umbilical cord is measured and the number of vessels counted and recorded
5. Sections of the cord are taken and preserved—they should not be taken from the placental insertion site
6. A membrane roll, also known as a jellyroll is taken and preserved by fixation
7. The adnexa are trimmed and the placental disc is weighed
8. The maternal surface is then examined after the placenta is turned over
9. If there are clots, they are measured and the number and size are recorded
10. The maternal surface is evaluated for completeness
11. The pathologist then slices the entire disc from decidua to chorionic plate to inspect and palpate the parenchyma
12. The color of the villous parenchyma is noted and recorded
13. Any lesions are measured and a description of them recorded as well as sampled for microscopic evaluation
14. If there are no lesions that need to be sampled and fixed, three cassettes are prepared from the following:
    a. One from the umbilical cord and membrane roll
    b. One randomly sectioned from the peripheral parenchyma, making sure that any atrophic areas are not sampled
    c. One randomly sectioned from the central parenchyma.[23]

---

[22] *Id.* at 705.

[23] J.M. Lage, M.D., *The Placenta*, *in* Pathology in Gynecology and Obstetrics 453 (1994).

The choice of tissue for the microscopic exam is dictated by what is observed at gross exam. Other than routine sampling, the pathologist will sample and fix any areas that seem to be important to study under the microscope. These areas may show, for instance, noninflammatory changes, acute inflammatory changes, infarction, intervillous thrombosis, chronic villitis, hemorrhage, thrombi, fibrin deposition, tumors, villous edema, erythroblastosis fetalis, and the like.[24] The stains that are used are generally hematoxylin-eosin-stained slides, but they may be special stains also. Cultures taken from the placenta are also grown out and evaluated in pathology. These may be viral or bacterial cultures. It is the better practice to submit a sample of the placenta for a viral culture, rather than swabbing the placental surface. If a viral culture is requested, the tissue should be obtained in a sterile manner and taken from the midportion of the placental disc or from the chorionic plate.[25]

§ 13.8   What Placental Pathology Can Tell Us

One thing is clear when dealing with the specialty of placental pathology—there is a great deal that is not known and cannot be known about how the placenta contributes, or does not contribute, to fetal well-being. This is true not only on a case-by-case basis but also when attempting to generalize. There can be disagreement among the placental pathology community about what a finding may mean with regard to its importance in causing dysfunction to the fetus. As stated, there can be no in vitro study of the placenta while the fetus is in utero, and the significance of a pathological finding after dysfunction has occurred is not always known. Some placental pathologists are willing to theorize, but the litigator must understand there is a difference between theory and fact.

One author has stated:

The placenta can no longer be the universal scapegoat for the unexplained perinatal death . . . It is positively detrimental to provide unsubstantiated placental causes for these deaths simply to satisfy the obstetrician or bolster the pathologist's ego. This change in attitude is nowhere more apparent than in the area of so-called "placental insufficiency," a term widely used in clinical practice, which has neither reliable diagnostic parameters nor specific or characteristic pathological features. Indeed, it has been argued that the term be discarded[26]

---

[24] C.M. Salafia & A.M. Vintzileos, *Why All Placentas Should Be Examined by a Pathologist in 1990,* 163 Am. J. Obstet. Gynecol. 1282, 1286 (No. 4, 1990).

[25] *College of American Pathologists Conference XIX on the Examination of the Placenta: Report of the Working Group on Indications for Placental Examination,* 115 Arch. Pathol. Lab. Med. 701, 704 (July 1991).

[26] D.I. Rushton, M.D., *Pathology of the Placenta, in* Textbook of Fetal and Perinatal Pathology, 161 (1991).

Another author states that:

> It is fanciful to assume that every adverse perinatal outcome is associated with an abnormal placenta, and equally fanciful to expect that every abnormal placenta will result in a poor perinatal outcome . . . . The full understanding of the relationship between placental disease and perinatal outcome has been hindered by the retrospective nature and inadequate sample size of many studies, as well as the lack of controls and of long-term follow-up.[27]

Some placental pathologists want to assign to every damaged child a placental cause. Whether this is from overzealousness for their specialty or the desire to assist another health care provider in litigation, it clearly occurs. There is presently a campaign in the United States to discover or redefine the causes of cerebral palsy to exclude the negligence of the health care provider. This campaign is not just on the part of placental pathologists but also advocated by obstetricians, other medical specialties, the insurance industry that must pay when a health care provider is required to compensate an injured child, and the lawsuit abuse lobby. There is no question that newborns are damaged by a cause other than negligence of a health care provider. Every attorney has the duty to attempt to exclude genetic, congenital, or unavoidable causes for the damage to a newborn before instituting suit. There is also no question that a certain percentage of damaged newborns are damaged as a direct and proximate result of the failure of health care providers to meet the standard of care in providing medical services to the maternal-fetal unit. Every attorney who practices medicolegal law also has the duty to vigorously represent newborns when they are injured by the negligence of a doctor, nurse, or other health care provider.

§ 13.9   The Placental Pathologist and the Litigation Process

Placental pathologists are often called to give testimony, either by deposition or at trial, to explain their findings on gross or microscopic exam. They may have done the original pathological exam, or the tissue may have been reviewed at the request of a party to the lawsuit. One significant problem that exists is that often adequate tissues from the placenta are not preserved. The placenta may not even have been sent to pathology for evaluation, but discarded after removal. The placental pathologist may be working with a handful of slides that the original pathologist preserved months or years before. So one problem that exists is having anything to review. The second problem is whether there is sufficient material for analysis and opinion. The third problem is the potential bias on the pathologist's part.

---

[27] T. MacPherson, *Fact and Fancy—What Can We Really Tell from the Placenta?*, 115 Arch. Pathol. Lab. Med. 672 (July 1991).

§ 13.10   What the Placental Pathologist Needs

Placental pathologists want as much information as you can provide for the basis of their opinions. If no placental tissue was preserved, obviously there is nothing the placental pathologist can examine. The placental pathologist wants to review the following:

1. The patient's entire medical record from conception to the present
2. How and when the placenta was examined, weighed, measured, fixed, stored, and the like
3. How and when the umbilical cord was measured, examined, fixed, stored, and the like
4. Any history of congenital abnormalities in the parent's family
5. Any slides or blocks of tissue that exist from the placenta or umbilical cord
6. Any photos of placental or umbilical tissue

§ 13.11   How the Defense Uses Placental Pathology

Placental pathologists are used increasingly to attempt to deny recovery to an injured newborn. Insurance carriers are enamored of their placental pathologists and some have set up regional task forces to defend birth injury cases.[28] The pathologist offers the opinion that there was some condition of abnormality to the placenta that, after examination by the "expert," clearly was not proximately caused by the medical care. This condition may be some placental abnormality in itself, or the placenta may reflect in its diary a fetal condition. The defense position will be either that the fetus was injured acutely before labor and delivery at a time that the fetal damage was unknowable, or that the injury was the result of a chronic problem that was likewise unknowable to the reasonable health care provider, or the result of some congenital process, such as a genetic defect. The defendant will utilize the placental pathologist to offer the opinion that the findings occurred as a result of such condition and to testify as to the time period in which the damage occurred.

---

[28] N.R. Schindler, *Importance of the Placenta and Cord in the Defense of Neurologically Impaired Infant Claims,* 115 Arch. Pathol. Lab. Med. 685 (July 1991).

§ 13.12   Placental Pathology and the Plaintiff's Case

The plaintiff can utilize a placental pathologist to negate the defense position outlined in § 13.11. The pathologist who is consulting with the plaintiff can evaluate the evidence and determine, among other things, whether:

1. The placenta was normal
2. Any abnormal findings caused the damage to the fetus
3. There was no proper harvesting of tissue to enable a pathologist to come to any proper scientific conclusions from the permanent specimens
4. The fixing, storing, and/or sampling of the placenta were inadequate and therefore no scientific conclusions can properly be drawn
5. The gross examination was not properly performed, including the weighing of the placenta
6. The report of the gross examination was inadequate, improperly done, and so forth
7. The conclusions from the microscopic examination are improper
8. The conclusions of the examining and/or consulting pathologist for the defense are insupportable scientifically
9. The umbilical cord was not examined and measured properly.

If the placental pathologist can so conclude, he or she would be called as a witness for the plaintiff to testify that there was no evidence that the injury to the fetus occurred prior to labor and delivery.

There is also an area of opinion that could be called for, in the proper case, that the placenta was fragile and barely capable of supporting the fetus until the stresses of labor and delivery. That is, there is no evidence that the fetus was permanently compromised before labor and delivery, but once the stress of labor started, the placenta could no longer function adequately because of its fragile state. In this type of case, the fetus has normal growth and other parameters but is acutely compromised during labor because of a failure of the health-care providers to adequately assess the labor and deliver the fetus before permanent damage occurred.

We must remember the limitations of the study of placental pathology and the potential bias of the members of that discipline. We must remember that many placental findings are normal and even the ones characterized as abnormal, or even severely abnormal, may not be the causative factor in the injury of a newborn. We must remember that the study of placental pathology is based, in many instances, on a retrospective guess as to the importance of a finding in a particular case.

SHOULDER DYSTOCIA

§ 13.13   Introduction to Shoulder Dystocia

"A sudden call to a gentlewoman in labor. The child's head delivered for a long time—but even with hard pulling from the midwife, the remarkably large shoulders prevented delivery. I have been called to many cases of this kind, in which the child was frequently lost."[29]

One purpose of this chapter is to attempt to assist the practicing malpractice trial attorney, counsel for the plaintiff or defendant, to determine whether a shoulder dystocia case has medicolegal merit. This is not an easy task. The discipline of law does not lend itself to answering these questions once and for all. There are so many variables that comparing two cases, five cases, 20 cases, or 85 cases is very difficult when you are attempting to define the characteristics that make a case winnable for either side. Nevertheless, this chapter attempts to begin this process on the subject of shoulder dystocia. A series of 85 cases taken from *Medical Malpractice Verdicts, Settlements and Experts,*[30] reported in that excellent publication from January 1986 through January 1994, are discussed and analyzed for their liability factors. As a caveat, when discussing the series of 85 cases, the reader must understand that this is a random sample. There has been no attempt, for example, to collect all brachial plexus cases for a year or several years in the entire United States, or to collect all the brachial plexus cases for a particular jurisdiction. That would be an impossible task. The series of cases are discussed only as a guideline. All of the defense verdicts reported for those years are included. All of the plaintiffs' verdicts or settlements that had identifiable factors set out in the case report were utilized. However, any case with shoulder dystocia with other injuries (such as cerebral palsy) was not included. This was an attempt to strictly define the database.

The reader is referred to Dr. James A. O'Leary's superb text entitled *Shoulder Dystocia and Birth Injury: Prevention and Treatment,* for an in-depth analysis of the medical issues concerning shoulder dystocia. Dr. O'Leary's text should be read by any attorney involved in shoulder dystocia case.

---

[29] W. Smellie, M.D., *Smellie's Treatise on the Theory and Practice of Midwifery* (1730) quoted in J.A. O'Leary, M.D., Shoulder Dystocia and Birth Injury: Prevention and Treatment 216 (1992) [hereinafter O'Leary].

[30] To obtain information on *Medical Malpractice Verdicts, Settlenents and Experts,* contact 901 Church Street, Nashville, TN 30723-3411; (615) 255-6288.

§ 13.14   Shoulder Dystocia

Shoulder dystocia simply means that the head of the fetus is delivered with the shoulder or shoulders impacted in the pelvis, whereby maneuvers must be performed to free up the impacted shoulder or shoulders and complete delivery of the fetus.

Once the fetal head is delivered, there is only a short period of time (four to six minutes) to deliver the rest of the fetus to avoid brain damage. The umbilical cord is often compressed during the time that shoulder dystocia is present. When freeing up the shoulder after delivery of the head, the Three Ps must be avoided: pulling, pushing, and pivoting of the neck.[31] There are three critical times in the care of a mother and her fetus that are significant to attempt to prevent complications from shoulder dystocia:

1.   Preconceptual period, considering medical factors that relate to the mother, for example, pre-pregnancy obesity.

2.   Prenatal period, for example, does the mother have gestational diabetes?

3.   Intrapartum period, for example, were mid-forceps used or is there an arrest of labor?[32]

The incidence of shoulder dystocia is less than 1 percent of all term deliveries and is probably 0.3 percent.[33] There were 4.14 million live births in the United States in 1991.[34] This calculates out to approximately 12,500 labors complicated with shoulder dystocia. This is obviously a large number of children at risk for injury and a significant medicolegal problem. There is a 35 percent risk of shoulder dystocia and 30 percent risk of perinatal death if the fetus is 4,500 grams or more and the second stage is greater than one hour.[35]

The strongest correlation of dystocia is generally seen by most physicians with fetal macrosomia or large fetal size.[36] A better way to define *fetal macrosomia* is an increase in body size in relation to head size.[37]

---

[31] O'Leary at 107.

[32] O'Leary at 11.

[33] O'Leary at 3.

[34] F.G. Cunningham, et al., Williams Obstetrics 3 (19th ed. 1993) [hereinafter Williams].

[35] R.A. Sak, M.D., *The Large Infant: A Study of Maternal, Obstetric, Fetal and Newborn Characteristics Including a Long-term Pediatric Follow-up,* Am. J. Obstetrics & Gynecology, 104: 194–204 (1969).

[36] O'Leary at 4.

[37] Williams at 510; O'Leary at 4.

§ 13.15   The Injuries from Shoulder Dystocia

The upper root brachial plexus palsy (Erb-Duchenne) occurs often from sudden traction to the arm. The clinical features after birth are that the arm is internally rotated at the shoulder and pronated at the forearm. Paralysis of the spinati, deltoid, biceps, brachialis, brachioradialis, and extensor carpi radialis is seen. There is minimal or absent sensory disturbance and the biceps and supinatur jerks are lost with the triceps preserved.[38]

Disturbance or palsy to the lower root of the brachial plexus (Klumpke's paralysis) is often as a result of a violent upward pull of the shoulder. The clinical features after birth are that the arm is flexed at the elbow, the forearm is supinated, the fingers extended, and there is edema and cyanosis of the hand. There is paralysis of the small muscles of the hand and the finger flexors. There is sensory loss of the ulnar aspects of the fingers, hand, and forearm and Horner's syndrome exists if the root is avulsed.[39]

The entire brachial plexus is commonly damaged and therefore there is a combination of Erb-Duchenne and Klumpke's.[40] The damages in a shoulder dystocia case are very significant. Often, these children are burdened with an extremity that just does not work. Sometimes there is some function present, but the reality is that any jury is sympathetic to these damaged children. In a strong shoulder dystocia case, the amount of damages awarded should be significant, because these children are required to travel through this life with a damaged, dysfunctional extremity that often is disfiguring. Even if there is some functional ability of the upper extremity, any dysfunction is significant.

§ 13.16   Dignam's Rules

The wise obstetrician follows Dignam's Rules. They are the following:

1. Prior consideration
2. Accurate knowledge
3. A well-conceived plan of action
4. Rapidity of execution.[41]

---

[38] J.H. Menkes, Textbook of Child Neurology 491 (4th ed. 1990).

[39] Id.

[40] Id.

[41] W.J. Dignam, *Difficulties in Delivery, Including Shoulder Dystocia and Malpresentation of the Fetus,* Clinical Obstetrics & Gynecology 19:3–12 (1976).

§ 13.17   Keys to Success

Dr. O'Leary, in his book, has synthesized from the literature what he terms the keys to success to guide practicing physicians and allow them to virtually eliminate obstetrician dystocia, or obstetrician distress. The keys are the following:

1. Ultrasound dating of pregnancy
2. Ultrasound recognition of the large for gestational age (LGA) infant at 32 to 34 weeks
3. Recognition of the platypelloid pelvis
4. Recognition of mild glucose intolerance
5. Routine induction of labor at 40 weeks using prostaglandin gel (routine induction at 41 weeks eliminates 64%, according to Smeltzer)
6. Liberal use of cesarean section in obese gravidas
7. Universal use of the McRoberts' position in high-risk patients
8. Cephalic replacement
9. Avoidance of midpelvic delivery of macrosomic infants
10. Cesarean section for diabetic patients when the estimated fetal weight is 4,000 grams or more.[42]

§ 13.18   Prenatal Case Factors

Prenatal shoulder dystocia case factors that the author has identified from his experience, in literature as well as in the 85 analyzed cases are set out below. The factors discussed in this section and in § 13.19 generally track the medical literature; however, they are the medicolegal factors identified. The legal system may emphasize one factor more than the medical field. There should be little, if any, divergence, however. The factors strictly taken from the 85 cases may also be different from those set out in this section and in § 13.19. Factors discussed in this section, if present, would suggest the possibility or probability of shoulder dystocia occurring. A simple analysis would be that the more factors present, the more probable a given shoulder dystocia case can be won. That is not always the case because one factor may catch the eye of a particular jury more than another equally important medical fact. There may be one incredibly important factor that decides the case, for example, mid-forceps delivery. Note that the author uses "frank diabetes" to describe a woman who had diabetes previous to the pregnancy. The factors set out in this section are the following:

---

[42] O'Leary at 73.

1. Diabetes
    a. Familial but none presently in the mother
    b. Gestational diabetes
    c. Frank diabetes (prepregnancy)
2. Previous big baby
3. Previous shoulder dystocia
4. Macrosomic fetus (greater than 8.8 pounds)
5. Obese mother before pregnancy
6. Excessive maternal weight gain
7. Abnormal pelvic structures.

The material for this list came from the author's experience, the 85 cases, as well as a general reading of Dr. O'Leary's textbook, particularly of Chapter 1.

§ 13.19   Intrapartum Case Factors

The following list likewise sets out the factors from the author's experience, the literature, and the 85 reviewed cases that an attorney would want to look at in a shoulder dystocia case with regard to the intrapartum period. The factors include the following:

1. Use of Pitocin
2. Post-term pregnancy
3. Fundal pressure
4. Use of mid-forceps
5. Mid-pelvic vacuum extraction
6. Arrest of labor
7. Prolonged second stage
8. Excessive traction
9. Diabetes
10. Large fetus
11. Maneuvers.

The material for this list likewise came from the author's experience, the 85 cases, as well as a general reading of Dr. O'Leary's textbook, particularly of Chapter 4. *Maneuvers* means the attempt by the obstetrician to complete delivery of the child by various methods to free up the impacted shoulder such as the Gunn-Zavanelli-O'Leary maneuver, McRoberts maneuver, the Hibbard maneuver, the Wood's Screw maneuver, and so forth. Pitocin is used (or abused) for induction as well as augmentation of labor and is a factor for several reasons, including the use of Pitocin in a labor that is arrested.

§ 13.20   Shoulder Dystocia Defense Position

In the author's opinion, for the defense to be successful, it must be able to prove to a jury that either:

1. The risk factors are not present
2. The risk factors may be present but are not known and should not be known
3. This occurrence just happened, was a sudden emergency, and the brachial plexus was sacrificed to preserve the child's life.

Two of the 85 cases reviewed utilized the defense that the brachial plexus injury occurred spontaneously while in utero during pregnancy or during normal labor and delivery.

The defense position can be succinctly enunciated, in the author's opinion, by the following statements:

1. There was an emergency with no data for macrosomic fetus during the prenatal or intrapartum period. The baby must be delivered immediately to prevent brain damage. The brachial plexus was sacrificed to save the child. The physician unexpectedly was presented with a macrosomic fetus with shoulder dystocia.
2. Shoulder dystocia occurred absent negligence and the standard of care was met by delivering doctor. This is not the same as item one, although it is similar. This is the defense position that the delivering doctor did not fall below the standard of care (for example, proper maneuvers were performed by the delivering doctor but the child's brachial plexus was still damaged, or the jury believes that the factors present in the prenatal and intrapartum period were not strong enough to believe the defendant should have known there was a large fetus and planned for a cesarean section or more controlled delivery). Maybe the doctor's conduct was not the highest, but it did not fall below the minimal level. This is the "squeaker" defense because these are very difficult calls for attorneys evaluating the case. If the defense has improperly evaluated the factors, the probability is that the jury will find against the defendant and award large damages.
3. Expulsive efforts and pushing caused the brachial plexus palsy to the fetus and no shoulder dystocia existed. This defense is available only if there is no evidence that the shoulder was impacted on the maternal pelvis. Of the 85 cases reviewed, two defense verdicts had this factor.
4. In a maneuver case with knowledge of the potential for shoulder dystocia, the physician makes a reasonable evaluation (in the defense's eyes) of the ability of the mother to deliver her child without damage. This is a corollary to item two. In this defense, the doctor is aware of the potential for a

macrosomic fetus, but believes that the fetus can be safely delivered vaginally. The ability of the defense to sustain its position depends on whether the risk factors are properly and adequately heeded and evaluated.

§ 13.21 Plaintiffs' Verdicts

The factors that recur the most when there was a plaintiff's verdict in the 85 cases reviewed are the following, in order of their frequency:

1. Use of forceps
2. Child greater than 8.8 pounds
3. Obese mother before pregnancy
4. Excessive traction
5. Diabetes (either frank, familial, or gestational)
6. Use of Pitocin
7. Arrest of labor or prolonged second stage labor
8. Mid-pelvic vacuum
9. Previous big baby
10. Fundal pressure
11. Post-dates pregnancy
12. Previous shoulder dystocia
13. Excessive maternal weight gain
14. Delivering maneuvers
15. Labor induction
16. Fetal heart rate monitor abnormal
17. Meconium.

These are the factors and their relationship to the other factors that appear in the pie chart in **Appendix 13–1** in **§ 13.24.** When the cases were published in *Medical Malpractice Verdicts, Settlements and Experts,* these are the factors that the attorneys or the publisher felt were the most significant. In looking at this data, the question arises of whether there is a cumulative effect; for instance, if you have forceps use, a fetus greater than 8.8 pounds, an obese mother, and excessive traction, should a jury give the plaintiff a verdict all the time? To answer these questions accurately and finally is impossible. Obviously, there are so many variables in each case. Attorneys who have litigated a number of shoulder dystocia cases will tell you that they get a feel for whether the plaintiff should get the verdict and those are the cases they accept. In the author's experience, previous shoulder dystocia, which is not that frequent a factor in the chart, is the single most important medicolegal factor in litigating a shoulder dystocia case when it exists. With previous shoulder dystocia, the plaintiff must have a verdict. The factor least likely to contribute to a plaintiff's verdict, in the absence of other factors present, is the delivering maneuvers case. Obviously from the chart, the factors such as fetal heart rate monitor abnormal or meconium are not seen as important factors mainly because they do not directly correlate to a large fetus. It does seem likely that the more factors from the chart that the plaintiffs have in their favor, the more likely a plaintiff's verdict will be had. However, there are some factors that are just so important, that either alone or in combination with one, two, or three other factors, should bring a verdict in for the plaintiff. As mentioned, previous shoulder dystocia is one of those factors. In an attempt to create a profile for the case factors that are so important, the author believes that the following profile is valid:

1. Previous shoulder dystocia
2. Mid-forceps or mid-pelvic vacuum extraction
3. Fetus greater than 8.8 pounds
4. Excessive traction
5. Diabetes or increased maternal weight gain
6. Fundal pressure
7. Previous big baby
8. Arrest of labor or prolonged second stage labor.

This is not to say that a plaintiff's verdict cannot be had in a maneuvers case. Obviously, that has occurred and can occur. An obese mother before pregnancy is a very important factor also. All of these factors are extremely important. However, there is no way to completely and accurately state that factor X with factor Y will translate into a plaintiff's verdict, but that factor X with factor Z will not. Each case must be evaluated on its own merits. A summary of the successful plaintiff's case is when one or more of the following occurs:

1. Failure to determine that the mother is carrying a large fetus
2. Signs and symptoms during the pregnancy suggestive of a macrosomic fetus
3. Failure to plan for the delivery either by cesarean section or having an experienced obstetrician who has delivered a fetus with shoulder dystocia present.

§ 13.22   Settlements

As mentioned in § 13.21, fetal heart rate monitor abnormalities and meconium are not significant medicolegal factors for shoulder dystocia. Further, there were only two case reports with a factor of suprapubic pressure being applied. Unlike fundal pressure, suprapubic pressure does not seem to be a violation of the standard of care if properly utilized. Fundal pressure is clearly a violation of the standard of care and should not be utilized. In the case reports citing maneuvers as a factor, half the reports of settlement were from cases that arose in New York City. Once that is adjusted for, maneuvers decreases in importance in the following chart, **Appendix 13–2** in **§ 13.25.** There were two reports of breech deliveries, but in the experience of the author, that is seldom seen. The factors that recur in the pie chart, **Appendix 13–2,** are the following, in their order of frequency:

1. Diabetes
2. Fetus greater than 8.8 pounds
3. Forceps or vacuum extraction
4. Maneuvers (this probably should be number eight or nine when adjusted for New York City cases)
5. Fundal pressure
6. Post-dates
7. Excessive traction
8. Increased maternal weight gain
9. Arrest of labor or prolonged second stage labor
10. Use of Pitocin
11. Obese mother before pregnancy
12. Previous big baby
13. Suprapubic pressure
14. Breech delivery
15. Fetal heart rate monitor abnormal
16. Meconium.

Not found as a factor in the 85 reported cases that were settled were the induction of labor or previous shoulder dystocia.

§ 13.23   Defense Verdicts

Based on **Appendix 13–3** in **§ 13.26,** the factors that recur the most in the defense verdicts of the 85 cases reviewed are the following, in their order of frequency:

1. Maneuvers
2. Baby greater than 8.8 pounds

3. Previous big baby

4. Increased maternal weight gain

5. Use of forceps

6. Diabetes

7. Obese mother before pregnancy

8. Use of Pitocin

9. Excessive traction

10. Fundal pressure

11. Previous dystocia

12. No shoulder dystocia

13. Suprapubic pressure

14. Baby less than 8.8 pounds

15. Arrest of labor or prolonged second stage labor

16. Poor maternal care

17. Vacuum extraction.

The factor of children greater than 8.8 pounds in defense verdicts so frequently is obvious: the overwhelming number of shoulder dystocia cases occur with big babies—no large fetus, no shoulder dystocia, no lawsuit. You would expect this factor to be frequent. In some shoulder dystocia cases, the fetus is less than 8.8 pounds, but these are a small part of the total. The factor of a previous big baby is an interesting one. The defense position is that if a woman has delivered big babies previously, her pelvis is tested for large fetuses and therefore the trial of labor is not below the standard of care. This is clearly a squeaker defense that cannot always carry the day. The factor of the use of forceps and its frequency is probably a reflection of the defense position and is probably supported by the medical records in the reported cases of the forceps being low or outlet forceps. Mid- or high forceps or mid-vacuum extraction is clearly not a favorable factor for the defense.

California led all states in defense verdicts, with 41 percent of the verdicts coming from that state. There was no apparent reason for this in the data reviewed by the author.

In a sense, nearly all of the brachial plexus cases are maneuver cases. In the final moments of delivery, when shoulder dystocia is a reality, maneuvers must be done to deliver the baby. Improperly applying excessive traction is a maneuver, even though it is below the standard of care. Maneuvers as a factor in defense verdicts occurred in 18.75 percent of the cases reviewed. Conversely, the factors of excessive traction, fundal pressure, and previous dystocia each occurred in only 4.6 percent of the defense verdicts.

Of the cases reviewed, the largest settlement was $2 million (New York State) and the smallest was $75,000 (Ohio). The largest verdict was $5 million (New York City) and the smallest was $150,000 (Amarillo, Texas). Clearly, if you have a plaintiff's maneuver case, you want to be in New York City (there were a significant number of maneuver cases) and if you are defending a shoulder dystocia case, you want to be in California.

What conclusions can be drawn by this chapter? There are no absolutes; the answers are tentative only. When will the plaintiff prevail; when will the defense? It is clear that there are a multitude of factors surrounding a shoulder dystocia case. Is the data reviewed from the 85 cases accurate? It is accurate to a point. The best way to answer this question is that the data seems right. In the author's experience, having litigated numerous shoulder dystocia cases, fundal pressure, use of forceps, obese mother, diabetes, mid-forceps delivery, and so forth are all bad for the defense. Conversely, a maneuver case that arose many years ago with no other factors present is bad for the plaintiff and good for the defense. There is no real way to answer these questions scientifically. Litigating this type of case is not merely a scientific endeavor.

§ 13.24   Appendix 13–1: Shoulder Dystocia
Plaintiffs' Verdicts

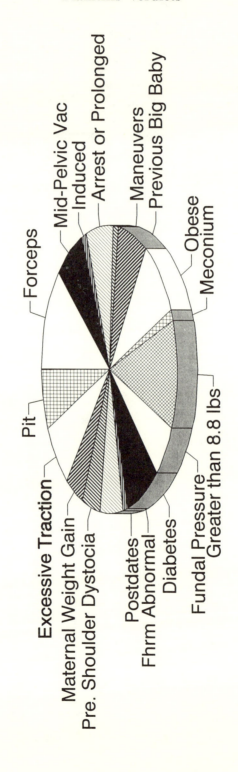

§ 13.25   Appendix 13–2: Shoulder Dystocia Settlements

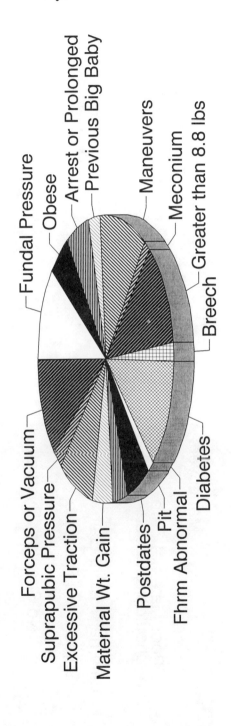

§ 13.26   Appendix 13–3: Shoulder Dystocia
Defense Verdicts

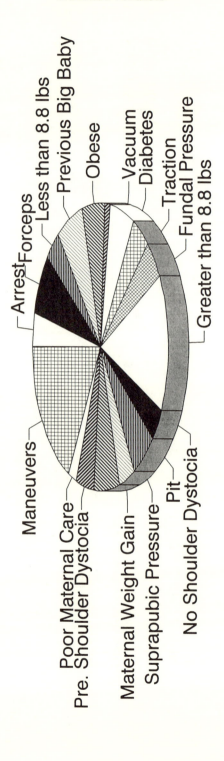

CHAPTER 14

ROUTINE CARE OF THE NEWBORN

C. Antonio Jesurun, M.D.

§ 14.1   Introduction

Infants have been delivered at home for centuries. Often, midwives or physicians would be called to the home to assist in the delivery of the child. Despite the recent arguments of lay midwives and consumers, the safest place to deliver an infant is in a hospital. Experienced and trained health care professionals are available should a calamity occur. Any hospital that has an obstetrical service is obligated to have competent personnel to evaluate and resuscitate newborn infants.

Physicians and nurses must be trained to attend the birth of an infant. They should have the equipment and support at their disposal to offer an infant the best opportunity for intact survival. A uniform training program has been developed through the American Academy of Pediatrics and the American Heart Association. After a day-long course in neonatal resuscitation, the attendee may be certified in neonatal resuscitation.

One of the standard reference texts for guidelines for care of the newborn infant was produced through a joint effort of the American Academy of Pediatrics and the American College of Obstetrics and Gynecology and published in 1992.[1]

§ 14.2   Levels of Pediatric Care

There are three levels of perinatal care as described in *Guidelines for Perinatal Care.*[2] In many states, health agencies review facilities available at many hospitals. To deliver a level of care requiring some degree of expertise, the hospital must meet specific standards established at a statewide level. These standards vary from state to state but are usually established by the state department of health.

---

[1] American Academy of Pediatrics & The American College of Obstetrics & Gynecology, Guidelines for Perinatal Care (3d ed. 1992). A new edition is expected to be published in 1996.

[2] American Academy of Pediatrics & The American College of Obstetricians & Gynecologists, Guidelines for Perinatal Care (3d ed. 1992).

Level I perinatal centers can provide for any normal labor, delivery, and nursery care. Consultation with Level II and III perinatal centers is encouraged for more complicated cases.

Level II perinatal centers care for common complications of pregnancy and, in general, serve as referral centers for Level I hospitals. Consultants and specialists are more available than at Level I centers. Level II centers have considerably more experience caring for sick mothers and newborns. Physicians and nurses are available around the clock to recognize and treat emergencies as they arise.

An intensive care nursery in a Level II perinatal center is staffed by physicians trained in neonatology, who are available for infants requiring specialized care. Respiratory support, such as mechanical ventilation, methods of delivering continuous positive airway pressure, and monitored oxygen, is available. Some major pediatric subspecialists are available for prompt consultation (surgery, cardiology, neurology, and infectious disease). Not all infants may be treated at a Level II center. When the attending physician feels more expertise is needed, referral is made to a Level III center.

A Level III perinatal center should have most subspecialties represented on its medical staff. A board-certified neonatologist administers the unit and is responsible for care delivered to newborn patients. The neonatologist should be certified by examination given by the American Board of Pediatrics Sub-Board of Neonatal-Perinatal Medicine after having completed fellowship training in neonatology. The most essential subspecialists that should be available for the sick newborn are pediatric cardiology, pediatric neurology, pediatric surgery, pediatric hematology, and genetics. Other subspecialties such as metabolic diseases, nephrology, dermatology, infectious disease, and gastroenterology are helpful.

Long-term respiratory management and treatment of other chronic diseases are best handled at Level III centers. Specialized diagnostic and treatment modalities are also more available at Level III centers.

While many Level II and III centers are staffed by university medical schools, many centers are staffed by physicians not affiliated with any university or medical school. Few community Level II and III hospitals have house staff. *House staff* are physicians in training, usually interns and residents. It is customary for pediatric training programs to assign interns and residents to the nursery and intensive care nursery on a rotating basis. The house staff may consist of interns and residents from various departments. Usually a second- or third-year pediatric resident directs the activities of other residents and interns (pediatric, surgical, obstetrical, anesthesia, family practice, or rotating). Most university centers have at least two board-certified or board-eligible neonatologists who directly supervise the house staff. Although many medical decisions are made by interns and residents, the attending neonatologist is directly responsible for the care delivered to the patients. Major decisions are made by the attending neonatologist on patient-care rounds or as dictated by the patient's condition.

In hospitals that have house staff, the pediatric resident attends all high-risk deliveries. The neonatologist attends the delivery as requested by the obstetrician or when a very complicated delivery is anticipated. The house staff usually takes call in the hospital overnight on a rotating basis, every third or fourth night, to attend high-risk deliveries and care for the patients in the intensive care nursery (Level II or III centers).

In centers where no in-house residents or neonatologists are available, the community physician or pediatrician must be contacted in anticipation of a high-risk delivery. There are times when the delivery of a sick newborn cannot wait for the arrival of a competent physician to take charge of the infant's care. There are, however, many instances where waiting is beneficial for the infant. All Level II and III centers should have competent personnel in-house for the resuscitation of the sick newborn.

More recently, *certified neonatal nurse practitioners* (CNNPs) (registered nurses with specific neonatal training) have taken the role of physician extender. These experienced nurses can perform many procedures under the supervision and direction of a neonatologist. These advanced nurse practitioners follow protocols and consult a physician for more complicated cases. A chart indicating the differences between Levels I, II, and III centers is helpful in comparing facilities, as seen in **Appendix 14–1** in § **14.23.**

§ 14.3   Risk Assessment and Risk Factors

Antenatal risk assessment is a sine que non for any perinatal center. Decisions are made based on complications that might be anticipated. Based on the list shown in **Appendix 14–2,** in § **14.24** an obstetrician may recognize maternal complications and elect to consult or to transfer the mother with the infant in utero.

It is preferable to transfer an infant inside the womb if a newborn complication is likely to occur and the birthing facilities are not appropriately equipped. Infants do not tolerate transfer well from one hospital to the other when in extremis.

Although the reasons are not entirely understood, it is felt that the outcome for mother and infant are superior if there is adequate prenatal care. Maternal diet, blood pressure, fetal growth, and infections can be properly monitored. Attempts should be made to identify abnormalities early to make appropriate intervention more effective.

An antepartum risk score[3] may be assigned to the pregnancy prior to the onset of labor. (See **Appendix 14–2** in § **14.24.**) Seventy percent of perinatal deaths occur in the group with a high-risk score.

Although some physicians state that 15 percent of all pregnancies carry significant risk,[4] this varies, depending on the population served in a particular

---

[3] I. Morrison, *Perinatal Morbidity and Antepartum Risk Scoring,* 53 OB/GYN 362 (1979).

[4] G. Avery, Neonatology, Pathophysiology and Management of the Newborn 33 (3d ed. 1987).

location. Intrapartum assessment is performed to anticipate maternal and fetal well-being. Using the list in **Appendix 14–3** in **§ 14.25** as a guideline, the pediatrician, anesthesiologist, neonatal nurse practitioner, nurse, or other competently trained personnel should be called to attend the delivery.

In the majority of cases, the obstetrician should personally communicate with the physician who plans to care for the infant in order to explain fully the maternal history. In complicated cases, the obstetrician/perinatologist will consult with the neonatologist to address anticipated maternal-fetal-neonatal complications. If time permits, the family should be informed as to the prognosis and therapeutic plan.

§ 14.4 Delivery

When the obstetrician feels delivery is imminent, the mother is taken to the delivery room. In low-risk situations the infant may be delivered in the labor suite or birthing room. The pediatrician is not called for routine uncomplicated deliveries.

The infant is delivered by the obstetrician and usually handed to the obstetrical nurse. In some hospitals a pediatric nurse, nurse anesthetist, or physician might be expected to assess and care for the infant in the delivery room. This person's only responsibility should be that of infant assessment and intervention, if necessary.

A prompt evaluation of the infant's condition is performed. If the infant is stable and requires no special care, then the mother may hold the infant. The infant must be kept warm to prevent hypothermia, hypoglycemia, and metabolic acidosis. After a short time the infant must then be taken to the observation or admitting nursery for continued observation.

Should the infant's condition in the delivery room require oxygen or resuscitation, this should be performed without hesitation. One can usually, but not always, stabilize a depressed infant (return vital functions such as heart rate and respirations) in five minutes.

§ 14.5 Assessment of the Infant

It has been said that passage through the birth canal is possibly the most important journey an infant will make. "Hospitals should ensure the availability of skilled personnel for perinatal emergencies . . . . At least one person capable of initiating neonatal resuscitation should be present at every delivery."[5]

---

[5] American Academy of Pediatrics & The American College of Obstetrics & Gynecology, Guidelines for Perinatal Care 4 (3d ed. 1992).

The *Guidelines for Perinatal Care* state that "Responsibility for identification and resuscitation of a distressed neonate should be assigned to a qualified individual, who may be a physician or an appropriately trained nurse-midwife, labor & delivery nurse, nurse anesthetist, nursery nurse, or respiratory therapist."[6] The evaluation of the infant involves objective assessment of vital signs and neurologic responses to the environment. This is universally performed in the delivery room at birth by use of the Apgar scoring system.[7]

The *Apgar score* ranges from 0 to 10. Zero indicates the absence of signs of life and 10 a perfectly breathing, oxygenating infant. In practice, very few infants should be assigned a score of 10, as there is normally *acrocyanosis* (blue hands and feet) present after birth. Infants with an Apgar score of 0 are usually not resuscitated and are considered stillborn. Occasionally, when a fetal heart rate has been previously recorded, a few successful attempts to revive the infant have been made with various neurological sequelae. The Apgar score is assigned at one and five minutes. Ten and 20-minute Apgar scores are helpful in describing the condition of a depressed infant with low one- and five-minute scores.

The person assigning the Apgar score should ideally be someone not involved with the delivery or resuscitation of the infant so as to be able to score the infant objectively. However, most of the time the pediatrician or obstetrician assigns the Apgar score, depending on the availability and experience of ancillary personnel.

The Apgar chart or scoring system is defined below:

Sign	0	1	2
Heart rate	Absent	Less than 100	Over 100
Respiratory effort	Absent	Weak, irregular	Good, crying
Muscle tone	Flaccid	Some flexion of extremities	Well flexed
Reflex irritability	No response	Grimace	Cough or sneeze
Color	Blue	Body pink, extremities blue	Completely pink

The one-minute Apgar score reflects the condition of the infant at birth. The score often is affected by obstetrical complications. An improvement in the five-minute Apgar score indicates improvement of the infant's cardiorespiratory system in response to resuscitation.

After the five-minute Apgar score has been assigned (seven or greater is considered stable), the mother is encouraged to hold the infant for a short time, for

[6] *Id.* at 84.

[7] Apgar, *Evaluation of the Newborn Infant's Second Report,* 168 JAMA 1985 (1958).

mother-to-infant attachment.[8] Problems may develop during this time if the infant is not observed for cyanosis and airway obstruction. After birth, the infant is taken to an admitting or transitional nursery, where experienced nurses observe and record the infant's many physiologic changes. **Appendix 14–4** in **§ 14.26** describes the normal changes in a newborn during the first 10 hours of life.

§ 14.6   Proper Equipment

Proper equipment is essential in every delivery room. A *radiant warmer* is an infant bed with an overhead heating element that controls the infant's temperature by a servo-control temperature probe. A bag and mask with appropriate size endotracheal tubes should be available, as well as an ample supply of oxygen (usually from a wall outlet). A stylet is sometimes needed to give the endotracheal tube stability during intubation. There may be a few occasions when a McGill forceps may be necessary to guide an endotracheal tube through the larynx.

Vacuum suction from a wall suction device is the most powerful of those available in the delivery room. The wall suction is connected to a small suction catheter. A bulb syringe or meconium aspirator device should also be available.

Warm infant blankets are useful in providing and maintaining heat for an infant who will be transported from the delivery room to the nursery.

A stethoscope is essential in assessing the neonatal heartbeat. Only a few resuscitation drugs are needed in the delivery room should standard resuscitative measures prove unsuccessful. These drugs are rarely needed except in extreme cases of neonatal depression. If drugs are needed to resuscitate the infant, that infant is seriously ill.

A list of equipment necessary for resuscitation that *always* should be in every delivery room follows:

1. Radiant warmer with temperature probe
2. Neonatal anesthesia or ambu bag to deliver 100 percent oxygen
3. Face masks (three various sizes)
4. Oxygen source (heated and humidified) with flow meter
5. Laryngoscope (sizes 0 and 1)
6. Stylet
7. Endotracheal tubes (sizes 2.5, 3.0, and 3.5)
8. Vacuum suction with catheters, bulb syringe, meconium aspirator device
9. Warm infant blankets
10. Stethoscope

---

[8] M. Klaus & A. Fanaroff, Care of the High-Risk Neonate 157 (2d ed. 1979).

11.   Resuscitation drugs, including IV fluid (D10 percent/water or D5 percent/water), 5 percent albumin, Narcan® neonatal, epinephrine (1:10,000).

§ 14.7   Assessment and Routine Care in Observation Nursery

The infant may remain under close observation, depending upon risk factors, for from four to as long as 6 hours. During this time, a disposition must be made by the physician as to whether to admit the infant to the normal nursery or to a special care unit. Level I or II perinatal centers may consolidate resources and locate the observation nursery in the same physical areas as the regular nursery. Level III centers usually have separate areas.

The nurse who makes the initial nursing assessment evaluates the well-being of the infant (see the nursing assessment form that is shown in **Appendix 14–5** in **§ 14.27**). All prenatal and obstetrical information must be delivered to the nursery so that a complete evaluation may take place.

The assessment by the admitting nurse in the observation nursery is essential in helping the physician admit the infant to the appropriate nursery. An experienced nurse may observe abnormal vital signs for a short period of time under the assumption that the patient will soon improve. The infant's physician is not usually present at the delivery of a normal infant. In a private practice setting, the physician's office is notified of the patient's birth and admission to the observation nursery. If, during the observation period, it is suspected that the patient's condition is abnormal, the nurse must contact the physician's office. Information is relayed directly to the physician who then decides if intervention, referral, or further observation is necessary.

§ 14.8   Temperature

One of the most important neonatal vital signs is that of body temperature. Newborn infants are born soaking wet with amniotic fluid. If the infant is not dried in the cool delivery room, the amniotic fluid will evaporate, thus cooling the infant. As infants have little ability to maintain body temperature, the infant's skin or core temperature may easily fall a few degrees centigrade.

The importance of keeping an infant in a warm environment is demonstrated in the graph in **Appendix 14–6** in **§ 14.28.** As the infant is placed in a suboptimum environment temperature, oxygen consumption increases.

Infants should be placed under a radiant warmer in the delivery room and immediately dried off, so that they may be examined naked and kept warm. A rectal temperature is not necessary as one may injure the rectum if care is not exercised. The core (rectal) temperature may be normal (37°C or 98.6°F) while the skin temperature might be low, thus giving one a false sense of security. A normal axillary or abdominal skin temperature is 36.5°C (97.7°F).

An infant should be kept in a thermoneutral environment. A *thermoneutral environment* is a controlled environment in which the infant can maintain body temperature using the least amount of oxygen.

Hypothermia (low temperature) is defined as a rectal or axillary temperature of less than 36.5°C (97.7°F). Infants with hypothermia should be placed in a radiant warmer or incubator. Hypothermia contributes to vasoconstriction, increased oxygen consumption, metabolic acidosis, and hypoglycemia. Many newborn disease states are aggravated by hypothermia.

Hyperthermia (elevated temperature) is a skin temperature greater than 37.5°C (99.5°F). The usual causes of hyperthermia in the first hours of life are a mother with fever or a radiant warming device that is malfunctioning or set improperly. The newborn infant tolerates hyperthermia even more poorly than hypothermia as it is very difficult for a neonate to dissipate heat.

§ 14.9   Respiration

All infants experience irregular respirations in utero. After birth, the infant must breathe regularly to sustain extrauterine life. The normal respiratory rate for a newborn ranges from 40 to 60 breaths per minute. Brief abnormalities of respiratory rate secondary to retained pulmonary fluid are not uncommon. Persistent and increasing *tachypnea* (fast respiratory rate) is cause for alarm and investigation. Unexplained respiratory distress is always cause for immediate concern. *Apnea* (cessation of respirations accompanied by cyanosis) is abnormal in infants of all gestational ages and requires special care for observation and evaluation.

There may be residual pulmonary fluid that is heard on inspiration with a stethoscope (*rales*). This is not necessarily indicative of pneumonia but may be normal pulmonary fluid that will be absorbed over a period of time.

The *Silverman score* (while used infrequently) was developed to assess a changing respiratory condition in the nursery. In contrast to an Apgar score, the higher the Silverman score, the worse the condition of the infant. **Appendix 14–7 in § 14.29** shows the Silverman Retraction Scoring System.

§ 14.10   Heart Rate

The cardiac examination is very basic to the evaluation of the infant. A normal heart rate for the neonate is between 120 and 160 beats per minute. *Bradycardia* (low heart rate) is usually defined as a heart rate of less than 100 beats per minute. Persistently low heart rates require evaluation of the patient's EKG and serum electrolytes. Persistently high heart rates greater than 220 beats per minute may indicate a cardiac conduction defect such as paroxysmal atrial tachycardia. Again, an EKG is helpful in diagnosis and treatment.

Heart murmurs are extremely common right after delivery. The hemodynamics of the infant's circulation changes from that of a fetal circulation to that of a normal newborn. Murmurs may not be hemodynamically significant, especially if found when examining an apparently healthy infant during the first 24 to 36 hours. Often the ductus arteriosus remains patent for as long as 48 hours and may not adversely affect a normal-term infant.

Vital signs such as temperature, heart rate, and respiratory rate are best recorded every 15 minutes for the first hour of life and then every four hours for the first 24 hours of life. Taking vital signs every eight hours after that is sufficient.

§ 14.11   Weight, Length, and Head Circumference

The birth weight, length, and head circumference are measurements of previous intrauterine growth and well-being. Perhaps head circumference is best correlated with the potential for mental development. Measurements of head circumference may be compared to that of other infants. Most measurements of a population may be placed on a curve with an average size or mean. Those that vary significantly from the mean may be abnormal. A head circumference that is greater than the 97th percentile or smaller than the third percentile is more than two standard deviations from the mean for age, sex, and gestation and is very suspect. Viral infections, chromosomal abnormalities, or severe growth retardation in utero may interfere with normal head growth and cause microcephaly (less than the third percentile). Microcephaly is associated with poor brain development and a small brain with mental retardation.

A head circumference two standard deviations greater than the mean suggest a central nervous system abnormality such as hydrocephalus. If the sutures are split and the anterior fontanelle bulging, a CT scan or neurosonogram can rule out hydrocephalus.

Thus the importance of the head circumference measurement is obvious. There are inconsistencies of measurement, as many infants are born with molded heads and overriding sutures. The head circumference, often called the fronto-occipital circumference (FOC), at birth may be smaller when molding is present. Multiple measurements made by different observers may lead to erroneous conclusions. Ideally, the physician should measure the head circumference at birth and upon discharge. In this way one of these measurements may be used as a baseline for comparison for future growth.

§ 14.12   Laboratory Evaluation

In most cases very little laboratory evaluation of the normal newborn is necessary. Some feel that all newborns should have a hematocrit drawn to assure the physician that the hematocrit is neither less than 45 vol% (*anemia*) nor more than 65 vol% (*polycythemia*). Anemia may indicate significant blood loss before delivery. Polycythemia may suggest prior intrauterine hypoxia or other medical complications.

An essential, yet simple, laboratory determination is the screening of the blood for *hypoglycemia* (serum glucose less than 40 mg%). A Chemstrip BG or Dextrostix determination is a screening method performed by placing a drop of blood on a reagent stick that changes color proportional to the level of blood glucose. Some institutions perform a serum glucose without using these two screening methods. It is important that hypoglycemia be avoided to prevent symptoms of possible central nervous system injury.

A complete blood count is indicated usually when there is a suspicion of infection or abnormality of the hematopoietic system. It is also important that the infant's physician determine the mother's recent serology test for syphilis. A recent serologic test for syphilis should be performed at the time of delivery or within the last month of pregnancy. If one cannot be ascertained, another serologic test for syphilis should be performed on the mother or the baby. Some hospitals have policies for mandatory HIV testing. This is not presently the rule because, in many states, the mother must give consent.

In all cases in which the mother's blood type is Rh negative or type O, a Coombs test should be performed on the infant or cord blood. A positive Coombs test may suggest careful observation for a serious incompatibility of blood leading to jaundice and anemia.

§ 14.13   Historical Data Collection and Assessment

The infant's physician routinely should gather historical data from the infant's chart, the pediatric nurse, the mother's chart, the mother, and the obstetrician. The obstetrician should have recorded all significant prenatal and perinatal information on the mother's chart. Copies of this information should then be transferred to the infant's chart for study and proper evaluation. The pediatrician must still obtain a maternal history, as occasionally some illnesses are not disclosed to or discovered by the obstetrician.

Maternal disease such as diabetes suggests that monitoring or screening of the infant's blood glucose is indicated. Infectious diseases contracted during pregnancy may explain abnormalities found during the physical examination of the newborn.

A medication and drug history is essential, as this information may also guide the examiner towards more careful observation. Otherwise, a history of illicit drug ingestion may not be obtained until after the infant manifests drug withdrawal. The abuse of cocaine and marijuana is endemic. Other drugs administered under the direction of a physician may lead to complications such as hormonal or metabolic abnormalities in the infant.

§ 14.14   Newborn Examination

The newborn examination by the physician must be performed within the first 12 to 18 hours of life in order to screen for abnormalities. It is unreasonable to expect the physician immediately to stop what he or she is doing in the office to examine what is reported as a normal newborn.

The initial newborn physical examination may be performed in five to 10 minutes. The infant should be completely naked so as to reveal any abnormalities.

The items listed below are merely guidelines to the physical examination of the newborn. The following should be recorded:

1. Heart rate
2. Respiratory rate
3. Temperature
4. Weight
5. Length
6. Head circumference.

External gross anomalies should be obvious, such as hydrocephalus, meningomyelocele, and abnormal limbs, digits, or abnormal facial features.

The examiner looks to whether the newborn is pink, jaundiced, plethoric, or pale, and whether the newborn is lethargic, active, sleepy, or alert. The skin is inspected for defects, nevi, staining, peeling, cracking, and ecchymoses. Molding of the head is common and usually not significant.

Fontanelles are usually flat and vary widely in size. The coronal and lambdoid sutures should not be separated unless there is hydrocephalus. It is not uncommon for the head to be asymmetrical because of intrauterine positioning or crowding. *Cephalhematomas* (collection of blood under the periosteum) are usually inconsequential as is swelling of the scalp (caput succedaneum). Occasionally a cephalhematoma may contribute to jaundice because of the excessive amount of blood sequestered.

An eye exam is performed to insure that the eyes are of normal size and structure. A *red reflex* (reflection of light from the retina) should be seen bilaterally. Difficulty in visualizing the red reflex may indicate retinal hemorrhage, cataracts, or an intrauterine viral infection.

It is important that both nares be patent (open). Anatomical obstruction of a nostril due to choanal atresia could impair respirations significantly.

The mouth is opened and inspected visually to rule out clefts in the hard and soft palate. Oral inclusion cysts and tooth buds are frequently found and are not significant. There should be no pharyngeal obstruction visible upon examination.

The neck should be examined to rule out lateral masses such as branchial cleft cysts, hematomas, or cystic hygromas. Goiters are found in the midline and are extremely rare.

The shape of the chest should be symmetrical. The clavicles should be palpated to rule out fractures from birth trauma. Although there may be rales bilaterally, this does not indicate pneumonia. Subcostal, xiphoid, and intercostal retractions are usually a sign of respiratory distress. This is manifest as sharp inward movements between and below the ribs. Unequal breath sounds or an asymmetrical chest may indicate a pneumothorax (collection of air in the chest) or other pulmonary pathology.

Auscultation of the heart may be very helpful. If the heart sounds are distant, a pneumothorax may be present on the left. Heart murmurs are very common and are frequently due to a benign ductus arteriosus. Some murmurs because of their location and radiation may be indicative of ventricular septal defects, most of which are not hemodynamically significant in the neonatal period. The femoral pulses should be palpated to check for *coarctation* (obstruction) of the aorta. The systolic, diastolic, and mean blood pressure should be recorded for each extremity.

The abdomen should first be inspected visually for distention and asymmetry due to masses. Patients with a diaphragmatic hernia characteristically have a scaphoid or flat abdomen as the abdominal contents may be in the thoracic cavity.

One can often feel the liver two to three centimeters below the costal margin. Rarely is the spleen tip palpable. The kidneys are difficult to feel as this examination requires that the examiner have some experience. The bladder is not usually palpated unless it is distended with urine. The majority of the abnormal abdominal masses are urinary tract in origin.

The umbilical cord should have two arteries and one vein, although a two-vessel cord is seen in .1 percent of births. Two-vessel cords may be associated with chromosomal, renal, and cardiac malformations. In this era of cost containment, watchful waiting is advised.

The male genitalia should be inspected for abnormalities. The foreskin should cover the glans. *Hypospadias* is a condition in which the urethral orifice is not found at the tip of the penis. It may be found anywhere along the shaft of the penis. In many cases of hypospadius the foreskin does not completely cover the glans and circumcision is contraindicated. The testes may be descended into the scrotum. Note should be made if the testes are either undescended or palpated in the inguinal canal at birth. Follow-up on an outpatient basis is warranted. If the testes do not descend by age two, surgical intervention may be necessary to place them in the scrotum.

The female genitalia may show prominent labia minora that may suggest prematurity. Hymenal or vaginal tags are asymptomatic and often regress. Withdrawal bleeding or a mucoid vaginal discharge are common in the female newborn. In cases of ambiguous genitalia, a large clitoris may in fact appear like a penis. Cases of congenital adrenal hyperplasia with virilization have gone unrecognized with serious consequences. Ambiguous genitalia are an indication for immediate chromosomal analysis.

A digital rectal exam is usually not necessary as patency is assured by the passage of meconium. With delayed passage of stool (greater than 24 hours), a digital examination is carefully performed to assure patency. The presence of a stool does not assure one that the entire gastrointestinal tract is patent as there may be meconium above and below atresias of the bowel.

Although the extremities should be symmetrical, there are many positional deformities of the arms, legs, and head that correct spontaneously. If there is intrauterine crowding or malpositioning, the head or face may be asymmetrical or the legs bowed.

The hips should be checked for dislocation, especially in cases of breech presentation. The spine should be palpated for occult spina bifida, especially if tufts of hair are present. Note should be made of any pilonidal dimples or sinus tracts.

§ 14.15   Neurological Exam

The neurological exam is perhaps the most important component of the physical examination. The infant's examination may be different depending on timing after birth, state of sleep, prematurity, postmaturity, feeding, or medication given to the mother or fetus.

The infant's activity level should be noted (quiet, hyperactive, or drowsy). The *tone* (resistance to passive movement of muscles) and ability to suck are important in assessing the integrity of the central nervous system. The maturity of the central nervous system will determine tone, with premature infants exhibiting less tone than term infants. A normal-term infant should exhibit flexion of all extremities such as the elbows, hips, and knees. Head lag should be minimal when pulling up both arms from a supine position. Asphyxia, chromosomal abnormalities, metabolic abnormalities, and serious disease states may affect tone. The term infant's ability to suck is essential to his or her well-being and is a reflection of central nervous system integrity. Without a strong sucking reflex, the ability to sustain caloric intake will be severely impaired.

The startle or Moro reflex should be elicited in all normal infants. Loud noises or the dropping of the infant's head back to the bed from two or three inches should alarm the infant. The infant should open both eyes and extend both arms outward. The arms are then withdrawn toward the midline and the infant cries. One of the reasons to elicit this reflex is to test for symmetry of neuromuscular activity. Infants with severe central nervous system abnormalities or depression may not exhibit this reflex. The reflex may be incomplete without crying or return of the arms to the chest. The incomplete Moro is not significant unless there is asymmetry of movement. If asymmetry occurs, then nerve injury, bone fracture, or central nervous system insult should be suspected.

The infant's cry should be evaluated. Some syndromes as well as central nervous system injury may be identified by eliciting a high-pitched cry. Infants who cry continuously or not at all are rare and definitely abnormal.

Although there are many more neurological reflexes that may be elicited, the above evaluation is the minimum for neurological assessment of the newborn. An excellent review of the newborn physical examination can be found in Scanlon's book, *A System of Newborn Physical Examination.*[9]

§ 14.16   Gestational Age Assessment

Gestational age assessment is important in identifying different groups of infants.[10] Two infants may weigh the same, yet have different gestational ages. The size of the infant may be a clue to underlying maternal or neonatal illness. Degrees of neurologic and physical criteria are graded to score the development of the infant. The total score correlates with gestational age (Dubowitz or Ballard exams). The Ballard exam sheet, as seen in **Appendix 14–8** in **§ 14.30,** demonstrates specific criteria and the method used for scoring.

Breast, ear, and genital development are also important criteria for measuring physical maturity. Physical characteristics such as skin texture, color, opacity, and swelling are graded.

Neuromuscular tone determines many of the results of the neurologic maturity examination. The infant's posture and ability to extend or flex the shoulder, hip, knee, wrist, and elbow are essential components of the neuromuscular examination. This part of the examination is affected by perinatal asphyxia or congenital neurologic abnormality.

§ 14.17   Routine Orders

Most normal infants do not require special orders by the physician. Routine orders vary from physician to physician. A sample of routine orders appears below and always includes the diagnoses suspected at delivery. This assists the nurse in his or her evaluation of the infant.

---

[9] J. Scanlon, A System of Newborn Physical Examination (1979).

[10] M. Klaus & A. Fanaroff, Care of the High-Risk Neonate 66 (2d ed. 1979).

Sample Routine Orders

1. Admit to observation nursery

2. Diagnosis: Term male/female, appropriate for gestational age

3. Condition: Good

4. Vitamin K, 1 mg. intramuscularly

5. Erythromycin, 1.0 percent, ophthalmic ointment or Tetracycline, 1 percent ophthalmic ointment or drops to both eyes

6. Triple dye to umbilical cord

7. Admission hematocrit and serum glucose (or Chemstrip BG or Dextrostix)

8. Report to physician if hematocrit greater than 65 percent or less than 45 percent.

9. Report to physician if Chemstrip less than 45mg. percent or greater than 160mg. percent

10. Maternal or infant serologic tests for syphilis on chart before discharge

11. Maternal type and Rh on chart

12. Infant's blood type, Coombs, and Rh on chart if mother is Rh negative, type O, or unknown

13. Routine formula feedings every four hours using mother's formula of choice

14. If breast-feeding, feed every three hours

15. Hepatitis B Vaccine 0.25cc/IM Recombivax® HB) after permit signed.

Vitamin K (phytonadione) should be administered to prevent hemorrhagic disease of the newborn. This disease is rare now that all hospitals administer this vitamin by injection to all newborn infants.

Eyedrops such as Erythromycin, or Tetracycline ointment, are placed in both eyes to prevent the maternal transmission of gonorrhea. Triple dye or other antiseptic agent is usually placed on the umbilical cord to prevent infection of the cord (*omphalitis*).

In 1992 there was considerable controversy regarding the statement made by the Committee on Infectious Diseases of the Academy of Pediatrics recommending universal Hepatitis B immunization.[11] While most of the controversy regarding efficacy has not been answered, the current standard is to immunize all infants at birth, followed by three boosters during the first year of life.

---

[11] Committee on Infectious Diseases of the Academy of Pediatrics, *Universal Hepatitis B Immunization,* 89 Pediatrics 795 (1992).

§ 14.18   Disposition and Assignment to Nursery

It is routine that after a six-to-eight-hour observation period the infant is transferred for continuing care to the regular nursery where the infant does not require such close monitoring. Upon transfer, the infant becomes the responsibility of the nurses in the regular nursery. Many observations are performed by nurses' aides, licensed vocational nurses, and the mother herself.

Vital signs such as temperature, heart rate, and respiratory rate are observed and recorded once every eight hours. Any deviations from the routine neonatal course (feedings, stooling, voiding) are recorded on nurses' notes and relayed verbally to the physician.

Appropriate interventions cannot be made if the physician does not monitor the infant's progress. Should an infant require frequent monitoring, more skilled observations, or treatment, the infant must be transferred to either an intermediate or intensive care nursery.

§ 14.19   Consultation

When the physician believes that more expert evaluation is needed, he or she consults the competent specialist of choice by personal communication, expressing the urgency of the consultation and informing the parents of the consultation. Infants requiring intensive care should have a board-eligible or board-certified neonatologist consultation to assure quality care. This is not possible in some communities in which a neonatologist is not available. Noncritical conditions do not demand immediate in-hospital consultation and may be evaluated on an outpatient basis.

§ 14.20   Transfer

The transfer of care of a newborn from one hospital or physician to another is time-consuming. Success usually depends on the time and persistence of the referring physician. Physicians are often familiar with admitting procedures required by the receiving hospital. Usually the hospital accepting the infant will send a transport team to assess and stabilize the infant before transfer.

One of the most common delays is administrative, as financial policies may determine admission to a hospital. This is a source of frustration for physicians caring for indigent patients. Other times, transfers are delayed because someone assumed the right call had been made, when in fact someone was waiting for a call that was never made. Federal requirements for patient transfer can be found in the *Guidelines for Perinatal Care*.[12]

§ 14.21   Early Discharge or Short Hospital Stay

A discharge physical exam should be made prior to the infant's leaving the hospital. The practice of filling out the admission and discharge physical examination papers on admission is not acceptable. This assumes that no changes may take place during hospitalization. Many normal changes in the physical exam do in fact take place. Some of these dictate further follow-up while others do not.

For many years the standard hospital stay for mother and child was 72 hours. In recent years, appeals for deviation from that standard have lead to much controversy for early discharge. Some consumer groups felt that the hospital was not a place for mothers and infants. These groups were responsible for pushing the medical establishment to ask "Why three days?" Pediatricians felt that indeed the routine discharge of infants who had no medical problems could be shortened. More recently, reimbursement policies by insurance companies have imposed shortened hospital stay policies upon physicians. Many managed care insurance companies have refused to pay for newborn and maternal hospitalization for more than 24 hours. Some insurance companies have pushed for hospital discharge as early as six hours after birth. One estimate showed a cost savings to insurers of four billion dollars a year by reducing newborn/maternal hospital stay.

The Committee on the Fetus & Newborn of the Academy of Pediatrics issued a statement in October 1995[13] outlining minimum criteria prior to newborn discharge. The statement reiterated the principle that the timing of the hospital discharge should be a decision between the physician and the family. The caveat for early discharge includes an examination by an experienced health care provider 48 hours after discharge. Many anecdotal reports of infants experiencing infection, jaundice, and dehydration have been associated with poor to absent follow-up or poor parental understanding of routine newborn care. The routine practice of early discharge prior to 72 hours has met with resistance from both the medical and legislative community. States such as Maryland and New Jersey passed laws mandating that insurance companies pay for a minimum two day hospital stay. There is no doubt that the struggle between payers and the medical establishment will continue as more studies are needed to demonstrate that changing the standard hospital stay is indeed safe.

---

[12] American Academy of Pediatrics & The American College of Obstetrics & Gynecology, Guidelines for Perinatal Care 245 (3d ed. 1992).

[13] Committee on the Fetus & Newborn of the American Academy of Pediatrics, *Hospital Stay for Healthy Term Newborns,* 96 Pediatrics 788 (1995).

An example of discharge orders may be the following:

1. Discharge to mother
2. Newborn screening before discharge and in two to four weeks
3. Mother to call physician's office for appointment for two-week check-up. If patient discharged at 24 to 36 hours of age, mother to call physician's office for physical exam 48 hours after discharge.

Some hospitals may have policies that stipulate to whom the infant may be discharged (mother, father, or foster parents with legal papers). The proper identification of these persons is essential. In many hospitals, the mother is issued an ID bracelet that matches the infant's ID bracelet. Upon discharge, she must present this bracelet to receive the infant. In some cases in which the mother is not recognized by the nursing staff, some additional form of maternal identification might be required.

§ 14.22   Newborn Screening

In some states a screening is performed on discharge. This sample is usually taken from blood by heel prick, collected on a filter paper form, and sent to the state department of health, and may screen for diseases such as hypothyroidism, galactosemia, phenylketonuria, congenital adrenal hyperplasia, or sickle cell disease. Different states may screen for different diseases depending on the frequency of the disease within the state. Some states require a second newborn screening to be performed at two to four weeks of age. The results of the newborn screening are usually mailed to the laboratory or office where the blood sample was taken. Results may take as long as two weeks to return. Some state health departments only phone the physician if the results are abnormal and then request another screening. It is not unusual to have multiple screenings performed. Only if one of the screenings is very abnormal is a venipuncture blood sample required for a specific test. The reason for two screenings is to aid identification of abnormal infants that may have been missed by the first screening. These screening tests are not diagnostic and, when results are abnormal, require close follow-up with diagnostic tests.[14] There is a potential for false negative results for phenylketonuria and galactosemia if the newborn screening is performed less than 24 hours of formula/breast feeding. While this may be a problem especially for infants with short hospital stays, the problem is circumvented by having a second test performed at two weeks of age.

---

[14]Three of the best references to the subject matter of this chapter are S. Aladjem, Perinatal Intensive Care (1977); S. Pierog, Medical Care of the Sick Newborn (2d ed. 1976); M. Zial, Assessment of the Newborn (1984).

§ 14.23 Appendix 14–1: Levels of Care

	Level I	Level II	Level III
Function	Risk assessment Management of uncomplicated perinatal care Stabilization of unexpected problems Initiation of maternal and neonatal transports Patient and community education Data collection and evaluation	General Level I plus: Diagnosis and treatment of selected high-risk pregnancies and neonatal problems Initiation and acceptance of maternal-fetal and neonatal transports Education of allied health personnel Residency education (affiliation)	Levels I and II plus: Diagnosis and treatment of all perinatal problems Acceptance and direction of maternal-fetal and neonatal transports Research and outcome surveillance Graduate and postgraduate education System management
Types of patients	Uncomplicated, emergency, and remedial problems such as lack of progress in labor, immediate resuscitation of depressed neonates, uterine atony, nursery care of large premature neonates (>2,000 g) without risk factors, physiologic jaundice	Level I plus: Selected problems such as pre-eclampsia, premature labor at 32 weeks and later, mild to moderate respiratory distress syndrome, suspected neonatal sepsis, hypoglycemia, neonates of diabetic mothers, hypoxia/ischemia without life-threatening sequelae	Levels I and II plus: Premature rupture of membranes or preterm labor at 24 to <32 weeks (500–1,500 g), severe maternal medical complications, pregnancy with concurrent cancer, complicated antenatal genetic problems, severe respiratory distress syndrome, sepsis, severe postasphyxia, symptomatic congenital cardiac and other systems disease, neonates with special needs (eg, hyperalimentation), prolonged mechanical ventilation

	Level I	Level II	Level III
Chief of service	One physician responsible for perinatal care (or codirectors from obstetrics and pediatrics)	Joint Planning: Ob: Board-certified obstetrician with special competence, special interest, experience, or training in maternal-fetal medicine Peds: Board-certified pediatrician with certification, special interest, experience, or training in neonatology	Codirectors: Ob: Full-time board-certified obstetrician with special competence in maternal-fetal medicine Peds: Full-time board-certified pediatrician with certification in neonatal medicine
Other physicians	Physician (or certified nurse-midwife) at all deliveries Anesthesia services Physician care for neonates	Level I plus: Board-certified director of anesthesia services Medical, surgical, radiology, pathology consultation	Levels I and II plus: Anesthesiologists with special training or experience in perinatal and pediatric anesthesia Obstetric and pediatric, medical and surgical subspecialists
Supervisory nurse	RN in charge of perinatal facilities	Separate head nurses with educational preparation and advanced skills for maternal-fetal neonatal services	Director/supervisor of perinatal services with educational preparation and advanced skills for maternal-fetal and neonatal services
Staff nurse/patient ratio	Normal labor 1:2 Second stage of labor 1:1 Oxytocin induction and augmentation 1:2 Cesarean delivery 1:1 Normal nursery 1:6 Admission nursery 1:4	Level I plus: Complicated labor/delivery 1:1 Intermediate nursery 1:2–3	Levels I and II plus: Intensive neonatal care 1:1–2 Critical care of unstable neonate >1:1

Source: American College of Obstetricians & Gynecologists, *Guidelines to Perinatal Care* 236–37, 3rd ed. Washington, DC, ACOG © 1992. Reprinted by permission.

§ 14.24   Appendix 14–2: Pregnancy Risk Factors*

		Score
A.	Prenatal Factors	
1.	Moderate to severe toxemia	10
2.	Chronic hypertension	10
3.	Moderate to severe renal disease	10
4.	Severe heart disease, Class II-IV	10
5.	History of eclampsia	5
6.	History of pyelitis	5
7.	Class I heart disease	5
8.	Mild toxemia	5
9.	Acute pyelonephritis	5
10.	History of cystitis	1
11.	Acute cystitis	1
12.	History of toxemia	1
B.	Intrapartum Factors	
1.	Moderate to severe toxemia	10
2.	Hydramnios or oligohydramnios	10
3.	Amnionitis	10
4.	Uterine rupture	10
5.	Mild toxemia	5
6.	Premature rupture of membrane > 12 hr	5
7.	Primary dysfunctional labor	5
8.	Secondary arrest of dilation	5
9.	Demerol > 300 g	5
10	$MgSO_4$ > 25 g	5
11.	Labor > 20 hr	5
12.	Second stage > 2-1/2 hr	5
13.	Clinical small pelvis	5
14.	Medical induction	5
15.	Precipitous labor < 3 hours	5
16.	Primary cesarean section	5
17.	Repeat cesarean section	5
18	Elective induction	1
19.	Prolonged latent phase	1

Source: Adapted from Hobel, C.J., Hyvarinen, M., Okada, C., Oh, W., *Prenatal and Intra-partum High-Risk Screening* at 2–4. Amer. J. Obstet. Gynecol. 117:1 (1973). Printed by permission from Mosby-Year Book, Inc.

20.	Uterine tetany	1
21.	Pitocin augmentation	1

C.   Neonatal Factors

1.	Prematurity > 2,000 g	10
2.	Apgar at 5 min > 5	10
3.	Resuscitation at birth	10
4.	Fetal anomalies	10
5.	Dysmaturity	5
6.	Prematurity 2,000–2,500 grams	5
7.	Apgar at 1 min < 5	5
8.	Feeding problem	1
9.	Multiple birth	1

§ 14.25   Appendix 14–3: Sample List of Perinatal Conditions that Increase the Risk for Neonatal Morbidity or Mortality*

Section A

Conditions Requiring Availability of Skilled Resuscitation at Delivery

1.   Fetal distress
  a.   Persistent late decelerations
  b.   Severe variable decelerations without baseline variability
  c.   Scalp pH < 7.25
  d.   Meconium-stained amniotic fluid
  e.   Cord prolapse
2.   Operative delivery
  a.   Cesarean delivery
  b.   Mid-forceps delivery
3.   Third trimester bleeding
4.   Multiple births
5.   Estimated birth weight < 1500 g
6.   Estimated gestational age < 34 weeks
7.   Breech presentation
8.   Prolonged, unusual, or difficult birth
9.   Insulin-dependent diabetes

---

*Source: Adapted from American College of Obstetricians & Gynecologists, Guidelines for Pre-natal Care 260–61 (2d ed. Washington, DC ACOG © 1983). Printed with permission.

10. Severe isoimmunization
11. Obstetrician's or pediatrician's request

Section B

Conditions Requiring an Immediate Assessment and Initiation of Care Plan

1. Major anomalies
2. Respiratory distress
3. Apgar score of 5 at 5 minutes
4. Signs of sedation in the neonate
5. Maternal infection
   a. Increased temperature
   b. Greater than 24 hours since rupture of membranes
   c. Foul-smelling amniotic fluid
6. Severe hypertensive disease
7. Suspected intrauterine fetal growth retardation, or excessive size
8. Class A diabetes
9. Maternal drug addiction
10. Oligohydramnios or hydramnios
11. Prematurity, postmaturity, dysmaturity
12. Previous fetal wastage/neonatal death
13. No prenatal care

§ 14.26   Appendix 14–4: Graph Showing Normal Changes in a Newborn

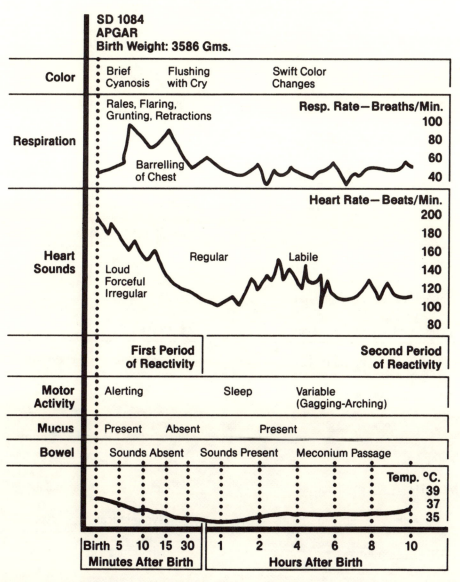

Graph showing normal changes in newborn for first 10 hours of life. *Source:* M.H. Klaus & A.A. Fanaroff, Care of the High-Risk Neonate 55. (W.B. Saunders Company, 2d ed. 1979). Reproduced with permission.

§ 14.27   Appendix 14–5: Infant Physical Assessment Form

INFANT PHYSICAL ASSESSMENT FORM

ADMISSION TIME _____ BIRTH DATE _____ TIME _____ BIRTH WT. _____

GM. GEST. AGE _____ APGARS _____ HEAD _____ CHEST _____ ABD. _____

LENGTH _____ TEMP. _____ PULSE _____ RESP. _____ BP:RA _____

RL _____ LA _____ LL _____

NORMAL FINDINGS   SIGNIFICANT FINDINGS

HEAD _____ molding _____ hair amount _____ lacerations _____ lesions

_____ forcep marks _____ bruising _____ hematoma _____ localized edema

FONTANELS

open/closed anterior _____ cm.x _____ cm.   _____ bulging

open/closed anterior _____ cm.x _____ cm.   _____ sunken

SUTURES _____ normal   _____ overriding _____ widened

EARS _____ normal _____ tubercles   _____ anomalous

_____ ear tags   _____ low-set ears

NOSE _____ patent nares   _____ flaring _____ nasal congestion

MOUTH _____ oral mucosal   _____ cleft lip _____ cleft palate

_____ teeth _____ Epstein's pearls   _____ asymmetrical _____ cyanosis

TONE _____ normal   _____ hypertonic _____ hypotonic

SUCK _____ strong _____ moderate   _____ weak _____ none

CRY   _____ strong _____ normal   _____ weak _____ high pitch

JAW   _____ normal   _____ small

NECK _____ normal/no masses   _____ masses

_____ clavicles intact   _____ clavicle/crepitation

CHEST

_____ normal _____ engorged breast   _____ barrel _____ sunken

_____ lung sounds equal/clear   _____ grunting _____ retraction

                                       breath sounds: _____ reduced

                                       _____ rhonchi/rales _____ murmur

                                       _____ abnormal heart sounds

ABDOMEN

_____ soft/no masses _____ stool   _____ distention _____ rigidity

_____ bowel sounds _____ 3-vessel cord _____ hernia _____ 2-vessel cord

UROGENITAL

_____ normal penis _____ normal scrotum _____ hyposadias _____ epispadias

_____ testes descended   _____ hematoma _____ hernia

_____ female normal _____ voided   _____ imperforate anus

                                       _____ hydrocele

EXTREMITIES

_____ normal digits _____ full ROM   _____ single palmar creases

_____ flexion _____ symmetrical   _____ webbing _____ cyanosis

                                       _____ uneven _____ extra digits

BACK

_____ spine straight   _____ curvature _____ hip click

_____ movement to both sides   _____ spinal defects

_____ R.N.

_____ DATE

DELIVERY ROOM INFORMATION

INFANT NEUROLOGICAL EXAM

To delivery room _____

Name: _____

Hours Postbirth _____ hours

Age: _____ D.O.B. _____

STATE: Active/Alert _____

Patient # _____

Lethargic _____

Asleep _____

Grp. & Rh _____ Gestation _____ date

TONE: Flexion of arms & legs _____

    sono _____ size _____

Symmetrical movements _____

Membranes: AROM/SROM Date _____

EYES: Abnormal movements _____

    Color _____ Time _____

If yes, explain _____

_____

Grav. _____ Para _____ Ab _____

Pupils equal/reactive _____

    X _____ visits

If no, explain _____

_____

Doctor: _____

Nurse: _____

PRIMARY   arm recoil _____

Anesthesia: _____

REACTIONS: leg recoil _____

Type of del.: _____

Grimace _____ Grasping _____

Forceps _____ Other _____

Attempts to hold head when

Epistiotomy _____ Placenta _____

lifted off mattress _____

Type of del. _____ Sex _____ Apgar __ / __

Sucking _____ rooting _____

Baby adm # _____ Wt # _____

Walking _____ Moro _____

    Gms _____

Babinski: Post./Neg. _____

BREAST/BOTTLE _____

OTHER: Tremors _____

Intrapartum

    Jerks _____ Irritability _____

Fetal monitoring: YES/NO

    Seizures _____

Significant patterns: _____   _____

_____   _____

Complications of Labor: _____

_____   _____

_____   _____

Complications of Delivery: _____

_____   _____

_____   _____

Complications of Pregnancy: _____

_____   _____

_____   _____

Maternal Drugs: Name/Time/Amt.   _____

_____   _____

_____   _____ R.N.

_____   _____ DATE

§ 14.28   Appendix 14–6: Graph Showing Effect of Environmental Temperature

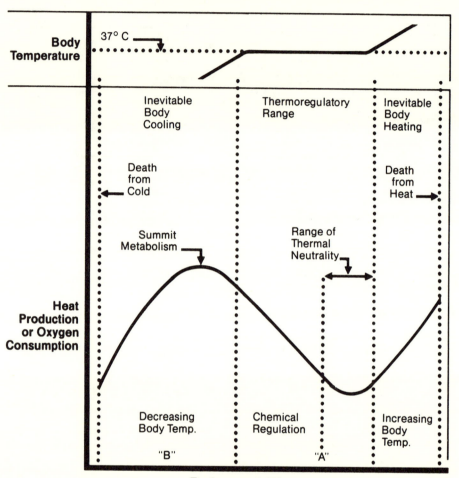

Environmental Temperature

Source: Effect of Environmental Temperature on Oxygen Consumption and Body Temperature, in M.H. Klaus & A.A. Fanaroff, Care of the High-Risk Neonate 97 (W.B. Saunders Company, 2d ed. 1979). Reproduced with permission.

§ 14.29 Appendix 14–7: Silverman Retraction

Observation of Retractions

	Grade 0	Grade One	Grade Two
Upper Chest	Synchronized	Lag on Inspiration	See-Saw
Lower Chest	No Retraction	Just Visible	Marked
Xipheid Retractions	None	Just Visible	Marked
Nares Dilation	None	Minimal	Marked
Expiratory Grunt	None	Stethoscope Only	Naked Ear

A score of 0 indicates absence of respiratory distress; a score of 10 indicates severe clinical distress. *Source:* Silverman, W.A., Anderson, D.H., *A Controlled Clinical Trial of Effects of Water Mist on Obstructive Respiratory Signs, Death Rate and Necropsy Findings Among Premature Infants.* Reproduced by permission of PEDIATRICS, vol. 17, page 1, copyright 1956.

§ 14.30   Appendix 14–8: Newborn Maturity Rating and Classification

NEUROMUSCULAR MATURITY

MATURITY RATING

score	weeks
-10	20
-5	22
0	24
5	26
10	28
15	30
20	32
25	34
30	36
35	38
40	40
45	42
50	44

PHYSICAL MATURITY

	-1	0	1	2	3	4	5
Skin	sticky friable transparent	gelatinous red, translucent	smooth pink, visible veins	superficial peeling &/or rash. few veins	cracking pale areas rare veins	parchment deep cracking no vessels	leathery cracked wrinkled
Lanugo	none	sparse	abundant	thinning	bald areas	mostly bald	
Plantar Surface	heel-toe 40-50 mm: -1 <40 mm: -2	>50mm no crease	faint red marks	anterior transverse crease only	creases ant. 2/3	creases over entire sole	
Breast	imperceptible	barely perceptible	flat areola no bud	stippled areola 1-2mm bud	raised areola 3-4mm bud	full areola 5-10mm bud	
Eye/Ear	lids fused loosely:-1 tightly:-2	lids open pinna flat stays folded	sl. curved pinna; soft; slow recoil	well-curved pinna; soft but ready recoil	formed &firm instant recoil	thick cartilage ear stiff	
Genitals male	scrotum flat, smooth	scrotum empty faint rugae	testes in upper canal rare rugae	testes descending few rugae	testes down good rugae	testes pendulous deep rugae	
Genitals female	clitoris prominent labia flat	prominent clitoris small labia minora	prominent clitoris enlarging minora	majora & minora equally prominent	majora large minora small	majora cover clitoris & minora	

Source: Ballard, J.L., Khoury, J.C., Wedig, K., Wang, L., Eilers-Walsman, B.L., Lipp, R., *New Ballard Score, expanded to include extremely premature infants,* Journal of Pediatrics 119(3):417–23 (1991). Reprinted with permission.

CHAPTER 15

COMPLAINT AND PAPER DISCOVERY IN LABOR AND DELIVERY

Michael D. Volk

§ 15.1   Goals of Complaints

Pleadings that are filed in a labor and delivery case must be succinct and concise. Counsel should let the defendant know the accusation without giving the entire plan away. If able to amend freely, the attorney should follow the rules of pleading in the jurisdiction but not plead too specifically until discovery has been completed. What follows in this chapter are some complaints for labor and delivery room cases, setting out both maternal and fetal injury, as well as some motions and other matters that may be helpful.

§ 15.2   Sample Complaint: Fetal Injury from Failure to Recognize Post-Maturity Syndrome

PLAINTIFFS' ORIGINAL COMPLAINT
TO THE HONORABLE JUDGE OF SAID COURT:

Now come the Plaintiffs, _____ and _____ Individually and as Next Friends of their Minor Child, _____ and complaining of _____ MATERNITY HOSPITAL and _____, M.D., Defendants herein. Plaintiffs would respectfully show the Court and Jury the following:

1. Plaintiffs are residents of the Country of _____, State of _____ and diversity jurisdiction exists between Plaintiffs and all Defendants.

2. Defendant _____ MATERNITY HOSPITAL is a business entity organized and doing business in the State of _____, with its principal place of business in _____ County, _____ where service will be had upon its hospital administrator. Defendant _____ MATERNITY HOSPITAL had in its employ physicians whose names are _____, M.D., and Defendant _____, M.D. Said physicians were agents, servants, and employees at the time of the acts complained of herein.

3. Defendants _____, M.D., and _____, M.D., are, and were at all times relevant to this lawsuit, physicians duly licensed to practice their profession in the State of _____, specializing in obstetrics and gynecology. Said Defendants have offices in _____ County, _____, and service of process will be had upon them there.

Claim is made against said defendants both individually and as agents, servants, and employees of Defendant _____ MATERNITY HOSPITAL.

4. All the acts complained of herein occurred within the _____ jurisdiction. The matter in controversy exceeds, exclusive of interest and costs, the sum of $10,000.00.

5.   Plaintiffs have fully satisfied the presuit requirements of § _____ of the code of the State of _____.

6.   Prior to _____, 19___, Plaintiff _____ was accepted as a paying patient by _____ MATERNITY HOSPITAL. In the late evening hours of _____, 19___, Plaintiff _____ went into labor significantly after her due date. Plaintiff _____ had been seen in Defendant's clinic on several occasions after her due date. On all occasions she was told that it was not time for the delivery and that her fetus was fine. When first admitted into Defendant Hospital, she was examined and put to bed rest by _____, M.D. Said agent, servant, or employee of Defendant Hospital did not examine or see Plaintiff _____ again although he was in Defendant Hospital for twelve (12) additional hours. Their child, the Minor Plaintiff _____, was delivered at approximately 7:21 P.M. on December 30, 1994. Defendants _____ MATERNITY HOSPITAL, _____, M.D. and _____, M.D., individually and as agents, servants, and employees of Defendant Hospital undertook to render medical services to the Plaintiffs, and in the course of rendering these medical services, committed acts and omitted to perform certain duties that constitute negligence as that term is defined by law. Defendants _____ and _____were chosen by Defendant Hospital to attend Plaintiff _____. Plaintiffs did not choose Defendants _____ or _____ and had no choice whatsoever as to whom their physicians would be. Defendant _____ and _____were Defendant hospital's doctor, not Plaintiffs' doctor. In particular, defendants failed to properly monitor Plaintiff's condition, and did not cause the timely performance of a Cesarean section, despite overwhelming signs of fetal distress as evidenced by decelerations of the fetal heart rate. A Cesarean section was finally performed, but at a time too late to prevent the Minor Plaintiff's brain damage. After his belated birth, the Minor Plaintiff _____ was transferred to the intensive care nursery at _____ Medical Center in _____, _____, by EMS.

7.   Defendants _____ and _____ individually and/or as agents, servants, and employees of Defendant _____ MATERNITY HOSPITAL, were negligent in the following acts of commission and omission in that they, and each of them:

a.   Failed to timely deliver Minor Plaintiff _____

b.   Failed to recognize that _____ was a high-risk infant because he was postmature

c.   Failed to properly monitor the progress of labor

d.   Failed to timely consult with other physicians

e.   Failed to timely perform a Cesarean section in the face of overwhelming fetal heart rate decelerations

f.   Failed to promptly and properly treat Plaintiffs

g.   Gave inadequate and dangerous orders

h.   Failed to give proper orders for the care of Plaintiff _____

i.   Failed to timely transfer Plaintiff _____ and her infant child to a hospital with proper facilities

j.   Utilized the drug pitocin when it was contraindicated by Plaintiff's small pelvis and lack of progression in labor.

k.   Failed to diagnose that Plaintiff's labor had not progressed in a satisfactory manner.

8.   Defendant _____ MATERNITY HOSPITAL by and through its agents, servants, employees, and representatives, nurses, allied medical personnel, and the doctors it employed, acting within the course and scope of their employment, were negligent and careless in their treatment of the Plaintiffs in the following acts of commission or omission in that said Defendant:

a.   Failed to timely intervene when the fetal distress of Minor Plaintiff _____ became obvious

b.   Failed to have adequate policies and procedures to protect the safety of the plaintiffs

c.   Failed to properly monitor the progress of labor

d.   Failed to properly notify Defendants _____ and _____ of the Plaintiffs' condition

e.   Failed to promptly and properly care for the Plaintiffs

f.   Failed to recognize that _____ was a high-risk infant because he was postmature

g.   Failed to timely consult with other physicians

h.   Failed to cause the timely performance of a cesarean section in the face of overwhelming fetal heart rate decelerations

i.   Gave inadequate and dangerous orders

j.   Failed to timely deliver _____

k.   Held themselves out as having all necessary facilities to care for Plaintiffs and other persons similarly situated as Plaintiffs

l. Represented that Defendant was able to provide all obstetrical and other services timely and adequately so that mother and child would not be endangered by a lack of facilities, equipment, and services

m. Ordered oxygen without a physician's order and without notifying any physician that oxygen was being utilized to allow a physician to determine why oxygen was needed

n. Allowed the drug pitocin to be utilized in spite of Plaintiff's small pelvis and failed labor

o. Increased the dosage of pitocin without an order

p. Increased the dosage of pitocin without notifying a physician

q. Failed to warn the Plaintiffs of the limited facilities available at Defendant _____ MATERNITY HOSPITAL

9. Further, Defendant _____ MATERNITY HOSPITAL misrepresented to the Plaintiffs that Defendant hospital was fully equipped to handle any and all obstetrical patients including well-trained physicians on the hospital premises at all times, including the ability to care for emergency Cesarean sections to preserve the health and well-being of mother and child.

Plaintiffs relied upon this representation and pursuant to that reliance entered into a contract with Defendant _____ MATERNITY HOSPITAL to deliver their first-born child. Said reliance was induced by Defendant hospital and plaintiffs' reliance was justified in that they were consumers and persons who did not have any medical training. Pursuant to that reliance, Plaintiffs delivered their first child at Defendant _____ MATERNITY HOSPITAL. The representations by Defendant were false in that Defendant hospital did not have all necessary facilities to perform an immediate Cesarean section to safeguard the health of mother and baby.

10. As a direct and proximate result of the negligence of the Defendants, the Minor Plaintiff sustained serious and permanent bodily injury, including, but not limited to, devastating brain damage, necessitating medical, surgical, and related care, and the reasonable expense thereof, and permanently impairing Plaintiff from engaging in normal family, social, recreational and wage-earning activities for the rest of his life. Great pain has been suffered and always will be suffered by the Minor Plaintiff. He has sustained ugly and cosmetic disfigurement that is permanent in nature and will cause him life-long humiliation, pain and suffering, anxiety, and embarrassment. His capacity to enjoy life in the future has been limited. He has required hospital and medical care, aid, and attention and he will require the same in the future. His ability to earn a living in the future has been drastically reduced. By reason of all the foregoing, Plaintiffs have been damaged in a sum in excess of the minimum jurisdictional limits of the Court. Further, the parent Plaintiffs have lost the joy of raising their son. They have suffered a loss of his society, affection, and help.

11. Plaintiffs demand trial by jury.

WHEREFORE, PREMISES CONSIDERED, Plaintiffs demand judgment against Defendants in a sum in excess of the minimum jurisdictional limits of this Court, costs of this action, and for such other and further relief as the Court may deem proper.

§ 15.3   Sample Complaint: Failure to Deliver Premature Infant

COMPLAINT
TO THE HONORABLE JUDGE OF SAID COURT:

Plaintiffs complain of Defendant and allege:

1.   This action is brought pursuant to the Federal Tort Claims Act and jurisdiction is founded upon such Act, 28 U.S.C. § 1346(b) *et seq.*

2.   On February 27, 1994, Plaintiffs filed their claim pursuant to 28 U.S.C. § 1346b *et seq.,* known as the Federal Tort Claims Act. This claim was received by the proper authorities and denied by letter dated _____, 19____. All statutory requirements have been met for filing this lawsuit.

3.   At all times relevant to this action, Plaintiff _____ was entitled to medical care and treatment at _____ Medical Center by virtue of the fact that her husband was assigned to _____ Medical Center as a member of the United States Armed Forces with the designated rank of _____.

4.   This action includes damages for wrongful death and is filed by Plaintiffs _____ and _____ as survivors of their deceased infant. _____, the decedent, died intestate, no administration of his estate is necessary and no application for administration has been filed. This action also includes damages for conscious pain and suffering endured by the decedent. This action also includes mental suffering or mental anguish and sorrow that Plaintiffs _____ and _____ suffered while witnessing the death of _____ at the hands of the Defendants in this lawsuit. Further, Plaintiffs seek damages pursuant to the Texas Supreme Court case of *Sanchez v. Shindler* that includes, but is not limited to, loss of companionship, affection, and society from their son, as well as lost consortium.

5.   On _____, 19____, Plaintiff _____ visited the Obstetrical Clinic at _____ Medical Center. She was diagnosed as being pregnant. From the aforesaid date until, and inclusive of _____, 19____, Plaintiff _____ experienced a medically complicated pregnancy that culminated in the wrongful vaginal traumatic breech extraction birth of the decedent, _____. _____ was admitted to _____ Medical Center on _____, 19_____ due to premature rupture of the

membranes and premature labor. During the course of her labor, Plaintiff received various tocolytic therapies to stop her labor and her unborn child, _____, received lung maturation therapy. The tocolytic therapies failed to stop Plaintiff's _____ labor. During the course of her labor, Plaintiff was not prepared for a Cesarean section, although it was determined that her premature unborn child was in a breech presentation. On _____, 19____ the deceased, _____ was delivered vaginally in a breech presentation by means of breech extraction utilizing baby Simpson forceps. The child's aftercoming head was stuck in his mother's vagina for approximately twenty (20) minutes. Defendant's agents, servants, and employees broke the decedent's neck by manipulation with the forceps. Said forceps were utilized by a second-year resident with little training in breech extraction of prematures, even though the chief of obstetrics was also present in the room. He died at eight (8) hours of life. The child was born asphyxiated and neurologically impaired.

6. Defendant UNITED STATES OF AMERICA, by and through their agents, servants, and employees was negligent and careless in the treatment of Plaintiff _____ and the deceased _____, in the following acts of commission and omission in that said Defendant:

1. Failed to timely diagnose and treat Plaintiff _____ as a high-risk pregnancy

2. Failed to timely diagnose and treat the deceased as a high-risk fetus

3. Failed to properly diagnose and treat Plaintiff's prenatal complications

4. Failed to take the necessary obstetrical precautions in the presence of premature labor

5. Failed to properly monitor the labor of Plaintiff

6. Failed to properly monitor the intrauterine condition of the deceased _____

7. Failed to adhere to acceptable obstetrical standards in the delivery of a premature infant in breech presentation by allowing an inadequately trained resident to deliver the decedent

8. Failed to perform a timely Cesarean section on the Plaintiff _____

9. Allowed the deceased, _____, to become physically traumatized and sustain intracranial hemorrhage, hypovolemic shock, birth asphxia, pneumothorax, and death as the result of the breech extraction delivery with the use of forceps

10. Broke the decedent's neck with forceps

7. As a direct and proximate result of said acts of negligence and medical mal-practice, the decedent suffered extreme pain and anguish from the time of his birth until the time of his death.

8. All the acts of said agents, servants, and employees of Defendant UNITED STATES OF AMERICA as alleged herein, both of commission and omission, were negligent and were committed by said agents, servants, and employees within the course and scope of their employment by the Defendant and were each and all a proximate cause or causes of the continued pain, suffering, and mental anguish of the decedent, his wrongful death and the continuing pain, suffering, mental anguish, loss of society, loss of consortium and other *Sanchez v. Shindler* damages of Plaintiffs, _____ and _____.

9. By reason of the aforesaid, Plaintiffs have sustained reasonable and necessary funeral expenses, including the costs of casket, headstone, and transportation of the remains of _____.

10. From the time Plaintiff _____ was taken to _____ Medical Center until the death of _____, Plaintiffs were in the vicinity and presence of _____ and were witnesses to and participants in his suffering and anguish as only parents can be. As a result of the aforesaid, permanent emotional and mental injury has been and always will be suffered by the Plaintiffs. The needless loss of his companionship, affection, consortium, comfort, and society has permanently injured the Plaintiffs.

11. By reason of all the foregoing, Plaintiffs have been damaged in a sum in excess of the minimum jurisdictional limits of this Court.

WHEREFORE, PREMISES CONSIDERED, Plaintiffs pray that Defendant be cited to appear and answer herein, and that upon final hearing and trial of this cause, Plaintiffs have judgment against Defendant in a sum in excess of the minimum jurisdictional limits of this court, together with interest thereon at the legal rate from the date of said judgment until paid, all costs of this suit, and all such other and further relief, both general and special, at law and in equity to which Plaintiffs may justly be entitled.

§ 15.4 Sample Complaint: Death of Fetus from Failure by Lay-Midwife to Transfer Mother

PLAINTIFFS' ORIGINAL PETITION
TO THE HONORABLE JUDGE OF SAID COURT:

Now come the Plaintiffs, _____ and his wife, _____, and complaining of _____, INC. and _____, Defendants herein. Plaintiffs would respectfully show the Court and Jury the following:

I.

Plaintiffs are residents of _____ County, _____. All the acts complained of herein occurred in _____ County, _____.

II.

Defendant _____, INC. is and was at all times relevant to this lawsuit a domestic corporation duly authorized and doing business in the State of _____ with its principal place of business at _____ Street, _____, and service of process will be had upon it there. Defendant _____ is and was at all times relevant to this lawsuit a lay-midwife practicing midwifery without any medical training in _____, State of _____ and is the owner and registered agent for _____, INC.[1] Service of process may be had upon her at the aforesaid address.

III.

This action includes damages for wrongful death and is filed by Plaintiffs _____ and _____ as survivors of their deceased infant. _____, the decedent, died intestate, no administration of his estate is necessary and no application for administration has been filed. This action also includes damages for conscious pain and suffering endured by the decedent. This action also includes mental suffering or mental anguish and sorrow that Plaintiffs _____ and _____ suffered while witnessing the death of _____ at the hands of the Defendants in this lawsuit. Further, Plaintiffs seek damages pursuant to the _____ Supreme Court case of *Sanchez v. Shindler* which includes, but is not limited to, loss of companionship, affection, and society from their son. In the early evening hours of _____, 19____, Plaintiff _____ was in early labor. Plaintiffs called Defendants, whereupon Defendant lay-midwife came to Plaintiffs' house, "examined" her and left after making a "diagnosis" of early labor. She was told to come to Defendants' place of business when her contractions were five minutes apart. In the early morning hours of _____, 19____, Plaintiff _____'s contractions became stronger and Plaintiff _____ again called Defendants and he was told to bring his wife to the offices of _____, INC. She was examined and sent home again with a diagnosis

---

[1] In some areas of the country, especially the southwestern United States, lay-midwives are allowed to deliver babies. A lay-midwife has very little or no medical training. They can deliver babies in some states because delivering babies is not defined as the practice of medicine. There is almost no regulation of lay-midwives. Every plaintiff's lawyer should understand the obligation to require such lay people, who are practicing one of the most dangerous aspects of medicine, to be accountable for their actions. It is virtually impossible to satisfy a judgment against a lay-midwife; however, counsel should recognize this as a pro bono duty to help eliminate the practice. The authors have seen many brain-damaged children resulting from delivery by lay-midwives. These tragedies could have been almost uniformly prevented. The cost to society and to these unfortunate, ill children is staggering.

of early labor. At approximately 8:00 A.M. on the morning of _____,
19____, Plaintiff _____ took his wife to the offices of _____,
INC. for the third time, whereupon she was examined and "admitted" to said
_____, INC. offices.

IV.

Plaintiffs _____ and _____ had previously contracted
with Defendants _____, INC. and _____ for prenatal care
and the delivery of their child. Further, at the time of the aforesaid contract Defendant
_____ misrepresented to Plaintiffs that _____, INC. was
fully equipped to handle and care for all kinds of obstetrical patients. Plaintiffs
_____ and _____ relied upon this representation. Said
reliance was induced by the Defendant _____ and Plaintiffs' reliance
was justified in that they were consumers and persons who did not have any medical
training.

V.

Pursuant to the aforesaid reliance, Plaintiff _____ remained at Defendant _____, INC. despite her nonprogression of labor, nonprogression
of cervical dilation, and the apparent fetal distress of her unborn son, _____.
Approximately four hours after the onset of the aforesaid labor complications, Defendant _____ took Plaintiff _____ to _____
General Hospital whereupon Plaintiff _____ underwent an emergency
Cesarean section. Said Cesarean section was done at a time too late to prevent the
subsequent death of Plaintiffs' son, from severe perinatal asphyxia, severe meconium
aspiration, severe respiratory distress syndrome and the further complications of
pneumothorax and pulmonary edema.

VI.

Defendants undertook to render medical services to the Plaintiff _____
at Defendant _____, INC. and in the course of rendering these medical
services committed acts and omitted to perform certain duties that constitute
negligence as the term is defined by law. In particular, Defendants failed to properly
monitor Plaintiff's condition and did not cause a timely referral and transfer of Plaintiff
_____ to a proper hospital and a licensed, qualified physician for
delivery, despite clear and overwhelming signs of nonprogressive labor and fetal
distress. Further, Defendants are not educated in medicine and should not be delivering
fetuses. Defendants were negligent in the following acts of commission and omission
in that they:

1. Failed to recognize that _____ was a high-risk infant thereby
causing his untimely death

2. Failed to properly monitor the progress of labor

3.   Failed to timely consult with any physician licensed

4.   Failed to timely intervene and transfer Plaintiff _____ to a qualified hospital or any hospital for delivery when fetal distress became obvious

5.   Failed to promptly and properly treat the Plaintiff

6.   Held themselves out as having all the necessary facilities to care for Plaintiff and other persons similarly situated as the Plaintiffs

7.   Represented falsely that the Defendants were able to provide all labor and delivery services timely and adequately so that mother and child would not be damaged by lack of facilities, equipment, services, and health care personnel

8.   Failed to warn Plaintiffs of the limited facilities available at _____, INC.

9.   Committed fraud on Plaintiffs by misrepresenting the level of services and care possible at the Defendant _____, INC.

10.   Failed to transfer Plaintiff to a hospital after being requested to do so by said Plaintiff

11.   Failed to have a physician immediately available to monitor the progress of Plaintiff's labor

VII.

As a direct and proximate result of the negligence of the Defendants, the minor child of the Plaintiffs' sustained bodily damage so serious as to cause his subsequent and untimely death. Said bodily damage was inclusive of, but not limited to, severe perinatal asphyxia, severe meconium aspiration, severe respiratory distress syndrome, pneumothorax, pneumomediastinum, and pulmonary edema, all of which necessitated medical, surgical, and related care, and the reasonable expense thereof. Great pain was suffered by the infant prior to his death. By reason of all the foregoing, Plaintiffs have been damaged in excess of the minimum jurisdictional limits of the Court. The parent Plaintiffs have lost the joy of raising their son. They have suffered a loss of his society, affection, and health. Plaintiffs are entitled to all damages as set out in the Texas Supreme Court case of *Sanchez v. Shindler.*

VIII.

Because of Defendants _____, INC. and _____'s conscious and reckless disregard for the health, safety, and well-being of Plaintiff and her unborn infant son, and because of the fraud perpetrated on the Plaintiffs, Defendants should be punished in a further reasonable sum as punitive damages.

IX.

Plaintiffs demand trial by jury.

WHEREFORE, PREMISES CONSIDERED, Plaintiffs pray to have judgment against the Defendants, jointly and severally, in a sum in excess of the minimum jurisdictional limits of this Court, punitive damages, costs of the action, and for such other further relief as the Court may deem proper.

§ 15.5 Sample Complaint: Failure to Perform Antenatal Testing

COMPLAINT[2]

1. Plaintiffs _____ and _____ were at all times material hereto husband and wife and residents of the City of _____, State of _____, and the parents of decedent _____.

2. Defendants _____, M.D., and _____, M.D., are and were at all times pertinent hereto physicians doing business and having their offices in _____, _____, holding themselves out as physicians and obstetric surgeons licensed to practice medicine.

3. Each Defendant was the principal or agent of each other Defendant at all times pertinent hereto and each Defendant was acting within the scope of his/its agency.

4. Plaintiff _____ was the father of decedent _____, and has been appointed Personal Representative of his Estate and, in that capacity brings this suit under the Wrongful Death Act, being § _____, code of _____.

5. Plaintiff _____ and her unborn twins were admitted and accepted as patients by _____ Hospital for care and treatment of approaching term pregnancy, and continued in the care of said hospital until discharge on or about _____, 19____.

6. In _____, 19____, Plaintiff _____ sought the medical services of Defendant _____, M.D. and _____, M.D. for herself and her unborn twins and was accepted by them as a patient, and continued as their patient during her pregnancy, including during her admission to _____ Hospital and during her delivery on _____, 19____ and thereafter until her last examination and treatment.

---

[2] This complaint was used in a case with Ms. Linda Atkinson of the Detroit, Michigan, firm of Philo, Atkinson, Steinberg, Walker & White.

7. At those times and thereafter, Defendants, and each of them, undertook for compensation the medical diagnosis, examination, care treatment, medication, observation, and attention to _____ and her unborn twins as to their general health and well-being and further to provide and furnish all necessary equipment, facilities, and personnel to treat, care for and attend them including, but not limited to physicians, surgeons, nurses, attendants, medication, surgery, testing, and equipment.

8. On or about _____, 19____, surgical delivery of Plaintiff's twins was indicated by medical signs, but delayed until _____, 19____, resulting in the death of decedent _____ *in utero.*

9. On or about _____, 19____, in connection with the diagnosis, care, observation, furnishing of equipment, surgery, examination, testing, and all other such treatment for Plaintiff, Defendants performed upon her procedures including, but not limited to Cesarean delivery, surgery, suturing, and other procedures incident to surgical delivery of her twin term fetuses and termination of her pregnancy, in the course of which her son, _____, was delivered mascerated and dead.

10. As a result of the negligence of the Defendants, and each of them, Plaintiff's decedent _____ suffered days of pain, and slow asphyxiation resulting in his death prior to delivery.

11. Defendants _____, M.D., and _____, M.D., jointly and severally, owed Plaintiffs the duty of reasonable care and the exercise of that degree of diligence, care, and skill ordinarily possessed by physicians and surgeons of similar training and experience, and conformity with the laws and statutes of the State of _____. Defendants' duties to Plaintiffs and the standard of care required that Defendants:

a. Provide for proper medical and surgical care for their obstetrical patient in anticipation of the absence of any of them at critical times in the clinical course of their patients

b. Perform thorough diagnostic testing, monitoring, and review of records when patients failed to progress in labor

c. Carefully and thoroughly diagnose patients' condition including performing a complete differential diagnosis to determine the status of the unborn twin fetuses *in utero*

d. Attend patients timely and prescribe a proper regimen of treatment, including immediate Cesarean delivery

e. Obtain prompt, timely, and thorough consultation for their patients

f. Treat the twin pregnancy of _____ as a high-risk pregnancy and intervene when it was necessary to do so to preserve the lives of both twins

12.   These acts of negligence of the Defendants and each of them were a proximate cause of the death of _____, and the injuries and damages of Plaintiffs _____ and _____

13.   The amount in controversy exceeds Ten Thousand ($10,000.00) Dollars.

14.   Plaintiff _____ on behalf of decedent has incurred medical, surgical, hospital and nursing expenses for his care and treatment prior to death, and has incurred funeral and burial and memorial expenses on his behalf. He has further suffered loss of his wife's services, and disruption of their marital relationship because of her injuries, and further, loss of his son's services and companionship by reason of his untimely death.

15.   Plaintiff _____ has suffered injury, mental and physical pain and suffering, loss of enjoyment of life, disruption of her marital relationship, and substantial medical, pharmaceutical, hospital, and surgical expenses. In addition, she has suffered loss of her son's services and companionship by reason of his untimely death.

WHEREFORE, Plaintiffs seek judgment against Defendants, jointly and severally, in whatever amount they are found to be entitled exclusive of costs, interest and attorneys' fees.

§ 15.6   Sample Complaint: Failure to Diagnose Hydatidiform Mole

PLAINTIFF'S ORIGINAL PETITION

Now comes _____, Plaintiff, complaining of _____, M.D., hereinafter called Defendant, and for cause of action would respectfully show the Court the following:

I.

Plaintiff is a resident of _____, _____.

The Defendant, _____, M.D., is a duly licensed physician and surgeon under the laws of the State of _____ and represents himself to the public as such. Defendant is regularly engaged in the practice of his profession in _____, _____, and will be served with citation at his office. The Defendant doctor undertook to provide medical treatment to the Plaintiff under such circumstances that a physician-patient relationship arose and Defendant doctor assumed the duty to exercise ordinary care in his diagnosis and treatment of the Plaintiff's conditions.

II.

On or about _____, 19____, in _____, _____,
Plaintiff employed Defendant doctor to diagnose and treat what she thought was her
pregnant condition and to provide her prenatal care. Plaintiff had missed her period.
On or about that date, Defendant doctor informed Plaintiff of his diagnosis that she
was pregnant. Plaintiff dutifully followed Defendant's instructions and returned for
examination on each occasion that Defendant instructed her to. Although Plaintiff
informed Defendant there was an absence of fetal movement, Defendant continued
to reassure Plaintiff that she was in fact pregnant.

III.

Thereafter, Plaintiff submitted herself for continuous treatment by Defendant for a
period of eight months and underwent prenatal care during this period. Plaintiff was
not pregnant but had an abnormal medical condition referred to as hydatidiform mole
that has become cancerous and metastasized to other parts of Plaintiff's body.

IV.

In diagnosing and treating Plaintiff as aforesaid, Defendant _____,
M.D., did not exercise the degree of skill and care or possess the degree of knowledge
ordinarily exercised and possessed by other physicians practicing in the same vicinity
in that: Defendant diagnosed Plaintiff's condition as that of a normal pregnancy, but
failed and neglected to make the diagnosis of hydatidiform mole, and was negligent
in the following respects in that said Defendant:

1. Failed to diagnose the Plaintiff's condition properly

2. Failed to properly examine Plaintiff and utilize proper and timely diagnostic
procedures

3. Failed to ever detect that the fundal height of Plaintiff's uterus was not consistent
with a diagnosis of pregnancy

4. Failed to recognize that his inability to palpate the fetal parts was a further
indication of the fact that Plaintiff was not pregnant

5. Failed to diagnose the fact that Plaintiff had toxemia of pregnancy

6. Failed to initiate prompt surgical removal of the hydatidiform mole before it
became cancerous and metastasized to other parts of Plaintiff's body

In connection with the foregoing, the Plaintiff alleges that each and every, all and
singular, of the foregoing acts and/or omissions were acts of negligence or were the
proximate cause of the injuries sustained by the Plaintiff.

VII.

As a direct and proximate result of Defendant's negligent acts, Plaintiff now has a cancerous condition which, in all probability, will result in her early and untimely death. Plaintiff has required massive medical care in an attempt to save her life which has caused her to lose her hair and to become nauseous and toxic. Further, Plaintiff has been caused great pain and suffering and mental anguish. These injuries to Plaintiff necessitated medical, surgical, and related care, and the reasonable expense thereof, and has permanently impaired Plaintiff from engaging in normal family, social, recreational, and wage-earning activities for the rest of her life. She has sustained ugly and cosmetic disfigurement. Her capacity to enjoy life in the future is minimal and she has likewise had a reduction in her ability to earn a living. By reason of all the foregoing, Plaintiff has been damaged in the sum in excess of Five Million Dollars ($5,000,000.00).

WHEREFORE, PREMISES CONSIDERED, Plaintiff prays that Defendant be cited to appear and answer herein, and upon a final hearing thereof, Plaintiffs have judgment against Defendant for Five Million Dollars ($5,000,000.00) with prejudgment and postjudgment interest, costs of court, and for such other and further relief, at law or in equity to which Plaintiff is justly entitled.

§ 15.7   Sample Complaint: Death of Mother and Fetus

COMPLAINT[3]

Plaintiff, by and through his attorneys undersigned, complains and alleges as follows:

I.

Plaintiff _____ is the widower of _____, deceased, and the father of his deceased infant son, _____.

II.

Defendants _____, M.D., _____, M.D., _____, M.D., and _____, M.D., are residents of _____ County, _____, are licensed to practice medicine in the State of _____, and, in fact, do practice medicine in _____ County, _____, and in particular, do practice medicine at _____ HOSPITAL, INC., a _____ corporation.

III.

Defendant _____ HOSPITAL, INC. is a _____ corporation organized and doing business in the State of _____, County of

---

[3] This complaint was used in a case with Mr. Leighton Rockafellow of Tucson, Arizona.

_____, and is licensed as a general hospital providing medical, surgical, and intensive care services to the public.

IV.

Defendants _____ 1–10's true names are unknown. Plaintiff requests leave of Court to add their names as they become known to Plaintiff. Defendants' true names are unknown, but Plaintiff requests leave to add their true names at such time as they become known.

V.

The actions complained of herein occurred within _____ County, State of _____, and, at all material and relevant times, the Plaintiff, the Plaintiff's decedents, and the Defendant physicians were residents of _____ County, _____.

VI.

On or about _____, 19___, Plaintiff's decedent _____ consulted with the Defendant _____, M.D., as a patient and was told by _____ that she was 11½ weeks pregnant. _____ agreed to become _____'s physician concerning that pregnancy and agreed to deliver her child at the _____ HOSPITAL, INC.

VII.

Thereafter, on _____, 19___, _____ was admitted into the Defendant hospital by Defendant _____ with a diagnosis of viral pneumonia. During said hospitalization, _____ was seen by Defendants and x-rays were taken by hospital personnel and read by Defendant _____.

VIII.

Thereafter, and before her admittance into labor on _____, 19___, _____ complained to the Defendants of being seriously ill. On _____, 19___ in the early morning hours, _____ was admitted into the Defendant hospital. Both she and her baby boy died that same day.

IX.

After prolonged labor with a fetal heart monitor showing numerous late decelerations, Defendant _____ informed both Plaintiff and his wife that their child was dead in utero. _____ then attempted to deliver the alleged deceased child vaginally after massive infusions of pitocin. During those attempts to deliver _____, the mother suffered cardiac and respiratory arrest and died.

X.

Their deaths were directly and proximately caused by the negligence of the Defendants, and each of them, by failing to properly diagnose and treat the decedent for the illness from which she was suffering at least from _____, 19____, up to and until the time of her death.

XI.

Decedent's death was a further proximate result of the negligence of the Defendant hospital by failing to adequately and properly screen the qualifications of the Defendant physicians prior to granting them staff privileges at the hospital and its failure to provide an adequate, trained, and attentive nursing staff.

XII.

Furthermore, the Defendants failed to properly consult with one another and failed to consult with other more qualified physicians, failed to timely transfer the decedents to a hospital that was better able to care for her, failed to adequately staff their facility, abandoned the decedents, failed to properly care for the decedents, failed to properly supervise the Defendants, failed to insist upon consultation with more qualified physicians, failed to recognize that the decedents were dangerously ill, failed to properly evaluate the decedent mother, failed to properly diagnose the decedent, failed to institute proper therapy for the decedent, allowed the administration of dangerous drugs without adequate safeguards to the decedent, gave inadequate orders and instructions, failed to properly monitor mother and child, and failed to perform necessary and proper laboratory and x-ray examinations, all said failures constituting negligence.

XIII.

As a direct and proximate result of the negligence of the Defendants, and each of them, as aforesaid and by reason of the wrongful deaths of mother and child, Plaintiff _____ has been deprived of the aid, association, support, income, protection, services, comfort, care, love, devotion, and society of the decedents. Plaintiff _____ has further incurred funeral and burial expenses for the decedents, has suffered mental anguish and sorrow, and claims damages by reason of the wrongful deaths of his wife and child pursuant to § _____, together with a sum to be determined by the Court and a Jury to be just and reasonable for exemplary damages.

XIV.

The complained of conduct of the Defendants, and each of them, was so outrageous as to make an award of exemplary damages appropriate to act as a deterrent to further outrageous behavior.

WHEREFORE, Plaintiff prays for Judgment against the Defendants, and each of them, as follows:

1. For compensatory damages in such an amount as will reasonably, completely, and adequately compensate the Plaintiff for all injuries, damages, and losses as aforesaid

2. For punitive damages in such an amount as will substantially deter the Defendants from further outrageous conduct in the future

3. For costs of suit necessarily and lawfully incurred herein

4. For such other and further relief as the Court deems just and proper in the premises

§ 15.8   Sample Complaint: Fetal and Maternal Injury from High Forceps Delivery

PLAINTIFFS' ORIGINAL PETITION
TO THE HONORABLE JUDGE OF SAID COURT:

Now comes the Plaintiff _____, a minor, by and through her mother and next friend _____ and complaining of _____ HOSPITAL, _____, M.D., and _____, M.D., Defendants herein. Plaintiff would respectfully show the Court and Jury the following:

I.

Plaintiff _____ and her mother are residents of the State of _____, County of _____, City of _____. Defendant _____ HOSPITAL is a business entity organized and doing business in the State of _____, with its principal place of business in _____, Texas where service may be had upon its hospital administrator.

Defendant _____, M.D., and _____, M.D. are and were at all times relevant to this lawsuit, physicians duly licensed to practice their profession in the State of _____. Said Defendants have their offices in _____, _____, and service of process will be had upon them there.

II.

All the acts complained of herein occurred within _____ County.

III.

Plaintiffs have fully satisfied the presuit requirements of § _____ of the code of the state of _____.

IV.

The mother and natural guardian of _____, _____, was taken care of during her prenatal period by Defendant _____, M.D. Defendant _____, permitted the pregnancy to go beyond 42 weeks and failed to take the necessary steps to assure the well-being of the mother and child. Eventually, _____ was admitted into Defendant _____ HOS-PITAL for the delivery of her child. Subsequent to her admission she was permitted to labor for a protracted period of time. The Defendants, jointly and severally, failed to adhere to the accepted principles of obstetrics and the management of her labor and delivery. Said Defendants further utilized forceps in a "high forceps" delivery and fractured the minor Plaintiff's skull.

V.

Defendants _____, M.D. and _____, M.D., individually and as agents, servants, employees, and representatives of Defendant _____ HOS-PITAL were negligent in acts of commission and omission in that they individually, and as agents, servants, representatives, and employees of Defendant _____ HOSPITAL failed to adhere to acceptable standards of medical practice in their treatment of the pregnancy and delivery of _____ and _____.

VI.

Defendant _____ HOSPITAL, by and through its agents, servants, employees, and representatives, nurses, allied medical personnel, and Defendants _____, M.D. and _____, M.D., acting within the course and scope of their employment, were negligent and careless in their treatment of Plaintiffs in acts of commission or omission in that said Defendants failed to adhere to acceptable standards of nursing and hospital practice in their treatment of the pregnancy and delivery of _____ and _____.

VII.

Further, _____ HOSPITAL and the Defendant physicians conspired to cover up their negligence by destroying the pertinent medical records in this case.

VIII.

As a direct and proximate result of the negligence of the Defendants, and all of them, the minor Plaintiff sustained serious and permanent bodily injury, including, but not limited to, brain damage, necessitating medical, surgical, and related care, and the reasonable expense thereof, and permanently impairing Plaintiff from engaging in normal family, social, recreational, and wage-earning activities for the rest of her life. Great pain has been suffered and always will be suffered by the minor Plaintiff. She has sustained ugly and cosmetic disfigurement, that is permanent in nature and will cause her life-long humiliation, pain, suffering, anxiety, and embarrassment. Her capacity to enjoy life in the past and in the future has been limited. She has required hospital and medical care, aid, and attention and will require the same in the future. Her ability to earn a living in the future has been severely and permanently impaired with a drastic, if not total, reduction in earning capacity.

IX.

By reason of all the foregoing, Plaintiffs have been damaged in a sum in excess of the minimum jurisdictional limits of the Court.

X.

Further, Defendant _____ HOSPITAL'S administration is, or should have been aware for many years, of below-standard obstetrical care being rendered at Defendant _____ HOSPITAL. Such substandard care, in light of all the circumstances surrounding medical care rendered at _____ HOS-PITAL, constitutes a conscious and heedless disregard for the welfare of the public at large, and the Plaintiff in specific, so as to further justify exemplary damages.

IX.

Plaintiffs demand trial by jury.

WHEREFORE, PREMISES CONSIDERED, Plaintiffs demand judgment against Defendants, jointly and severally, in a sum in excess of the minimum jurisdictional limits of this Court, exemplary damages, costs of this action and for such other and further relief as the Court may deem proper.

§ 15.9 Goals of Interrogatories

The next section is a relatively extensive set of interrogatories. This set of interrogatories can be used in nearly every labor and delivery room case to find out some essential facts about the defendant, his or her background, some of the operative facts of the physician-patient relationship, and what experts the defendant will call. The utilization of these interrogatories will allow counsel to have baseline data to use to prepare for the deposition of the defendant.

§ 15.10 Standard Interrogatories to Defendant in Labor and Delivery Room Case

INTERROGATORIES PROPOUNDED TO DEFENDANT DOCTOR[4]

1. State the full name, current address, telephone number, and office, title, and capacity or position of each person answering or assisting in answering these Interrogatories on behalf of Defendant.

---

[4] These interrogatories are taken from two cases the authors had with Ms. Linda Atkinson of the Detroit, Michigan firm of Philo, Atkinson, Steinberg, Walker & White and Mr. Leighton Rockafellow who practices in Tucson, Arizona.

2. Has Defendant ever been known by any other name?

3. If so, for each other name, state:

    a. The name in full

    b. The inclusive date he or she was known by that name.

4. What is the date and place of Defendant's birth?

5. Has Defendant ever been associated or in partnership with any other medical practitioner?

6. If so, for each such person, state:

    a. His or her name, address, specialty, and qualifications

    b. The nature of Defendant's business relationship to him or her

    c. The inclusive dates of the relationship

    d. The reason for termination of the relationship.

7. What is the name and address of each medical school of which Defendant is a graduate, and the inclusive dates of attendance at each school?

8. What is the name and address of each undergraduate college which Defendant attended and the inclusive dates of attendance at each college?

9. What is the name and address of the medical institution at which Defendant served his or her internship, and the inclusive dates of internship?

10. In what states is Defendant now, or has Defendant ever been, licensed to practice medicine, and in what year did he or she receive his or her license to practice in each such state?

11. Has Defendant ever been licensed to practice medicine in any other country, other than the United States?

12. If so, give the name of each such country and the inclusive dates of licensing.

13. Has Defendant ever had a medical license suspended, revoked, or terminated in any state or country?

14. If so, for each such license, indicate:

    a. The state or authority which granted it

    b. Whether it was suspended, revoked, terminated, or otherwise restricted, indicating which

    c. The date it was suspended, revoked, or terminated

    d. The reason it was suspended, revoked, or terminated, and whether it was ever reinstated or renewed and if so, on what date.

15. Has Defendant confined his or her medical practice to any particular specialty or specialties?

16. If so, state:

    a. The name of each specialty

    b. The inclusive dates of practice in each specialty.

17. Has Defendant had training in a medical specialty?

18. If so, for each such training, state:

    a. The name of the specialty involved

    b. The name and address of each institution in which Defendant trained

    c. The inclusive dates of Defendant's training.

19. Is Defendant now or has he or she ever been a member or diplomate of any specialty board?

20. If so, for each specialty board, state:

    a. The name and address of the specialty board

    b. The inclusive dates of membership

    c. If no longer a member, state the reason for termination of membership

    d. The qualifications required in order to take the membership examination

    e. The date Defendant qualified to take the membership examination

    f. The number of times the examination was taken and the dates thereof

    g. The place the examination was taken

    h. The full names of the oral examiners.

21. Is Defendant, or has Defendant ever been, a member of any medical society, association, or organization?

22. If so, for each association, society, or organization, please state:

    a. Its name and address

    b. The inclusive dates of membership

    c. Whether Defendant ever held any office and, if so, the name of the office and the inclusive dates such office was held.

23. Does Defendant have, or has Defendant ever had, any staff privileges at or associated with any hospital?

24. If so, for each hospital, state:

    a. Its name and address

    b. A description of each staff privilege granted to Defendant

    c. The inclusive dates each such privilege was held by Defendant.

25. Has Defendant ever had any staff privileges denied, restricted, or revoked at any hospital?

26. If so, for each such privilege, state:

    a. A description

    b. Whether it was revoked or curtailed, and if curtailed, in what way

    c. The date it was revoked or curtailed

    d. The reason it was revoked or curtailed

    e. The name of the disciplinary body that revoked or curtailed it.

27. Has Defendant ever held a position or office in any hospital?

28. If so, for each position or office, please state:

    a. Its name or designation

    b. The duties and privileges attached to it

    c. The name and address of the hospital at which it was held

    d. The inclusive dates it was held.

29. Has Defendant ever been connected in a teaching capacity with any medical institution?

30. If so, for each institution, state:

   a. Its name and address

   b. A description or designation of each position held, and the inclusive dates thereof

   c. The name of each subject taught by Defendant.

31. Has Defendant ever written or contributed to a medical textbook?

32. If so, for each such textbook, please state:

   a. Its title

   b. If Defendant was a coauthor, the name and address of each other author

   c. The name and address of the publisher

   d. The date of original publication and of each reprint or subsequent edition

   e. If Defendant was a coauthor, identify part authored

   f. Whether it is a prescribed book in a medical school.

33. Has Defendant ever written or contributed to a medical paper or article?

34. If so, for each paper or article, please state:

   a. Its title

   b. The subject matter

   c. The date and place of each publication

   d. The title, edition, and name and address of the publisher of each printed publication in which it has appeared

   e. The name and address of each other person who contributed

   f. If defendant was a coauthor, identify which part was contributed.

35. Has Defendant ever had any experience or training as a medical member of any branch of the armed forces?

36. If so, please indicate:

    a. The branch of the service

    b. The inclusive dates

    c. A description of the experience or training received.

37. At any time in Defendant's medical career, has he or she received any award or honor?

38. If so, for each award or honor, please state:

    a. A description or designation

    b. The name and address of the institution for which it came

    c. The achievement for which it was given

    d. The date and place received.

39. Please state with specificity the fact of the Defendant's involvement directly or indirectly in the:

    a. Evaluation and testing

    b. Diagnosis

    c. Consultation

    d. Treatment

    e. Hospitalization

    f. Surgery

of _____ and her unborn child prior to _____,
19____.

40. With reference to Interrogatory No. 39, was Defendant assisted in the role by any other doctor, and if so, identify the doctor by stating the name and current address of such person and what care was given Plaintiffs by the assistant.

41. Describe completely and specifically each procedure, medical service, evaluation, or test which was followed or performed on or rendered to _____

by Defendant or by someone on Defendant's behalf and for each such procedure, medical service, evaluation, or test, please state:

    a. The name of the person or persons performing such procedure

    b. The exact time and date each person or persons performed such procedure or rendered such service

    c. The common name of each procedure, medical service, evaluation, or test

    d. The purpose for each procedure, medical service, evaluation, or test

    e. The result(s) of each procedure, medical service, evaluation, or test

    f. The name of the person or persons authorizing the conduct of each procedure, medical service, evaluation, or test identified in subpart (c) above, if other than the person identified in subpart (a).

42. Describe completely and specifically each and every ultrasound, fetal activity, or other fetal monitoring test, evaluation, or examination performed on _____ and her unborn child and for each, please provide the same information required in Interrogatory 41.

43. With respect to each person identified in Defendant's answer to Interrogatory No. 42, please state the exact and complete nature of the relationship between Defendant and each such person.

44. State the full name, current address, job title, and capacity or other qualification of each person known to this Defendant as having knowledge of the facts involved in the incidents that are the subject of this lawsuit.

45. With regard to each expert witness Defendant expects to call at trial, please state:

    a. His or her name and address

    b. His or her qualification or, in lieu thereof, attach a curriculum vitae to answers

    c. The subject matter on which he or she is expected to testify

    d. The substance of facts and opinions to which the expert is expected to testify

    e. A summary of the grounds for each opinion

    f. Whether a written report has been furnished, and if so, from which expert. Attach a copy of any reports rendered.

46. State precisely the name of textbooks, treatises, or other articles or works that will be utilized:

    a. By each expert witness called by this Defendant and indicate which material will be used by which witness

    b. To otherwise substantiate Defendant's contentions herein.

47. Name by author, title, and publisher all books, texts, treatises, and articles that Defendant contends are authoritative on the subject of:

    a. Diagnosis and treatment of labor

    b. Fetal complications in a pregnant woman

    c. Proper and timely fetal monitoring, testing and evaluation, including ultrasound

    d. Treatment of labor complications by Cesarean delivery.

48. Name by author, title, and publisher, and date of publication for each book, text, treatise and article that Defendant consulted specifically during the course of _____'s pregnancy and labor.

49. Please state whether Defendant had any insurance agreements which might provide Defendant with coverage as to the occurrence set forth in Plaintiffs' Complaint.

50. If so, please provide:

    a. The policy number of any primary coverage available and the inclusive dates of coverage

    b. The policy limits of any primary coverage available

    c. The complete name and address of the insurance company issuing the above described policy

    d. The claim number and file of the insurance carrier defending this case

    e. Whether or not you are being represented under a reservation of rights and, if so, the reason for said reservation

    f. Whether or not any excess, supplemental, or umbrella insurance coverage is available, and if so:

    i.   The policy number of each excess policy

    ii.   The policy limits of each excess policy

    iii.   The name and address of each excess insurance carrier.

51.   Please state whether or not any of the insurance companies listed in any answers to the preceding Interrogatory have claimed or are claiming that insurance coverage for the occurrence described in Plaintiff's Complaint is excluded for any reason.

52.   If the answer to the preceding Interrogatory is in the affirmative, state the nature of the exclusion being claimed.

53.   Have you ever been a named Defendant in any medical malpractice action other than the instant case? If so, please provide the following information:

a.   The case caption, specifically identifying Plaintiff and Plaintiffs and all named Defendants, including the county and state that the case was filed in and the number of the case, including the approximate date the case was filed.

b.   Provide the name, address, and telephone number of the Plaintiff's attorney, as well as the name, address, and telephone number of the attorney for each Defendant named in (a.) above.

c.   Provide a brief description of Plaintiff's claim against you in any lawsuit identified above.

d.   Provide a brief description of the ultimate disposition of any lawsuit identified above, including any amount of money paid in settlement or to satisfy a Judgment.

54.   Have disciplinary proceedings ever been taken against you by the State Board of Medical Examiners? If the answer is affirmative, please provide the following information:

a.   The date of the disciplinary action

b.   The reason for the disciplinary action

c.   The result of the disciplinary action and the actual discipline you were given by the State Board of Medical Examiners

d.   The name, address, and telephone number of the complaining party that initiated the disciplinary proceedings.

55.   Have you ever served as a panel member in any medical malpractice panel hearings? If the answer is affirmative, please provide the following information:

a.   The case caption of the case in which you served as a panel member, including the county, the state, the number, names of all Plaintiffs, names of all Defendants, and names, addresses, and telephone numbers of the attorneys involved for the Plaintiffs and/or the Defendants.

b.   The names, addresses, and telephone numbers of the other panel members.

c.   A brief description of Plaintiff's claim against the Defendants.

d.   The disposition of the panel hearing.

56.   List specifically and in detail each and every exhibit you propose to utilize at the trial in this matter. This Interrogatory is directed both to exhibits you intend to use at the time of trial and exhibits you may use.

57.   With reference to the exhibits listed in the previous Interrogatory, please state the source of the exhibit, the nature of the exhibit, that is, whether said exhibit is documentary, a picture, or other, who prepared each exhibit, and the date on which same was prepared.

58.   Please state the title, author, edition, and publisher of every textbook dealing with obstetrics, pediatrics, neonatology, and neurology of the newborn you owned at the time _____ was your patient and for the five years preceding your first contact with this patient.

59.   Please state the name of each medical journal that you subscribed to or received free of charge at the time _____ was your patient and for the five years preceding your first contact with this patient.

§ 15.11   Sample Deposition on Written Questions to Prove up Treating Physician's Medical Records

DIRECT QUESTIONS TO BE PROPOUNDED TO THE WITNESS, CUSTODIAN OF RECORDS FOR TREATING PHYSICIAN[5]

1.   Please state your full name, occupation, and official title.

ANSWER _____

---

[5] This is a standard form used by attorneys in Texas. Many firms use something similar. This was taken from a case the authors had and was filed and used by a defense firm.

2. Have you been served with a subpoena duces tecum for the production of medical records pertaining to _____?

ANSWER _____

3. Has _____ been treated or examined by Dr. _____?

ANSWER _____

4. Has Dr. _____ complied, made, or caused to be made any notes, records, or other written documents and reports of the examination and treatment of said patient?

ANSWER _____

5. Were the entries on these notes, records, and reports made at the time or shortly after the time of the transaction recorded on these entries?

ANSWER _____

6. Were these notes, records, and reports made or caused to be made by Dr. _____ in the regular course of business as a doctor and physician?

ANSWER _____

7. In the regular course of business of Dr. _____, did the person who signed the records and reports either have personal knowledge of the entries shown on the records and reports or obtain the information to make the entries from sources who have such personal knowledge?

ANSWER _____

8. Are these notes, records, and reports under your care, supervision, direction, custody, and control?

ANSWER _____

9. Were these records kept as described in the preceding question?

ANSWER _____

10. Please hand exact duplicates of the medical records pertaining to _____ _____ or the originals thereof for photocopying to the Notary Public taking your deposition for attachment to this deposition. Have you done as requested? If not, why not?

ANSWER _____

§ 15.12   Sample Motion to Require Defendant's Examining Doctor to Render Report

TO THE HONORABLE JUDGE OF SAID COURT:

Now come the Plaintiffs, by and through their undersigned counsel and would respectfully show the following:

1. On _____, 19____, the minor Plaintiff in the above-styled and numbered cause was seen by Dr. _____, a pediatric neurologist pursuant to a Motion ordered by this Honorable Court.

2. To the date of the filing of this Motion, Plaintiffs have not received a report from Dr. _____.

3. This case is set for jury selection on _____, 19____, 30 days from the date this Motion is being filed.

4. This Honorable Court ordered that upon completion of the examination and tests, the Defendants will furnish to Plaintiffs' counsel copies of all test results and medical reports.

5. When Dr. _____ examined the minor Plaintiff on _____ _____, 19____, he ordered *no* tests of any kind even though he was empowered to order a wide variety of tests by this Court's order. In other words, Dr. _____ did not order any genetic or metabolic tests of any kind whatsoever.

6. Plaintiffs request the Court to order defense counsel to either turn over the report that they have from Dr. _____ or obtain a report promptly. If Plaintiffs' counsel have to wait until after _____, 19____, jury selection will be upon us.

    WHEREFORE, PREMISES CONSIDERED, Plaintiffs pray that this Motion be granted and the defendant and his counsel be Ordered to obtain a report from Dr. _____ at a time no later than set by the Court.

§ 15.13   Sample Motion for Plaintiffs' Counsel to Be Present at Medical Examinations of Client

TO THE HONORABLE JUDGE OF SAID COURT:

Now come the Plaintiffs, by and through their undersigned counsel, and move the Court as follows:

1. Defendant _____, M.D., has asked for a Rule 35 physical examination of the brain-damaged minor child who is the subject of this lawsuit.

2. Plaintiffs have agreed to a physical examination by a pediatric neurologist with the provision that no invasive procedures be done to the child.

3. Because of the nature of this case, it is important that Plaintiffs' counsel be present at any examination and testing of the minor Plaintiff or discussion of their child with the parent Plaintiffs. There is a tendency for physicians to want to assist other physicians in malpractice cases. This is well known by all and part of this tendency is the "conspiracy of silence" that existed in the past and still exists, for the most part, today. This is not to say that a physician requested by Defendant or ordered by the Court would not want to be honest and fair, but the tendency would be to want to help the Defendants in this case because they are health care providers and are being sued in a malpractice case.

4. Mr. Justice Douglas, while dissenting in a case, specifically addressed this question. A bus driver was allegedly operating his vehicle so dangerously that Plaintiffs' counsel asked for a Rule 35 physical examination to test the physical well-being of the Defendant driver. Mr. Justice Douglas in his dissent, tells us the following:

> Once patients "are turned over to the medical or psychiatric clinics for an analysis of their physical well-being and the condition of their psyche, the effective trial will be held there and not before the jury. There are no lawyers in those clinics to stop the doctors from probing this organ or that one, to halt a further inquiry, to object to a line of questioning. And there is no judge to sit as arbitrator. The doctor or the psychiatrist has a holiday in the privacy of his office. The Defendant is at the doctor or psychiatrist's mercy; and his report may overawe or confuse the jury and prevent a fair trial." *Schlagenhauf v. Holder*, 379 U.S. 104, 13 L.E.D. 2d 152, 85 S.Ct. 234 (1964).

While in *Schlagenhauf* it was the Plaintiff asking for a physical examination of a Defendant, Mr. Justice Douglas' remarks are well taken. It is extremely important that Plaintiffs be allowed to have counsel present.

5. A recent case recognized that Plaintiffs' counsel should be allowed to be present at the medical examination of a Plaintiff by a defense expert. *Jakubowski v. Lengen*, 45 N.Y.S.2d 612 (1982). A copy of said case is appended hereto as Exhibit "A" and made a part hereof for all purposes. The Court stated that there was good ground for a party insisting that his doctor or attorney be present at any examination, because this practice reduces the possibility of misleading medical reports. The Court further stated that the presence of the Plaintiff's attorney at an examination may well be as important as their presence at an oral deposition, and that a physician selected by a Defendant is not necessarily a disinterested, impartial medical expert, indifferent to the conflicting interests of the parties. Further, the Court reasoned that Plaintiffs' counsel should be present to guarantee that the defense doctor does not interrogate the Plaintiffs on liability questions in an attempt to seek damaging admissions, a practice frequently done.

6.   In the interest of justice, Plaintiffs move the Court to allow Plaintiffs' counsel to be present at any Rule 35 examination of the child or any discussion by any Rule 35 physician with the parents.

WHEREFORE, PREMISES CONSIDERED, Plaintiffs pray that Plaintiffs' counsel be allowed to attend any physical examination ordered by this Court.

CHAPTER 16

EXAMINATION OF THE EXPERTS IN A MERITORIOUS LABOR AND DELIVERY CASE WITH RESULTING FETAL INJURY

Michael D. Volk

§ 16.1   Theory of Cross-Examination of Defendant Doctor in Labor and Delivery Room Case

Counsel should not take the defendant doctor's deposition until after gathering all the records, performing the preliminary investigation, and completing a thorough workup of the medical facts. Many courts will not allow more than one opportunity to depose a defendant doctor, and counsel must be prepared.

The purposes of deposing the defendant fall into three broad categories:

1.   To evaluate the defendant and determine how he or she will present in front of a jury
2.   To find out the defendant's side of the case and learn all the operative facts that are within the defendant's knowledge
3.   To obtain testimony that can be used for impeachment.

There are two avenues of impeachment that the attorney should consider when deposing the defendant. One is intended to obtain material to impeach the defendant at a later point in the litigation, and the other is to obtain material for immediate impeachment as well as possible later impeachment.

The preparation for and taking of a deposition are serious matters and should not be taken lightly. Deposition preparation cannot begin 30 minutes before the deposition. Remember that while counsel is sizing up the defendant, the defendant is sizing up counsel. There are no hard and fast rules for preparing and taking a deposition of a defendant doctor or cross-examining at trial. This chapter provides examples of certain types of examination both at deposition or examination before trial and at trial that are intended to illustrate various techniques.

In this chapter, the illustrations relate to that very vital period of time known as labor and delivery, when events move rapidly. Often, defendant doctors attempt to defend themselves by saying events moved too quickly. However, they are being well paid to think quickly. The attorney for a plaintiff in a labor and delivery room case must graphically illustrate this process.

§ 16.2   Cross-Examination of Defendant Doctor: Preliminary Matters in a Labor and Delivery Room Case

The purpose of examination on preliminary matters is the same as in any other type of lawsuit: to place the witness and inquire about background. Counsel should have a Medline search run on the defendant to get any and all articles written or contributed to. Counsel should also check the *Dictionary of Medical Specialists* for biographical information. The following is a partial transcript of a discovery deposition that shows a typical, generic set of preliminary questions to place the witness.

Q. State your name.
A. Dr. Henry Moore.
Q. What is your business or occupation?
A. Doctor of medicine.
Q. What is your professional address?
A. My professional address is 1402 Medical Drive, Glendale, Arizona.
Q. Has your lawyer explained to you the purpose of this deposition today?
A. Yes.
Q. Has he explained to you that you are under oath, just like you are testifying in front of a judge and jury?
A. Yes.
Q. Have you ever had your deposition taken before?
A. Yes.
Q. On how many occasions?
A. Once before.
Q. What was that occasion?
A. I was sued by a patient for the brain damage of her child.
Q. Please explain to me the facts of that case.

Counsel should make sure that the defendant tells the name of the patient involved in the prior litigation, who the defendant's attorney was, the attorney for the patient, where the action was filed, and the result.

Q. If I ask you any questions that you don't understand or you would like me to repeat or rephrase, please go ahead and tell me that you would like a question rephrased or repeated.
A. Okay.
Q. Give me some idea of your background and education experience starting with college and working forward.
A. I went to the University of Texas. I graduated there in 1965 with a B.S. in chemistry. In 1966 I went to the University of Texas at Galveston Medical School for four years. I then did a rotating internship at Brooke Army Medical Center and a residency in obstetrics and gynecology at that same institution. I am in private practice today and have been since I finished my residency and military service.
Q. Are you board certified?
A. Yes.
Q. When did you become board certified?
A. 1978.
Q. How many times did you take the board examination?
A. Twice.
Q. I take it you failed the board examination the first time?
A. Yes.
Q. Have you ever practiced with any partners or associates?
A. No, I have always been in practice by myself.
Q. During the course of your residency, tell me the names of the individuals responsible for your training in obstetrics.

Counsel should find out as much as possible, including the names of all professors. Many of them will have written articles or books which shed light on the defendant's medical care in the case.

Q. What journals of obstetrics do you subscribe to?
A. I have subscriptions to the *Journal of Obstetrics and Gynecology* and the *Survey of Obstetrics and Gynecology*.
Q. What textbooks of obstetrics do you presently own?
A. *Williams Obstetrics*.
Q. Is *Williams Obstetrics* a standard reference?
A. I don't know if you would consider it a fairly standard reference, but it is one of the books that people read.
Q. Do you read it at all?
A. I have read the book before, yes.
Q. Did you use it in the course of your training?
A. Yes.
Q. What hospitals do you presently have privileges at?
A. I have privileges at Glendale Memorial Hospital, Mercy Hospital, and Southern Methodist Hospital.
Q. Have you ever had your privileges suspended, revoked, or curtailed at any hospital?
A. No.

Obviously, there may be areas that need to be explored further. For instance, if hospital privileges have been revoked, counsel must inquire into this topic fully.

§ 16.3 —Failure to Perform Timely Cesarean Section

In the testimony used here as an example, the examination regarding the failure to perform a timely cesarean section was a lengthy one. It concerned a case wherein there were sufficient signs to perform a cesarean section on a primigravida when her child was showing signs of fetal compromise during labor.

Q. You performed a vaginal exam?
A. A vaginal exam was done, that's correct.
Q. You noted that the head had not yet become engaged but looked like it was going to?
A. Well, now, I didn't say that.
Q. Minus one to zero—
A. Station. The head was down, but certainly was not unengaged in the pelvis at this point.
Q. What does *plus one* mean, if that were to be referred to?
A. In determining the descent of the fetus, we refer to the ischial area spines as zero station. Usually everything below that is considered a plus station. And, of course, this is a very coarse method of grading, because it's based on, obviously, estimating, from the exam.

Q. Engagement is when the widest diameter of the head, then, in a vertex presentation, passes the ischial spine?

A. Usually when the head is at about a minus one to zero station, the head by that time is usually well engaged. If it's at a high minus station, generally it's unengaged.

Q. There would be no reason to push a baby from the abdomen if the head were engaged, would there?

A. For what reason?

Q. To push the baby's head down and engage it.

A. Well, are you saying was there reason to do that? I don't know of anybody that does that.

Q. It's not good practice to do that, is it?

A. Well, to be honest with you, I have never seen it done.

There was evidence that this doctor had pushed on the mother's abdomen to try to bring the fetus down into a deliverable position. This maneuver has been encountered on numerous occasions in numerous cases according to testimony by the parents and other relatives. However no doctor or nurse ever seems to admit to doing it.

Q. In your note in the nurses' notes, I don't see any recordation of position of the vertex. Did you determine the position?

A. I don't recollect whether the position was determined or not.

Q. Were you concerned that there was eight to nine centimeters dilation and complete effacement at 8:00 A.M. and yet the head was still at minus one?

A. The assessment that I made was that this lady seemed to have progressed well in labor up to this point. She was at this point having adequate contractions. And from that exam, because there was not a lot of molding, I still felt that there certainly was a chance this lady was going to deliver vaginally.

The defendant has shown a lack of knowledge about this baby's station and presentation.

Q. In people like Mrs. Gorham who go on to develop ineffectual contractions, what is the differential diagnosis of that condition? One, I guess, is that you're dealing with an inadequate pelvis?

A. That's one possibility.

Q. Basically the primagravida pelvis has never been tested to determine how adequate it is for the passage of a child, whereby in a multigravida, the pelvis has been tested and you have a little better idea on the capacity?

A. One has had a baby and one has not. That's correct.

The concept of a tested pelvis is an important one. The next questions deal with decelerations. Any attorney dealing in a labor and delivery case must understand decelerations and their significance. Many obstetricians will attempt to confuse the issues as this defendant attempted.

Q. Are decelerations ominous on the fetal heart rate monitor?

A. Decelerations are very difficult, mainly because there are decelerations and there are decelerations. A lot of it depends on, of course, the stage of labor.

Q. Tell me at what stage of labor decelerations are a warning flag?

A. In terms of outcome, I think certainly if a patient were in very early labor, let's say for example, and were having, let's say severe, very severe decelerations, very early in labor, that can be a sign, for example, of obviously pending problems.

Q. How do you define severe decelerations?

A. Depending, again, on the situation. The problem with assessing the ultimate impact on the fetus of decelerations, a lot of it will depend on how long the decelerations are going to go on. Not so much how severe they are, but for how long a period of time.

Q. What do decelerations tell the physician?

A. The problem with decelerations is that many times they are nonspecific, meaning the umbilical cord could be lying right up against the head and every time the lady has a contraction, the fetal heart tones decelerate.

It could mean the head is down in the pelvis and every time she has a good contraction or she's trying to push, you get a deceleration. So there's many reasons for decelerations.

Obviously, some decelerations can mean that the fetus is not being adequately oxygenated also.

Q. Is there a difference between early decelerations and late decelerations in terms of how the physician interprets those?

A. Most people tend to associate late decelerations with placental insufficiency. The placenta is not supporting this baby if you're getting late decelerations and those are usually considered to be repeated late decelerations.

Q. How about early decelerations?

A. Again, you know, depending on the progress of the patient and the situation, it's very hard to say because sometimes patients will have decelerations for a while and then stop having them. Sometimes the decelerations go away.

Q. What do the textbooks say about early decelerations or whatever material you are reading in an attempt to increase your medical knowledge?

A. Again, in this respect, I think most of my assessment of decelerations is based on experience. I'm not sure I can say there is a textbook somewhere written that describes the way you should interpret every deceleration.

This testimony came from a physician who had graduated from his residency only two years previously.

Q. You do not know the distinction between early decelerations and late decelerations? Is that what you're telling the jury?

A. No, that's not what I'm telling you.

Q. Doctor, you stated that the normal fetal heart rate is between 110 and 180, unlike what I understand to be a normal fetal heart rate of 120 to 160. What standard reference, textbook, journal, article, or professor of obstetrics did you utilize to arrive at a broader range of normal than what is in at least

Williams Textbook of Obstetrics in defining what is and is not normal for a fetal heart rate?

A.   Somewhere, somebody may have written that 180 is. I don't know.

Q.   The answer to my question is, today you're not able to tell this jury what textbook, medical textbook, or what journal articles support the proposition that the normal fetal heart rate is 110 to 180. At least today, you're not able to do it?

A.   Would you repeat the question?

Q.   At least today you're telling this jury that you are unable to tell them what obstetrical textbook or journal article supports your contention that the normal fetal heart rate is 110 to 180?

A.   What I'm saying is that—would you repeat the question one more time?

After a recess, the witness answered the question.

A.   No, I'm not.

Q.   What measurements did you make of Mrs. Gorham's pelvis to determine that it was of adequate size?

A.   I did a clinical assessment of the adequacy of her pelvis.

Q.   How did you go about doing that?

A.   It's based on doing a lot of exams before.

Q.   Tell me what measurements you took to determine the adequacy of the pelvis.

A.   There are no number measurements taken.

Q.   Tell me what you did.

A.   What I did, I examined her as an obstetrician/gynecologist who had done lots of deliveries before and said this lady had an adequate pelvis.

Q.   Tell me where you put your hand and what you felt and how you felt it.

A.   It takes years and years of doing it. You just have to keep doing it over and over again and base it on your experience.

Q.   Doesn't take years and years to tell the jury how you did it.

A.   Well, I'm sorry. It's an assessment made by an experienced gynecologist.

Q.   You took your hand and put it into Mrs. Gorham's vagina, did you not?

A.   That's right.

Q.   What was the first assessment you took of the size of the pelvis and how did you do it?

A.   What I did, of course, I examined her and felt for the head where it was, got an idea of just basically how big the pelvis felt, the adequacy of the pelvis.

Q.   I'm asking how you did that. What bones did you touch and how did you determine the significance of touching the various bones?

A.   When I do an exam I reach for the sacral promontory. Usually if I can't reach it, of course, that's a good sign that this lady has an adequate AP diameter of the pelvis.

Q.   What other measurements did you take other than the AP?

A.   Usually at this time what I feel for next is how prominent the ischial spines are.

Q.   Do you make any measurements?

A. No.

Q. Do you measure the distance between ischial spines?

A. No.

Q. Any other measurements that you took clinically?

A. Usually what I depend on is those measurements.

Q. To your recollection, you didn't determine the position of the head?

A. To my recollection, I did not determine the position of the head.

Q. After you finished your assessment at 8:00, what did you make of the nurse's reporting that there were decelerations two times before you came?

A. That's in the labor record?

This defendant should have had a better command of the medical record.

Q. What we have labeled previously 1-B, the labor and delivery record.

A. Looking back from my recollection, looking at the fetal heart tracing, again I'm not sure specifically what they are referring to here, so I'm not sure exactly what part of the tracing—it's not marked or anything, since they just put decelerations. I'm not sure I remember what part. I mean, I reviewed—in reviewing it there may have been some decelerations, but I don't specifically know which ones, if they were referring to specific decelerations here in their notes or what.

Q. Did the nurses discuss with you any concern about decelerations on the tracing?

A. Right now, I don't recall any specific discussions.

Q. How low did the pulse rate drop on those decelerations, do you recall?

A. The problem is, I do not know what—I couldn't tell you specifically what decelerations they were referring to on here. I mean, unless we look on the fetal heart tracing and correlate that specifically with a deceleration they were referring to, I can't say. I don't know.

Q. The next notation that's made here would have been made by the nurses at 8:35, and they have a note in here, "Fetal heart decelerations noted. Dr. Moore notified." Were you notified?

A. Yes.

Q. At the 8:35 entry, there's an indication that oxygen was started at five liters per mask, but I don't see an order for that. Did you order that or did the nurses just begin it on their own?

A. The nurses probably started it on their own. I don't specifically recall ordering the oxygen.

Q. What would the oxygen have been started for? What were the nurses concerned about?

A. Many times, again, depending on the hospital, many times when the patients start to have decelerations, the nurses will start oxygen and try to eliminate these decelerations by positioning the patient usually one way or the other.

Q. Was there a legitimate reason why oxygen might be of assistance to the mother and the fetus in that situation?

A. Whenever you have decelerations sometimes people start oxygen with the idea that this is certainly not going to hurt the patient or the baby and may increase the level of the oxygen in the mother's—I should say it will increase the amount of circulating oxygen that the mother has available.

Q. In turn, increasing the amount of oxygen available to the fetus?

A. Yes, that's the idea.

The previous questions show significant problems developing with this labor. The next questions concerned the inordinate delay in performing the cesarean section, and the failure to plan ahead.

Q. Then on your third entry on Plaintiffs' Exhibit Number 1-C, can you read that entry that is timed 11:00?

A. "Cervix still eight to nine centimeters. No further progress. Fetal heart tones dropping." That's what the little arrow means. "80 beats per minute with contractions. Plan, cesarean section. Failure to progress with fetal distress."

Q. What steps did you have to take before you could get Mrs. Gorham to the operating room for her cesarean section?

A. The way the hospital operates, we needed to notify certain people in terms of getting everything ready. We had to notify the person who was the nurse anesthetist on call to come in. And the nurses had to call somebody that would assist on a cesarean section to come in and assist me.

Q. What other things needed to be done?

A. Of course, a Foley catheter had to be placed. The abdomen had to be shaved. The patient had to have ether—her husband had to sign a consent form for the surgery.

Q. You had not, then, at least at 10:00 A.M., you had not made arrangements for the provision of possibly having to do an emergency C-section?

A. The arrangements we had made included having typed and crossed her earlier. This is the thing that generally takes the longest time to do, just because they don't have a blood bank.

Q. You had typed and crossmatched her at 9:00, had you not?

A. I don't recall when the order was written.

DEFENDANT'S ATTORNEY: Blood was drawn at 8:35.

Q. So at 8:35 at least, you had some reason to suspect you might have to perform a cesarean section in your own mind?

A. And again, this was preparing—the main reason again, we tend to order blood more often just because it takes us anywhere from an hour to an hour and a half to get it. So even if we suspect there may be a chance, we would usually type and cross the patient early on.

Q. At 8:10 when you wrote the order, was it with the anticipation of the possibility that a cesarean section would be performed?

A. It was in anticipation that a cesarean section would be done, because this lady may not have an adequate pelvis, probably failure to progress at that point.

Q. So at least at 8:10 you were aware it was possible that this mother and child would have problems and would require a cesarean section?

A. We were thinking that she would not deliver vaginally at that point.

§ 16.4   —Failure to Recognize Abnormal Monitor Tracings with Resulting Asphyxia

The fetal monitor tracings in any labor and delivery room case are *very* important. The monitor can graphically display the swings in the fetal heart rate that show the child is in trouble. The attorney must go over the tracings panel by panel with the witness.

> Q. The fetal monitoring record you have before you, Doctor, how many minutes is each of those pages, if you know? Is every two blocks one minute?

Counsel must establish this at the outset because machines differ in their rate.

> A. Three blocks, 11 minutes.
> Q. Why was fetal monitoring started on Mrs. Gorham?
> A. Just about every physician on the staff felt most comfortable when every single patient was monitored in labor.
> Q. What is the purpose of monitoring them?
> A. Mainly to have a good record of exactly what's going on.
> Q. The hope is that careful monitoring and early detection of abnormalities will result in the prevention of brain damage to some infants?
> A. That's the ideal. But like any other method in medicine, it has its limitations and there's no one who can stand before you who can say that if every single baby is monitored there will be no asphyxia ever.
> Q. Alternatively, most everybody, at least most experts in the area, concede that some cases of fetal asphyxia can be prevented.
> A. That's the hope, with the monitor, that you can pick it up.
> Q. You wouldn't do a useless procedure on every patient that came into the hospital, would you?
> A. I don't think most doctors would do a useless procedure.
> Q. On block 42150, what is the baseline fetal heart rate?
> A. On this one, the baseline is varying somewhere between 150, 160 with what looks like a reasonable amount of fetal heart variability on there.
> Q. Are there some segments, though, that appear to lack variability?
> A. Not more so than any other tracing would vary. Again, the problem can be— sometimes variability seems to come and go at times, and this would be what I would consider average.
> Q. Then on the bottom of 42150, what are those units called, contractions? What are we looking at on the hills that appear there?
> A. What we're looking at is the external monitor's indication of the uterine activity. And again, the problem being on the external monitor, this is more to gauge the frequency of the contractions.
> Q. And their duration rather than their strength?
> A. That's correct.
> Q. How long does the first contraction last?
> A. The first contraction, from the beginning, seems to last a little over a minute.

Q. Through 42173 and 42174, the pages we have turned, do the tracings look relatively normal?

A. She's having what appear to be fairly good contractions at intervals with no evidence of any compromise of the fetus.

Q. At 42265, is there a deceleration there?

A. A little tiny bit of a deceleration occurs. If this is the peak of the contraction, she has a momentary deceleration and then it goes right back up again.

Q. That deceleration, is that an early or late or variable deceleration?

A. I would call that a variable deceleration.

Q. At 42266, is there a deceleration?

A. Again, she has—I'm not sure you can interpret that. I think that's part of the fetal heart variability that's going on.

Q. At 42271, you see a drop in the fetal heart rate from 170 to about 130?

A. A short variable, probably.

Q. Where does it arise in terms of the contractions?

A. Again, it's very hard to tell just because of the shape of the contraction. But it looks like if you drew the line it would be basically at the peak of the contraction and go away.

Q. The next few pages we see some interference?

A. I think again this is probably just some artifact on the machine from the tracing.

Q. Then at 42293 and -4, there's a dramatic drop in pulse rate that someone has been kind enough to circle, isn't there?

A. Again, I don't know whether—I can't tell you whether circled meant they moved, or what. That would make me disagree with what you're saying, if you look at the shape of the previous uterine contraction, it's nice and smooth. And this one, all of a sudden everything goes off the tracing. The uterine contraction monitor goes off and is trailing out here and totally off up here. And so again, because it was circled does not mean that the fetal heart tone actually got that low.

Afterward, a doctor will testify that the leads for the machine are not placed properly so the abnormal tracings are *artifact*. A labor full of artifact is an unmonitored labor.

Q. The nurse circled it so you would know it wasn't working properly?

A. [Silence by the witness.]

Q. In any case, the rate drops, if it is not an artifact, drops down almost to 40, does it not?

A. Again—

Q. Assuming it is not an artifact?

A. I don't know that we can assume that.

Q. Let's not assume it. Let's ask you, what is the lowest reading that the bottom line of that tracing drops to?

A. It looks like it dropped to 50.

Q. Actually a little less than 50?

A. 47.

Q. How long a period of time is there between when the line drops and when the line comes back up?

A. There appears to be a minute, a minute and 20 seconds.

This is a massive deceleration. The defendant is still trying to say it is artifact. At trial, this panel was turned into a poster exhibit to illustrate graphically the deceleration.

Q. Then on the next page, 14 and 15, are the pulse rates down in the range of 30?

A. No. Again, what I would say, if at this point we totally lost the tracing— because as you see, everything following it is pure artifact, and there's no way possible that I think you could interpret it being that way just because of what follows it.

Q. Again, artifact, what I have yellowed in on 14. Is that right?

A. I think, you know, from what I'm seeing and everything that follows it, just because the machine has a circuit to start scribbling when it loses a signal, starts scribbling.

Q. In this case it started scribbling in the area of 30?

A. It lost a signal somewhere back here.

Q. Can it lose a signal if the rate gets too low, fetal heart rate?

A. I don't know if it can—I'm not familiar with the electronics enough to be able to say whether it does that or not.

Q. At 42315, the Pitocin is started. Is that right?

In the face of an abnormal fetal heart rate, the doctor definitely should not have ordered Pitocin.

A. That's correct.

Q. And an internal lead?

A. Internal lead was placed right there.

Q. Actually the Pitocin is started a little bit before that. Cervix is eight to nine centimeters dilated?

A. That's what we have recorded.

Q. Was the Pitocin started to dilate the cervix further?

A. Well, the Pitocin was given in hopes of better contractions getting this lady to full dilation.

Q. Wasn't the cervix almost fully dilated already?

A. It was eight to nine centimeters dilated.

Q. That's what you were taught during your residency, you put somebody on Pitocin who is almost virtually fully dilated already?

A. Again, given the situation, this lady had reached eight to nine centimeters and was not having adequate contractions.

Q. At 24 and 25 you now have your internal monitor on, do you not?

A. Yes.

Q. After you start your Pitocin with an internal monitor, on the third uterine contraction, what does the pulse rate drop to?

A. She has a drop to 70 and then recovers. Seems to recover fairly rapidly and go back up.

Q. Did you think that was an encouraging sign for this child's brain right after you started Pitocin that a pulse rate dropped on an accurate internal monitor to less than 70?

A. [No answer given.]

Q. Did you come to the opinion this was in the best welfare of the child, immediately after starting Pitocin, to have a fetal heart rate of less than 70 on the fourth or fifth contraction after starting Pitocin? Did you interpret that as a sign her utero placental function was good and she could tolerate Pitocin in ever-increasing dosages?

A. I interpreted that as this lady had, again, this lady was—had a good contraction, which obviously put some head compression on the fetus. There was a quick recovery and this was not a late—certainly not a late deceleration.

Q. It's an early deceleration, isn't it?

A. It's a variable deceleration.

Q. If you look, it starts right at the beginning of the uterine contraction.

A. According to what I was taught, you can line up when the contraction starts, and it starts right with the contraction and recovers right at the end, this is a variable deceleration.

Q. So you thought this was just the head being compressed. You weren't worried about cord compression, about whether the placental function was intact?

A. Cord compression was a possibility, head compression was a possibility, at that point.

Q. At 9:30 A.M., was it your opinion when the pulse rate dropped on Pitocin to less than 60 that that was a sign of a thriving fetus getting ready to come into the world fully equipped to handle the functions of life?

A. My assessment at that point was she was having a better quality labor. Probably she was—the head was being compressed, but then again it was going down and coming right back up again and then again, this was followed immediately by good fetal heart variability on the internal lead.

Q. So you were taught head compressions associated with Pitocin with rates dropping in the range of 40, 50 were a sign of thriving intrauterine environment?

A. More important than that—well, the important thing, the fetal heart was dropping, she was recovering on the internal lead, she had good beat to beat variability, very acceptable variability, and there was every sign to think this baby at this point was still oxygenating well.

Q. At 9:40 the pulse rate drops down to 90 during a uterine contraction. Did you again feel this was a sign of a thriving, healthy baby who was not having any degree of hypoxia, or you could assure the family was not having any degree of hypoxia?

A. Again, at this point, this patient had still—right immediately after that contraction had good fetal heart variability.

Q. How about this youngster's nice variability, as I have yellowed in, after these protracted periods of fetal heart rate less than 50? What happens to variability after that at this tracing? Is that nice and variable?

A. She seems to have a decrease in the fetal heart variability at that point, and I waited to see what's going to keep happening at this point.

Q. What is the most ominous sign of lack of the connection between the child's vagal system in the brain because of hypoxia?

A. The most ominous signs are the late decelerations.

Q. Not loss of variability?

A. Again, they go hand in hand. If there were late decelerations, to me at that point, again sometimes you see one without the other. You can see loss of fetal heart variability without late deceleration. Sometimes you'll see late decelerations. And again, depending on the situation, you may develop some loss of variability.

Q. Tell me if I'm correct. Loss of variability is a sign that the child can be so hypoxic that they can no longer even respond to the hypoxia with a variation in their heartbeat, and consequently you get a tracing that shows loss of beat to beat variability?

A. Okay. Ultimately, what one has to do to put this in context is how long is this going on? Are we talking about short periods of loss of variability, with again return to variability or whether it's a continued loss of variability.

Q. But it's the final sign. If you get a child whose brain is totally wiped out by hypoxia, what you see is a total lack of variability on the tracing. He no longer has a brain that can respond. Is that the theory?

A. Depending on the events leading up to it. And in this case, all we had were variable decelerations leading up to it, all of which had recovered, there had basically been no significant change in the baseline, baseline was running more or less what it was running when this lady walked into the hospital.

Q. In response to the diminished beat to beat variability, you increased the amounts of Pitocin given to Mrs. Gorham, didn't you?

A. The increase in the Pitocin was not done because there was a short period of loss of variability. It was done, again, because we were looking at her contractions and trying to get her in the best pattern of labor possible.

Q. Dr. Moore, at some point in here, you decided to perform a cesarean section. Is that correct?

A. That's correct.

Q. What factors caused you to decide to have this lady delivered by cesarean section?

A. When it became apparent at this point, at the point that this lady was not going to deliver vaginally in spite of the adequate contractions she was getting, she was not going to deliver vaginally in spite of the adequate contractions she was getting, she was not going to deliver vaginally and what appeared to be the continued variable decelerations at that point with no real hope at that point of really being able to get her delivered vaginally.

Q. Let's see if I understand you correctly. You thought she wasn't progressing any further, she had continued variable decelerations and you decided to do the cesarean section?

A.   That's correct.

Q.   Would you agree with me the reason why you at that point decided to perform the cesarean section, you wanted to make sure you would do what you could to ensure the fetus's well-being?

A.   At that point, we didn't feel that it was appropriate to proceed any further because she was continuing to have decelerations. Even though at this point the baby was recovering after each one, we didn't want to reach a point where we would compromise the fetus.

Q.   What information did you have at 9:00 when you decided to perform the cesarean section that you didn't have at 7:00 or 8:30 o'clock?

A.   I think the information was that at this point the lady had not made any further progress in labor, which to me at that point was the most significant thing, she had not—she was not at a point where we could even attempt a vaginal delivery by getting her to push or anything like that, and felt that the most appropriate thing at that point would be to go ahead and deliver her by C-section at that point.

§ 16.5   Direct Examination of Prior Treating Physician Used to Fix Liability on Defendant for Abnormal Labor Pattern, Abnormal Fetal Heart Rate Pattern, and Failure to Perform Stat Cesarean Section

The following is a partial transcript from the deposition of a treating house physician. This physician took care of the laboring mother immediately before the physician involved in §§ 16.2 to 16.4, and this testimony was used to help fix liability against the subsequent treating physician.

Q.   When you reviewed the clinic record, were you aware of the fact that you were dealing with a postdate baby?

A.   That's right, certainly.

Q.   What did the nurse note as the presenting part on Mrs. Gorham when you examined her at 9:00 P.M.?

A.   She didn't note it, as you can see there. There's no indication of whether it was vertex or breech.

Q.   That's important for you to know, isn't it?

A.   I checked her at the same time, so I would have noticed if it was breech or not.

Q.   I understand that, but what I'm saying, as you sit there today, you don't know what the presenting part of this child was?

A.   Certainly we know what the presenting part was.

Q.   How do you know that?

A.   Because it's delivered as a vertex.

Q.   How do you know that?

A.   If you look at the operative note, you can see that.

Q.   Why don't you turn to the operative note and tell me where it—

A. It should have been.

Q. I understand that. Tell me where Dr. Moore notes the presenting part of the baby when he opened this lady's abdomen up.

A. Okay. I stand corrected.

Q. There's no—to make it easy for you, there's nowhere in this chart ever by any doctor or any nurse a notation on the presenting part of this child and as you sit there today, you don't know what it was, do you?

A. Not according to the record, no.

Q. What was the station when you signed off the case?

A. Station at the time I left was minus one station.

Q. What does that mean to you, Doctor, a minus one station?

A. It means that the head has descended down to one centimeter within the reference point, the spines.

Q. I understand that. Did the fact that she was a minus one station after this amount of labor, did that concern you at all?

A. Between a minus one and zero station, it's within normal variation.

Q. Where does it say minus one, zero?

A. Minus one, I would be happy with that.

Q. No one ever said that this baby was at zero station ever, did they?

A. Okay. Well, I'll be happy with minus one.

Q. What I'm saying, my question is: No one ever said this baby was at a zero station. Correct?

A. That's right.

Q. Do you see after the notation "Gorham 10:43 A.M." a deceleration?

A. It's another variable with a quick return to the baseline with no shoulder. Again, it's not an ominous variable deceleration.

Q. Heart rate down to 60?

A. Down to 60, but then back up immediately to the baseline.

Q. Is that followed by—

A. Good variability for about two minutes.

Q. Then what?

A. Another variable.

Q. Down to 40.

A. Down to 50 at least.

Q. How is the shoulder on that?

A. It's flattened out a little bit, but again you have to put it in context with the previous ones and the one that followed, which shows a normal return to baseline.

Q. When the shoulders flatten out, is that an ominous sign?

A. That shows that the baby is probably becoming hypoxic.

Q. Why don't you continue reading the strip?

A. What would go against that is the fact that previous—not previous, but following contractions showed normal return to baseline.

Q. Then what happened?

A. Baseline here between 160 and 170.

Q. Is there a late deceleration?

A. This is still a variable.

Q. Variable deceleration?

A. Right.

Q. Incidentally, this deceleration between panel 43 and 44 where you said it flattened out a little bit, what type of deceleration is that?

A. Still I would call it a variable deceleration, just by the appearance of it. There was a sudden decrease in the fetal heart rate and then a return. I can't say what's happening. I can't relate it as far as being early or late because I'm not sure what's going on with the contraction. The machine was just not picking up this contraction.

Q. Then we were at 42194?

A. Okay, this lasts for—

Q. The one that's circled?

A. About a minute and a half until it completely returns to baseline.

Q. When the baby's heart rate gets down to 50 or 60, is that dangerous to the fetus?

A. Not if it returns immediately. If it stays prolonged and repetitive, it can be.

Q. We have seen repetitive decelerations?

A. Repetitive but not that severe.

Q. So your opinion is they are not that severe?

A. Yes, that is my opinion.

Q. Does it continue on—

A. If you pick out an isolated deceleration, it is severe, but overall—

Q. Until the end of this strip, do they continue and get more frequent?

A. Not more frequent, but you can see them occurring with almost each contraction for a period of about—looks like about 10 minutes here.

Q. You are aware that they had to resuscitate this baby in the delivery room?

A. I'm aware they found meconium which would require resuscitation.

Q. Obviously at one point in time Dr. Moore decided to take this baby by section, but the feeling I get from your testimony so far is that everything seemed to be chugging along okay.

A. No, at this point apparently the lady was not progressing. She stayed the same.

Q. She never really progressed?

A. She got up to eight to nine, but beyond that she didn't change.

Q. What does the minus one station mean to you? Does it mean to you that the baby has not descended and is not going to be delivered vaginally?

A. It means you need to watch closely. If she hasn't progressed beyond that period of time she probably won't deliver vaginally.

Q. When would you have intervened if you had stayed in charge of this patient and performed a cesarean section?

A. When I saw the more ominous contractions toward the end of the labor. Certainly by 8:30, I would begin to prepare this lady for cesarean section on the basis of this variable deceleration.

Q. That's the one with the late component?

A. Yes. In other words, if this didn't improve, I think you should be ready to deliver the lady by cesarean section.

Q. How long would be an acceptable period of time?

A.   If this became repetitive with each contraction, probably at that point.

Q.   What I mean is, how long does it take? Let's say Dr. Moore says at 8:30, "I don't like this, I'm going to deliver this lady by section," what is the acceptable time period to get the baby out of there?

A.   I'd say as long as it returns to the baseline sharply, I would estimate probably 30 to 40 minutes should be it.

Q.   So the baby, in your opinion, should have been delivered before 9:30?

A.   Sometime after 8:30. I can't really say.

Q.   What I want to know is how long should a doctor be standing down there? There's a period of time when it's not right anymore. The patient has got to have the baby out. I mean is it 20 minutes, 30 minutes, five hours that they can wait for an emergency cesarean section? How long a period of time?

A.   Well, it depends. If you need to do an emergency cesarean section, you do it with local anesthetic, then you have blood available as backup if you should need it. Rarely do you need it, but occasionally you might. Most institutions, even if we have a nurse anesthetist in the hospital, like at Greenwood, it takes, you know—we cannot do it in five minutes. They may be doing another case. They may have only one team doing an appendectomy downstairs.

   In fact, that happened a few weeks ago. We had a crash cesarean section. The cord prolapsed and the team was occupied doing a surgical, general surgical case and they could not come up and help us.

Q.   What did you do?

A.   So we did do the cesarean section with a local anesthetic and the team came in later. You do what you have to do under the circumstance.

Q.   I understand. Let's say that you want to wait for blood and you want to wait for anesthesia. How long is the maximum permissible time to wait?

A.   I'd say 40 minutes or so. Between 40 minutes and 50 minutes up to an hour.

§ 16.6   Direct Examination of Treating Neonatologist

Sometimes a subsequent treating physician can be used to fix the fetus's condition on delivery showing that the child was asphyxiated during labor and delivery. The following trial transcript illustrates this:

Q.   Please look at your physician's record of the newborn infant. Your admission diagnosis was asphyxiated newborn. Is that correct?

A.   Asphyxiated newborn, correct.

Q.   Can you tell the jury what *asphyxiated* means?

A.   *Asphyxiated* means a deprivation of oxygen supply to the tissues.

Q.   To lay people, does it mean that the baby didn't get enough oxygen?

A.   That's correct.

Q.   That asphyxiation occurred before you saw the child?

A.   Yes.

Q.   Your second admission diagnosis was meconium aspiration. Is that correct?

A. That's correct.

Q. Tell the jury what meconium aspiration is.

A. Meconium is the first stool that a baby passes. It's a very thick, dark green tenacious material that has a lot of bile acids and other compounds in it. In stressful situations in utero the baby will pass this stool into the amniotic fluid where it becomes dissolved. Then as the baby is deprived of oxygen, he will actually begin to take deep gasping respirations in utero, and that meconium and amniotic fluid mixture may then be drawn down into the lungs themselves.

Q. By aspiration, you mean that process of drawing down meconium mixed with amniotic fluid into the baby's lungs?

A. Yes.

Q. Your records state that the child had decreased activity. Can you tell the jury what you mean by *decreased activity?*

A. Well, this would be a baby who is not in the normal vigorous posture that a newborn experiences after being delivered. A newborn is very agitated at being delivered, being brought out in the cold, cruel world having to experience all the outside stimuli. A child frequently protests very vehemently about this. This baby was not protesting.

Q. What significance did that have for you?

A. The child had a central nervous system that was depressed for one reason or another.

Q. Can that central nervous system be depressed because of a lack of oxygen?

A. It can.

Q. Did you think this child's central nervous system was depressed because of a lack of oxygen during labor and delivery?

A. At the initial physical and evaluation of the patient, there were several considerations at that time. Along with asphyxia, a metabolic derangement that can occur manifests as a lack of activity.

Q. You got those laboratory tests to check whether there was any metabolic problem, didn't you?

A. We did.

Q. There wasn't any metabolic problem, was there?

A. We found none.

Q. Looking back on this now, that decreased activity was because of a central nervous system problem because of a lack of oxygen, wasn't it?

A. That would be my opinion, yes.

Q. Your physical exam showed molding with full but not bulging fontanelles. What did that mean to you?

A. Molding of the head means that the sutures are overlapping. In the presence of labor this would indicate the head was attempting to fit through the pelvis. The fact that the fontanelle was full rather than depressed means that the patient was not in an obvious dehydrated state. The fact it was not bulging meant there was no grossly apparent increase in the intracranial pressure.

Q. What was the significance of the molding?

A. To me it meant the head had attempted to mold itself to the contour of the pelvis during labor.

Q. The next abnormality was increased AP diameter. What is that?

A. That is the description of a child whose lungs are trapping air on the inside much the same as an older person with emphysema. The air that would normally be expired is incomplete and remains inside the lungs.

Q. Why would that be incomplete?

A. It could be incomplete for a variety of reasons. There would be something acting as an obstructive force to the outflow of air from the lungs.

Q. In this child, you suspected the meconium the child had aspirated was acting as a barrier to the air flowing out of the lungs?

A. That was my diagnosis at that time, yes.

Q. You said there was decreased breathing with rales?

A. The decrease in the breath sounds means we could not physically hear with a stethoscope the normal character of breath sounds indicating good air exchange in there. The rhonchi are very coarse breath sounds indicating there is some material in the airways much the same as the bubbling of water in a pipe or a plastic tube. Rales are very fine sounds that we hear much like the crinkling of Saran wrap, clear paper as it comes off something, indicating there is some fluid present in the alveoli spaces of the lungs.

Q. Did that all confirm your admission diagnosis of meconium aspiration?

A. The increased AP diameter, the decreased breath sounds and the rhonchi were strongly suspicious of a child who had a syndrome such as meconium aspiration going on. The chest X-rays were interpreted by us to be compatible with that even though we were in disagreement with the radiologist.

Q. The radiologist said there were minimal infiltrates. Did you read the X-ray yourself?

A. Yes.

Q. Did you feel like there were more than minimal infiltrates?

A. In my own mind it was more of a mild to moderate infiltrated pattern consistent with an aspiration syndrome, which I don't believe they alluded to.

Q. I'm going to show you what's been marked P-2.

[Deposition exhibit marked, P-2.]

Q. That's the first day of your progress notes. You say that the child was born by emergency cesarean section for severe decelerations. Is that correct?

A. That's true.

Q. Would that have been possibly Dr. Redleg who told you that?

A. Yes.

Q. And you also said heavy meconium staining?

A. Yes.

Q. That evening the child began to have some twitching which you interpreted as seizures. Is that correct?

A. Yes, that's true.

Q. You put the child on Phenobarbital, which is a medication for the seizures?

A. Yes.

Q. Then the 5th of August your notes show the child was very rigid with tight flexor position. Will you please explain to the jury what that is?

A. A flexor position is where the baby's major joints, that is, the knees, the elbows, the shoulders, and the hips are flexed. They are contracted. They are not extended or straight out.

Q. What does that mean to you?

A. Very tight flexor position is seen in children who have central nervous system irritation for one reason or another.

Q. I have marked as P-4 the report of the CT scan. Correct me if I'm wrong, but what this actually tells you is that the child did not have any congenital lesions inside of his brain, that is, he was not damaged as he developed in utero. He did not get some congenital defect or deficit.

A. None that could be discerned by the study.

    [Deposition exhibit marked, P-5.]

Q. What I have marked as P-5 is a report of an EEG taken on one day of life when Dr. Harris read this as an abnormal record?

A. Yes.

Q. Did this correlate and fit with your clinical diagnosis of seizures at that point in time?

A. It did.

Q. Your discharge summary states that the child's condition on discharge was that he was a stable baby. Is that correct?

A. That's true.

Q. That, of course, is stable within the child's own parameters?

A. That's true.

Q. That is to say, the child had suffered some insult and was on a medication to stop him from having convulsions?

A. That is true.

Q. Let's look at the summary of labor and delivery. Do you see that the child was suctioned?

A. Yes.

Q. He was given oxygen?

A. Yes.

Q. Are both of those things done to every newborn that is delivered?

A. Not necessarily.

Q. Is almost every newborn suctioned?

A. Yes.

Q. Is every noncompromised newborn given oxygen in the delivery room?

A. No.

Q. Does every noncompromised newborn have a laryngoscope passed?

A. No.

Q. Is that also checked?

A. Yes.

Q. What is a laryngoscope and how is it used on a baby?

A. It's an instrument that assists the physician in visualizing the trachea of the patient.

Q. You use that sometimes to pass an endotracheal tube of a baby?

A. Yes.

Q. You see the child had an endotracheal tube passed?

A. I see it has an endotracheal something. I don't know whether that means suctioned or whether a tube was placed.

Q. Does every newborn child have endotracheal suction or a tube passed?

A. No.

Q. Do you see there was also positive pressure by mask checked?

A. Yes.

Q. Would that lead you to believe that before that child was delivered that that child got his asphyxiation before he was delivered?

A. By virtue of those findings, the fact the child's Apgar at one minute was two and at five minutes was three, it would indicate to me that he had suffered an asphyxiating event sometime prior to his delivery.

Q. Do you see where it says "heavily meconium-stained"?

A. Yes.

Q. Does it say "slight cry"?

A. Yes.

Q. What does *slight cry* mean to you as a neonatologist?

A. That he was nonvigorous.

Q. Are most newborns fairly vigorous?

A. Most.

Q. This is the sheet of the nursery room record at Glendale Hospital before the child was transferred.

A. That's correct.

Q. Do you see I have marked in yellow, "cyanotic color"?

A. Yes.

Q. What does *cyanotic color* mean?

A. Means the patient was not pink.

Q. What does that mean to you as a neonatologist?

A. It means he had an insufficient supply of oxygen in the blood of the tissues that were being observed.

Q. Do you see it says "slight cry"?

A. Yes.

Q. So we know the child still has a slight cry in the nursery before he is taken to Newton Hospital.

A. That is the way it is recorded.

Q. Do you see that the child was said to be very flaccid?

A. Yes.

Q. Tell me what that means to you.

A. Means a lack of muscle tone in the patient.

Q. What does that signify to you?

A. It means the central nervous system is depressed.

Q. That can be from a lack of oxygen?

A. From a variety of factors of which lack of oxygen is one.

Q. In this child, you would suspect it probably was a lack of oxygen?

A. It would be high on my list.

Q. That would be top on your list, wouldn't it?

A. I have no idea about any medications that this mother received or anything else, so I would be—it would be difficult for me to render an opinion without knowing those things.

Q. It would be pretty high up on your list?

A. It would be high on my list.

Q. Do you see there—is that "lavage" or "gavage"?

A. "Lavage" is the way I interpreted it.

Q. —with water. Large amount of meconium fluids obtained. Do you see that?

A. Yes, sir.

Q. What is *lavage*? What does that mean?

A. There's no indication as to what was lavaged, so I would assume it would be the stomach which would be the typical place of removing a potential source of further damage to the baby. Very frequently they will have meconium-stained fluid in their lungs. They can vomit and aspirate after they are born and compound the problem. This would be an attempt to remove that factor.

Q. This would be some confirmation of your diagnosis that the child had meconium aspiration?

A. It would be supportive, yes.

Q. I mean, that came from his stomach or his lungs?

A. I strongly suspect it came from his stomach.

Q. When you discharged this child, you put this child on Phenobarbital twice a day?

A. Yes, I did. I think I put him on that prior to discharge.

Q. That was eight milligrams every 12 hours?

A. I believe that's it.

Q. The reason why you ordered the Phenobarbital?

A. To prevent any further seizures at home.

Q. Did Dr. Redleg transfer every baby that's born at Glendale Memorial Hospital to your care at Newton Hospital at this time?

A. Not every patient, no.

Q. Babies are transferred because they are sick. Isn't that correct?

A. That was true, yes.

§ 16.7 Theory of Direct Examination of the Plaintiff's Expert on Liability

In most medical malpractice cases, the plaintiff's case-in-chief stands or falls with the expert called to the witness stand by the plaintiff. The jury should be apprised fully of the expert's qualifications so that they have the opportunity to understand that they should listen to the expert witness. One should not allow counsel for the defendant to stipulate as to the expert's qualifications. **Section 16.8** is part of a direct examination of a plaintiff's expert in a failure to perform timely a cesarean section with resulting brain damage.

§ 16.8   Direct Examination of the Plaintiff's Expert: Preliminary Matters

Counsel must, of course, show the background and training of any expert called by the plaintiff. This must be thorough but not overdone. The jury must understand that the expert is not a "hired gun," but an extremely well-qualified physician who practices in the same field as the defendant. Some attorneys like to tightly control the direct examination; others prefer open-ended questions so that the jury hears the doctor, not the attorney, testify. The latter procedure is recommended.

Q. Would you please state your name?
A. Robert L. Martin.
Q. Sir, do you practice a profession?
A. Yes.
Q. What is that?
A. Medicine.
Q. Can you tell me a little bit about your background, where you were born and grew up?
A. Yes. I was born in New York City and grew up in these environs.
Q. Can you tell us when you were born?
A. August 12, 1940.
Q. Can you tell the jury where you went to undergraduate school?
A. Yes. Harvard University.
Q. Where you went to medical school, please.
A. Harvard University.
Q. After your medical school, did you engage in any kind of further training?
A. Yes. I had an extensive postgraduate training.
Q. Will you please tell the jury about that.
A. Yes. I was a rotating intern at the Massachusetts General Hospital in Boston, then a surgical resident at the New York Hospital and Cornell Medical Center. Then I spent four years as a resident in obstetrics and gynecology at the Women's Hospital in New York City.
Q. Will you just tell the jury briefly what the function of a residency is?
A. A residency is postgraduate training after medical school in a specialty in the field of medicine.
Q. Doctor, can you tell us what states you are licensed in?
A. New York, Virginia, and Pennsylvania.
Q. Is your license on file with the appropriate authorities here in Virginia?
A. Yes.
Q. Have you published any journals or medical journals, articles, or books?
A. Yes.
Q. Can you tell us about how many?
A. I think there are 15 or 16 articles and two books.
Q. Were those articles pertaining to obstetrics?
A. Yes.

Q. Please tell us a little about those publications.

The witness describes them and briefly relates how they prepare him for his testimony. Counsel for the plaintiff should be intimately familiar with the expert's publications.

Q. Can you tell us if you belong to any specialty organizations?
A. Yes. I belong to the American Medical Association, the Virginia State and County Medical Societies, the American College of Surgeons, the American College of Obstetricians and Gynecologists, the Virginia Gynecological Society, the Virginia Academy of Medicine, and various other rather minor groups.
Q. Are you board certified in Obstetrics and Gynecology?
A. Yes. I am.
Q. How does a physician become board certified?
A. One submits to a searching two-part examination, the first part of which is a written examination, and then after two years of practice in the specialty one takes the oral examination.
Q. When were you certified?
A. 1970.
Q. Have you ever held any teaching positions?
A. Yes.
Q. Will you tell the jury about those, please.
A. I have been assistant clinical professor of obstetrics and gynecology at the University of Virginia since 1967.

Counsel can expand as need be on this line of questioning.

Q. Do you know the specialty of Drs. Johnson and Irwin?
A. Yes.
Q. What is that specialty?
A. Obstetrics and gynecology.
Q. Is that the same specialty as yours?
A. Yes.
Q. Is their education, training, background, and experience approximately the same as yours or different?
A. Quite similar.
Q. Are the standards of good medical practice or accepted medical treatment the same for obstetricians like you and Johnson and Irwin all over the United States?
A. Absolutely.
Q. Is there some type of minimum fundamental standard that all doctors like yourself must meet?
A. Certainly.
Q. Are you knowledgeable about that standard for doctors like yourself and Dr. Irwin and Dr. Johnson in 1980?

A. Yes.

Q. Doctor, are you involved in daily practice with patients?

A. Yes.

Q. Obstetrical patients?

A. Yes.

Q. How long have you been doing that?

A. Since I entered private practice.

Q. Have you in the past assisted lawyers, judges, and juries and helped them understand the medical issues in the case?

A. Yes, I have.

Q. Why is that?

A. In order to—

DEFENSE ATTORNEY: I object to the question, as to its relevance.

Q. Go ahead.

A. In order to clear some of the mystery from the interface between the law and medicine.

In a case alleging that the defendant's failure to perform a cesarean section resulted in injury to the infant, the court affirmed a directed verdict in favor of the defendant obstetrician, explaining that the causation testimony of the plaintiff's expert was properly excluded. The plaintiff in *Levesque v. Regional Medical Center Board*[1] alleged that the disorders suffered by her infant son included right hemiparesis, severe mental retardation, epilepsy, optic nerve hypoplasia, and cerebral palsy. The plaintiff offered the testimony of an OB/GYN that the infant's disorders were caused by the defendant's failure to perform a cesarean section. Plaintiff's expert admitted on cross-examination that he had no expert knowledge of the causes of any of the infant's problems as follows:

Q. You would agree with me, Dr. Engel, that you are not an expert on the causes of hemiparesis?

A. That's correct.

Q. You agree with me, Dr. Engel, that you are not an expert on the causes of cerebral palsy?

A. That's correct.

Q. You would agree with me, Dr. Engel, that you are not familiar with the eye or [the] visual problem known as optic nerve hypoplasia?

A. That's correct.

Q. That you have never studied it?

A. That's correct.

Q. That you do not know what causes it?

A. That's correct.

The court explained that an expert may testify only as to matters within his training and experience and that it is error for the trial court to allow an expert

---

[1] 612 So. 2d 445 (Ala. 1993).

witness to testify to matters outside his expertise. Although the plaintiff's expert was an expert in the OB/GYN field, he admitted that he had no knowledge of the causes of epilepsy, hemiparesis, cerebral palsy, or optic nerve hypoplasia from which to render an expert opinion.

The court went on to explain that even if the plaintiff's expert qualified as an expert on the issue of causation, plaintiff's case would fail. The questions posed to the expert elicited only the answer that the defendant's actions "probably could have" caused the injuries. This response falls short, the court explained, when measured by the standard by which evidence of proximate cause is tested.

Similarly, in the case of *Romero ex rel. Romero v. United States,*[2] the court found the plaintiff's expert to be unqualified to testify as an expert. The plaintiff's case alleged medical malpractice relating to the neonatal care of her infant son who was later diagnosed with severe general hypertonicity and cerebral palsy and had spastic quadriplegia due to intracranial hemorrhage. The court explained:

In a medical malpractice case, a plaintiff must prove through the testimony of experts in the particular field that the medical treatment received fell below the degree of care ordinarily exercised in the same circumstances by a physician having the degree of learning and skill ordinarily possessed by practitioners in the same speciality and locality.

A medical expert is not qualified as a witness unless it shows that he is familiar with the standards required of physicians under similar circumstances. Dr. Leviss, plaintiff's expert obstetrician, does not render care to newborn infants. Dr. Leviss admitted that he has not received any formal training in the area of the premature infant, and that he does not hold himself out to be an expert in the area of neonatology.[3]

In *Koontz v. Ferber,*[4] the court held that the plaintiffs did not show that the trial court abused its discretion in excluding a deposition passage in which one of plaintiffs' doctors stated his opinion that the reading "'minus 5 base excess' *may* reflect any 'metabolic acidosis'. . . ."[5] "The court concluded that [t]he physician's opinion that the lab reading 'may' reflect acidosis is not the same as an opinion, to a reasonable degree of medical certainty, that the lab reading *does* reflect acidosis."[6]

---

[2] 806 F. Supp. 569 (E.D. Va. 1992), *aff'd,* 2 F.3d 1149 (4th Cir. 1993).

[3] *Id.* (citations omitted).

[4] 870 S.W.2d 885 (Mo. Ct. App. 1993).

[5] *Id.* at 890.

[6] *Id.*

§ 16.9   —Failure to Perform Timely Cesarean Section

Once the doctor's background has been placed in front of the jury, counsel should ask if the physician is prepared to render an opinion and should then elicit the opinion.

Q.   Doctor, today are you prepared to render an opinion on the care of the mother and the child in the Sanchez case?

A.   Yes, I am.

Q.   Doctor, I would ask you, for any of your opinions, to base them on a reasonable degree of medical probability, based upon your education, training, and experience, and minimal fundamental standards of care for doctors like yourself, Dr. Irwin, and Dr. Johnson in 1980.

A.   I understand.

Q.   And any answers or opinions you give today will be based on that standard. Can we have that agreement?

A.   Yes, we may.

Q.   Thank you sir. What materials have you reviewed before your deposition today?

This line of questioning makes for smoother testimony. A litany of standard questions is avoided.

A.   [Witness states materials reviewed.] I have reviewed the record of admission of Maria Sanchez to Brown Memorial Hospital of January 25, 1980.

I have reviewed the antepartum records of Maria Sanchez with Drs. Irwin and Johnson.

I have reviewed the record of admission of the infant female Sanchez at Brown Memorial Hospital of January 25, 1980.

I have reviewed the autopsy report from the County of Maricopa office of the medical examiner re Bertha Sanchez, signed by John T. Goodwin, M.D., and dated May 18, 1980.

I have reviewed the oral deposition of William Irwin, M.D., which is dated September 22, 1982.

And I have reviewed the oral deposition of Henry Johnson, M.D., which is dated September 22, 1982.

Q.   First of all, tell me, in your opinion, how this pregnancy should have been managed.

A.   The standard of care would demand that in the face of a family history of diabetes, this woman should have been submitted to the appropriate testing for gestational diabetes during her pregnancy, that is, a glucose tolerance test. And, further, in that her menstrual cycles were notoriously irregular, she should have had at least two ultrasound examinations during the pregnancy in order to confirm the calculated expected date of confinement.

Q.   Doctor, why is that? Will you explain to the jury why that would be important?

A.   When we calculate an expected date of confinement from the date of the last regular menstrual period, it is based on the assumption that the woman has her menstrual periods every 28 days. If she does not, if she is grossly irregular in her menstrual cycles, then the calculation which we use is invalid and, at best, only a very rough guide. Therefore, more refined methods of defining the expected date of confinement are necessary. And in this particular case the ultrasound would be that more refined method.

Q. Was that the standard sort of thing doctors were doing in 1980?

A. Absolutely.

Q. Can you tell us, if you could, in kind of a summary form, any departures from the standard of care as you know it and as we have defined it today in the care that Drs. Johnson and Irwin afforded Maria Sanchez and her child?

DEFENSE ATTORNEY: Let me object to the form of the question as including the conduct of both doctors and therefore being a multiple question. If the doctor would like to testify as to each of the particular doctors, I have no objection.

Q. Doctor, I think that is a good objection. I wonder if you would answer that question talking about either Dr. Johnson or Dr. Irwin first and then about the other.

A. Yes, I will deal with Dr. Johnson first. When the patient was admitted in labor on January 25, 1980, at 6 A.M., Dr. Johnson saw her at 6:15 A.M. At that time the nurse's notes indicate that the variability on the fetal heart monitor was apparently minimal. And Dr. Johnson was privy to these data or informations when he saw the patient.

He ruptured the membranes at 6:15 A.M., obtained what is said to be moderate amount heavy meconium-stained fluid. An internal fetal scalp monitor was applied, and virtually immediately adverse fetal heart patterns appeared on the fetal heart monitor and tape.

In addition, Drs. Johnson and Irwin had sent Mrs. Sanchez for an X-ray pelvimetry on December 6 which had demonstrated clearly a flat pelvis.

With the combination of a flat pelvis, a woman who was $42\frac{1}{2}$ weeks pregnant, a woman whose stature was very small at 4 feet 8 inches tall, a woman who has meconium in the amniotic fluid and adverse deceleration patterns on the monitor, this woman should have had a cesarean section at 6:15 A.M. or shortly thereafter. And Dr. Johnson's failure to carry out cesarean at that time and in an ongoing manner thereafter was a deviation and a departure from the customary standard of good and acceptable obstetrical practice.

Many attorneys versed in medico-legal matters often forget that an expert's testimony has to be translated into ordinary English so that the jury can understand. If the jury does not understand, the plaintiff is in trouble.

Q. Doctor, let's define some things for the jury now.

You said, I think the first thing I wrote down was that the variability was minimal as noted by the nurse. First of all, is that also your opinion from reading the fetal heart strip?

A. No.

Q. Can you tell us what your reading of the heart strip was?

A. The external fetal heart monitoring tapes, which ran only some 15 or 20 minutes, are somewhat difficult to interpret. But they appear to show some subtle late decelerations. However, more to the point, one cannot make a comment on variability based on an external fetal heart monitor and tracing.

Q. Can you tell me or define for the jury so they can understand it, because they are not doctors—and of course we are not doctors, the lawyers in this case—will you define *late decelerations* for us?

A. Yes. These are slowings of the fetal heart which begin about halfway through the contraction or pain. They have a rather shallow, uniform configuration when one looks at them on fetal heart monitoring tapes. They look like little saucers. Then the slowing persists past the end of the contraction and only resumes itself at the normal rate when the contraction is well over by 30 seconds or so.

Q. What is the importance of this event called late deceleration on the fetal monitor strip?

A. Persistent, repetitive late decelerations are evidence of what is called uteroplacental insufficiency, which is another way of saying that the child is simply not getting enough oxygen from the mother.

Q. You also used the term "meconium." Would you explain to the jury what that is?

A. Yes. Meconium is the content of the fetal intestine, the fetal feces, as it were.

Q. What significance or importance does that have in this case, if any?

A. When the fetus passes meconium into its sac in the uterus, that is regarded generally as an ominous sign for the state of fetal health and, at the very least, demands an increased intensive surveillance of the child with a prejudice to immediate delivery by the most expeditious and least traumatic route possible. In other words, when one sees meconium in the amniotic sac, one is constrained to assume that the child is undergoing some serious compromise of its health.

Q. And you said—you used the term "internal fetal monitor."

A. Yes. That is an apparatus which consists of an electrode which is gently screwed into the child's scalp. It records a continuous cardiogram, electrocardiogram from the child. This cardiogram is converted in a computer into a series of blips on a fetal heart monitoring tape which is moving across a drum, so that one can see the rate of the heart from instant to instant.

Q. You also used a term "X-ray pelvimetry." I think you defined that as an X-ray.

A. Yes. It is an X-ray of the bones of the pelvis or the bones of the birth canal simply to investigate whether or not there is adequate room in this pelvis for the child to pass through.

Q. I think you then said that she had a "flat pelvis." I wonder if you would explain that to the jury.

A. Yes. That is a pelvis in which the diameter of the ring of bones—and the pelvis is nothing more than a solid ring of bones through which the child's head and body must pass. In this particular case the ring was flattened from front to back. It was as if someone had put the patient in a vice between her abdomen and her back and tightened the vice so that the ring of bones flattened from front to back.

Q. Why is that important?

A. Because this would indicate that the head was too large to pass through the ring of bones.

Q. When you say head, you mean the head of the fetus?

A. Yes. That would constitute a condition known as cephalopelvic disproportion, which means that the head is disproportionately large to the ring of bones.

Q. What is the treatment for cephalopelvic disproportion?

A. Cesarean section.

Q. You also mentioned that she was 42½ weeks.

A. Yes.

Q. Would you explain to the jury what you meant by that.

A. Yes. She was 42½ weeks from the first day of her last regular menstrual period. Normally, a pregnancy lasts approximately 40 weeks. When it passes the 42nd week, we call that condition postdatism. And it is universally acknowledged that women who are postdate, and their children particularly, are at risk for various insults and compromises during the remainder of the pregnancy, labor, and delivery. In other words, postdate—or babies of postdate women are notoriously fragile and vulnerable to any kind of insult or injury.

Q. Doctor, can you tell us physiologically why postdatism is a concern for obstetrics?

A. It is felt that the placenta, the organ which transmits oxygen and nutrients to the child and removes toxic waste products or byproducts from the child during the pregnancy, begins to age or to flag or pale in its function following the 42nd week. Therefore, the child is or may be deprived of oxygen and/or nutrients and becomes, as I say, in effect, a chronically sick person.

Q. Doctor, I wonder if you can, now that we have defined some terms so the jury understands them, I wonder if you can kind of put this together for the jury so that they can understand, in your opinion, the failure to meet the standard of care by Dr. Johnson in this case.

A. The departures or violations of the standard of care with respect to Dr. Johnson, as I indicated earlier, were based on the failure, his failure, to apprehend the significance of the 42½ week gestation as a serious risk factor and his failure to apprehend again the significance, taken together, of this 42½ week pregnancy, which as I explained earlier places the woman or at least her child at risk, in combination with the X-ray pelvimetry which had been carried out on 21 January, which showed that this was a flat pelvis and a child of average size would not pass through this pelvis, that there was, in effect, cephalopelvic disproportion.

   Those factors in combination with the presence of meconium in the amniotic fluid, which as I explained earlier is an ominous sign for the state of fetal health, and the adverse or alarming patterns on the fetal heart monitoring tape, which was moving along with an internal monitor in place, all of these factors acting together mandated cesarean section at 6:15 or immediately thereafter. The failure to carry out cesarean section at that time was, in my opinion, a flagrant and conspicuous violation of the standard of care.

From what I see from the medical records, any physician, any average, prudent, practicing physicians being confronted with these various risk factors at 6:15 A.M. should have and would have taken the appropriate course of action, namely, carrying out cesarean section. Therefore, one is inexorably and inevitably led to believe that in fact Dr. Johnson did not apprehend the significance of these factors in that he failed to act appropriately.

Q. What steps should Dr. Johnson have taken to adhere to standards of good obstetrical practice as they existed in 1980?

A. Quite simply, Dr. Johnson should have proceeded to cesarean section at 6:15 or shortly thereafter, and his failure to do so was a violation of the standard of care.

Q. Do you have an opinion as to whether or not the departures from standards of good medical practice by Dr. Johnson were a cause of the injuries and subsequent death of Bertha Sanchez?

A. Yes, I do.

Q. What is that?

A. My opinion is that these were the cause of her death.

Q. Let's talk about Dr. Irwin for a minute. What steps should Dr. Irwin have taken to adhere to standards of good obstetrical practice as they existed in 1980?

A. Well, Dr. Irwin was aware of the results of the X-ray pelvimetry and in that regard should have proceeded to have Mrs. Sanchez admitted to the hospital on 24 January when he saw her, with an eye to carrying out elective cesarean section at that time.

Q. Why would that be important?

A. Mrs. Sanchez had had a non-stress test on 15 December which had shown a healthy child. There was the chance to give this mother and father a healthy baby. She was 4 feet 8 inches tall. She had what was clearly an inadequate, flattened pelvis, and there was a strong presumption of cephalopelvic disproportion, and that this child was not going to negotiate that birth canal safely. And in combination with the state of postdatism, she was then $42\frac{1}{2}$ weeks on 23 January, and the state of cephalopelvic disproportion, she should have been admitted to the hospital while this child was still healthy and the cesarean section done.

Q. Doctor, would you define for the jury the term you used, which was a *non-stress test?*

A. Yes. That is a test which involves putting an external fetal heart monitor on a woman and picking up the fetal heart rate from moment to moment. And by means of examining the tracing with respect to its reaction to fetal movements, one can tell whether the child is healthy or not. If there is an acceleration, a speeding up, of the fetal heart rate with the movements of the child, generally we consider the child in good health at that moment.

Q. Were there, in fact, such accelerations?

A. Yes, there were.

Q. Do you have an opinion as to whether or not the departures from standards of good medical practice by Dr. Irwin were a cause of the injuries and subsequent death of Bertha Sanchez?

A. Yes, I do.

Q. What is that opinion?

A. My opinion is that they were the cause of her death

Q. Doctor, you told us about 6:15 to 6:30. Can you tell us what happened after that, what the subsequent course of events was?

A. Well, quite simply, there was—

DEFENSE ATTORNEY: I object to the form of the question in that the doctor was not shown to have been present. If he wants to express an opinion based on his review of the records as to what may have occurred, he is permitted to testify in that manner, but not as to what happened.

Q. Doctor, the medical records are in front of you, aren't they?

A. Yes, they are.

Q. What is a medical record compiled for? What is the purpose of it?

A. It is compiled mainly to aid those who participate in the care of any particular patient. And many people participate in the care of patients, including nurses, laboratory technicians, doctors, residents, and so on. Everyone must be privy to the information and the data being gathered in the course of managing the patient.

Q. Do people rely on what they see in the medical record?

A. Absolutely.

Q. What I want you to do is by using the medical record, to define the subsequent course of events with this child. Let me ask you first some kind of definition questions. Will you explain to the jury what *station* is?

A. Yes. *Station* is the relationship of the leading part of the head, of the child's head as it comes down the birth canal, to two landmarks in the bony pelvis, in the birth canal, which is called the ischial spines. If the head is a certain number of centimeters above the line between these two landmarks, that is called minus station; and if the head is below these landmarks, it is called the plus station.

Q. What is the significance of minus station and plus station?

A. The minus station indicates that the head is not truly engaged into the birth canal. That is to say, it is not settled securely into the birth canal and the largest diameters of the head have not passed through the opening of the birth canal. That is what engagement is about. In this particular case the head was at the minus 3 station when this woman came in in labor. That is, again, another indication of cephalopelvic disproportion, the failure to engage the head.

Q. Did her station ever get to the point where the head was engaged?

A. No. The station never proceeded past the minus 2 or minus 1 station, somewhere between minus 2 and minus 1, so the head was never engaged.

Q. What is *effacement?*

A. *Effacement* is progressive thinning of the cervix, the neck of the womb, prior to dilatation of the cervix.

Q. Can you tell us whether or not Maria Sanchez was ever effaced fully or 100 percent?

A. She was never fully effaced, no. The effacement proceeded to 90 percent.

Q. Does that have any particular importance in this discussion?

A. Yes. It would indicate that the head simply never settled securely against the cervix to fully efface it, since the head was held up or obstructed by the very small diameters of the pelvis.

Q. Can you tell us what *dilatation* is?

A. Yes. That is simply the opening of the cervix or the neck of the womb. The cervix progressively opens and has to allow the head to then descend through the birth canal.

Q. Can you tell us what Maria Sanchez's dilatation was?

A. Yes. It remained at approximately three centimeters throughout the course of this labor.

Q. What is fully dilated, how many centimeters?

A. Ten centimeters dilated.

Q. The fact that she was only three centimeters, does that have some importance in this case?

A. Yes. The fact that it remained at three centimeters further confirmed that there was, in fact, cephalopelvic disproportion here.

Q. Let's—I wonder if you could get out your copies of the external fetal monitor and internal fetal monitor in this case.

A. Do you want the non-stress test or the actual monitoring in the hospital?

Q. I think we have talked about the non-stress test. In your opinion, from reading the non-stress test, is that a normal non-stress test?

A. It was perfectly normal and reassuring.

Q. Let's go to the monitor strip taken in the hospital.

A. Yes.

Q. Let's, first of all, define some terms. Then I'm going to ask you to go through the strip and give us your opinion of what it tells you and what it—what significance it has in this case. All right?

A. Yes.

Q. Now, will you explain to the jury just very briefly, explain to the jury exactly how this machine works physiologically.

A. Well, the external monitor consists of two parts, one called a toco, which is simply a diaphragm, which records the contractions of the uterus. The other is an ultrasound apparatus, which picks up the motion of the fetal heart and translates that through a computer into an instant heart rate. And it is put on a moving drum so that what one finally sees is simply a squiggly line for the instant heart rate.

Q. Is that put on paper by the machine then?

A. Yes, the paper is on a drum, and the paper is then saved and we end up with long strips such as what we have here.

Q. I wonder if you can define for the jury what *variability is.*

A. Yes. That's the difference in the fetal heart rate from one instant to another. And there are two kinds of variability, what are called long-term variability and short-term variability.

Q. And you know the next question. Could you define *long-term* and *short-term* for us?

A. *Long-term variability* are the gross swings of the fetal heart rate. And generally one sees between two and six of those cycles, as it were, per minute.

Short-term variability is the instant or at least the variation in the instant rate from moment to moment. And this averages, oh, perhaps between two and three beats per minute.

The heart rate of the child is never the same from one minute to the next, or at least it never should be the same. If it is, then the child is considered to be seriously ill. But from moment to moment, it varies two or three beats a minute, and that is called the short-term variability.

Q. What I would like to do is to go through this strip and talk about variability. I wonder, is there some way that you can tell the jury which panel we are talking about? Are they numbered?

A. The panels are numbered below. We start here with panel 63.

Q. In your reading and analysis of the strip, are there problems with variability?

A. Yes. From the moment that the internal monitor was applied at panel 68, there is definitely decreased variability, that is, short-term variability. The long-term variability appears to be preserved.

Q. What is the importance of decrease in short-term variability?

A. This indicates some compromise of the child if it persists, which it did in this particular case.

Q. How long does it persist?

A. Short-term variability diminution or reduction here appears to persist throughout the entire tracing, which goes to panel 152.

Q. Please define for us again a deceleration.

A. Yes. Those are slowings of the fetal heart beat, lasting less than two minutes.

Q. Would you tell us what importance that has to a child in utero?

A. If the deceleration patterns are of the type which is considered ominous, then the child's health is clearly imperiled.

Q. What types of patterns are considered ominous?

A. Late decelerations, particularly with decreased variability, and late decelerations which are persistent and repetitive are considered to be ominous. Variable decelerations are also ominous if there is reduced variability and if they are of the sort which last perhaps longer than 60 seconds or plunge to a rate of 70 or less.

Q. Can you tell us how often Maria Sanchez was having contractions when she came to the hospital by reading the monitor strip?

A. Yes. The contractions were every two minutes.

Q. Is there any significance in this case to her having contractions every two minutes?

A. She was obviously in good labor.

Q. Would you characterize this labor as mild, moderate, strong?

A. It would be a moderate to strong labor, yes.

Q. Did she ever contract, at least from the records, any less than about every two minutes?

A. No.

This is important because the defendants testified that the child was never in danger because the mother was never really in labor.

Q. What is significant in the monitor strip?

A. Quite simply, the panels throughout the entire tracing show reduced short-term or beat to beat variability. And there seems to be no alleviating of that phenomenon anywhere in these panels.

   And secondly, there is a pattern of repetitive, persistent late decelerations here which, again, are evident throughout the entire tracing from beginning to end.

Q. Can you show us when the first late deceleration shows up on the strip?

A. Yes. In panel 80 there is a late deceleration. And thereafter there are simply repetitive persistent late decelerations.

Q. Doctor, I am going to show you a poster exhibit that has been blown up for the jury. It has panels 80 through a portion of 83. I wonder if you could mark on this any late decelerations.

A. Yes.

Q. In red.

A. Yes. Right here, right here, here, here. Those four would be late decelerations. Some more subtle than others, but they are all late decelerations.

Q. Should a physician trained like Dr. Johnson and like yourself, should that physician be able to understand that those are late decelerations?

A. Yes.

Q. Doctor, does the portion of the strip in the poster show the machine working properly?

A. Oh, yes.

Q. And is that an adequate and accurate representation of the fetal heart rate and the contraction pattern?

A. Yes.

Q. And is it then your testimony that throughout the rest of the strip to the end of the strip, there is short-term variability loss and late decelerations?

A. Yes, there is a considerable or significant loss or at least reduction in short-term variability, and there are persistent, repetitive late decelerations.

Q. Doctor, we have talked about—I think you defined meconium for us. Will you tell us what importance it has to this case?

A. The meconium simply was a confirmatory of evidence that the child was compromised, that it was undergoing an ongoing hypoxic insult. That is to say, it was not getting enough oxygen from the mother throughout the entire labor. And, as I said, the presence of meconium merely confirmed what was clearly evident from the fetal heart monitoring tapes themselves. I don't know what else these doctors needed to realize this baby needed to be born.

Q. Doctor, there was some medication given to Mrs. Sanchez called Demerol.

A. Yes.

Q. Is that a narcotic?

A. Yes, it is.

Q. Can you tell us whether the administration of that medication has any importance to what we are discussing here and this case?

A. Yes, Demerol is a narcotic. It gains access to the child's circulation by going across the placenta, and it would act as a serious depressant to the vital centers of the child once the child is delivered.

Q. Doctor, can you tell the jury what *across the placenta* means?

A. Yes. The circulation of the mother has an interface with the circulation of the child. At that interface various substances cross over from one to the other. In this particular case the Demerol would go from the mother's circulation, through the placenta, into the child's circulation.

Q. Doctor, does this record reflect what the nurses were informing Dr. Johnson about?

A. Yes, it does.

Q. Can you tell us whether or not the nurses seemed to be in touch with Dr. Johnson or whether they failed to communicate with him what was going on with the patient?

A. No, the nurse's notes indicate that Dr. Johnson was notified regarding the events which were transpiring here, when he was not actually physically present.

Q. Can you tell us whether or not the labor progress chart shows whether or not Dr. Johnson came in and examined the patient?

A. Yes, he did on a number of occasions.

Q. In keeping with standards of good medical practice as they existed in 1980 and based upon your education, training, experience, and reasonable medical probability, when should Maria Sanchez and her child have had the C-section performed?

A. At 6:15 or shortly thereafter when the pattern on the internal monitor confirmed that there was significant fetal compromise and when it was already known that there was cephalopelvic disproportion based on the X-ray pelvimetry and on the fact that this woman had come in in labor with the head at a minus 3 station, clearly unengaged, and in fact virtually floating.

Q. And would you define *floating* for me, please?

A. Yes. The head is moving freely over the birth canal but has not entered the birth canal.

Q. Doctor, do you have an opinion whether or not Bertha Sanchez suffered an injury during the prenatal and labor and delivery course of her mother?

A. There is no question that the child suffered an injury at some time during this labor.

Q. Do you have an opinion of what kind of injury she suffered?

A. Yes, it was a hypoxic injury to the central nervous system.

Q. *Hypoxia* is what?

A. A reduction in oxygen.

Q. How does the fetus get oxygen?

A. Through the placenta from the mother.

Q. Can you tell the jury as an obstetrician what the mechanism of injury would have been?

A. There was a deficiency or a defective transfer of oxygen through the placenta to the child.

Q. When the non-stress test was done on January 21st, do you have an opinion whether or not the child was receiving the right amount of oxygen at that time?

A. Yes, I do.

Q. What is that opinion?
A. The child was receiving adequate oxygen and was in good health.
Q. Do you have an opinion as an obstetrician when this injury occurred?
A. Yes.
Q. Just what is that opinion?
A. It was clearly sometime after the non-stress test of 21 January since the non-stress test was indicative of a healthy fetus.
Q. Do you have an opinion when the hypoxia occurred?
A. Sometime between the non-stress testing of 21 January and the admission to the hospital. And there is no question that the asphyxia was aggravated, enlarged upon, and exaggerated during this labor.
Q. In adhering to standards of good obstetrical practice as they existed in 1980, would a physician be obligated to know that brain damage for an infant could occur from attempting to deliver Bertha Sanchez through her mother's abnormally small pelvis?
A. Yes, it could.
Q. And would a physician be so obligated to know that this could occur?
A. Yes.
Q. How long has this type of information been available to the medical profession?
A. This particular information has been known to the medical profession for hundreds of years.
Q. Is there any other accepted way other than cesarean section to solve Maria's condition in order to prevent brain damage to her child?
A. No.

In *Riley v. Koneru,*[7] the plaintiff's expert testified that, in his opinion, the defendant should have performed an ultrasound examination to determine whether a condition known as hydramnios was present; that the defendant should have hospitalized plaintiff when he discovered that the fetus was lying horizontally in the womb; and that he should have evaluated the plaintiff when she complained of lack of fetal movement, cramping, and spotting. Finally, it was the plaintiff's expert's opinion that the defendant's failure to perform an immediate cesarean section on the plaintiff deviated from the standard of care and resulted in the fetus's death.

The jury returned a verdict in favor of the plaintiff. On appeal, the defendant argued that the plaintiff failed to establish the applicable standard of care since the expert had evaluated the defendant's conduct against a higher standard of care than that imposed by state law. The defendant referred to the following testimony:

The best medicine is practiced by following the standard of care. . . . [T]he highest degree of knowledge then contributes to the standard of care.

---

[7] 593 N.E.2d 788 (Ill. App. Ct. 1992).

* * *

... equating standard of care with what I consider to be good medical practice based on current information to optimize outcomes. . . . My understanding is, of standard of care, is what [plaintiff's attorney] and I describe as good obstetrical practice based on scientific evidence to optimize outcome.[8]

The appellate court found that it was not error to allow plaintiff's expert's testimony and affirmed the verdict of the jury. The statements referred to by the defendant were statements made during cross-examination. The court stated that the questioning was an attempt to have the expert recharacterize his direct testimony in which he established the standard of care with regard to obstetrics, but that the expert's responses do not evince a retreat from his opinion of the standard of care or of the defendant's violation of that standard.

§ 16.10   Theory of Cross-Examination of the Defendant's Expert: Failure to Perform Timely Cesarean Section

There are two basic styles to cross-examination of the defendant's expert. The first one is to learn the opinions of the expert in order to prepare to blunt them for trial. The second one is a full-blown attempt to vigorously cross-examine the expert and shake the foundations of his or her opinions and the defendant's case.

In the first method of cross-examination, questions that revolve around the central theme of discovering all of the experts' opinions and everything that they are going to testify to is the goal. The basic approach is to ask the expert to set out, in list form, a summary of the opinion. A thorough questioning on each item of the list follows with questioning on the facts and basis for each opinion. The deposition is concluded by asking whether *all* opinions have been expressed.

In the second method, counsel must be armed with material to impeach the defendant's opinion. This can take the form of evidence from the case, such as depositions or medical records, articles from the general medical literature, and textbooks and articles written by the expert or the defendant.

§ 16.11   Cross-Examination of Defendant's Expert

The following transcript represents a portion of the deposition of a well-published expert for a defendant.

---

[8] *Id.*

Q. Please state your name.
A. Charles Johnson.
Q. How old are you?
A. 39.
Q. Where do you live?
A. I live in Los Angeles, California.
Q. Please give me a little bit of your educational background.
A. I went to San Fernando Valley State College and I graduated in 1969 with a B.S. Degree. I went to medical school at the University of California in Los Angeles and graduated in 1978. I then did an internship at Orange County Medical Center and a residency in obstetrics and gynecology at the same institution.
Q. What did you do after you finished your residency?
A. I did a two-year fellowship in maternal-fetal medicine or perinatology at the University of California Irvine Medical Center. I completed that in 1979.
Q. Do you limit your practice to any speciality?
A. I limit it to obstetrics and I further limit it to high-risk obstetrics.
Q. Are you board certified?
A. Yes, in obstetrics and gynecology and maternal-fetal medicine.
Q. Now, have you had an opportunity to review the entire prenatal record?
A. Yes.
Q. Okay. And would you explain for the jury what a prenatal record is?
A. It's a record of the patient's care prior to the onset of labor during her pregnancy.
Q. Would it be accurate to say that it monitors the development of the fetus to the extent that the physician can observe it?
A. Yes.
Q. In your evaluation of the prenatal record, did you find anything to indicate that this was not a normally developing fetus?
A. Not specifically, no.
Q. Did you find anything nonspecific that concerned you?
A. With respect to the possibility of a problem with the fetus, the fact that the patient did go beyond her due date could have indicated that there was a problem with the development of the fetus.
Q. I note that you're looking at some records. Are those some handwritten notes that you have made?
A. That's correct.
Q. And were they made by you at the time you were reviewing this matter?
A. Yes.
Q. Is that the only record you have that was authored by you regarding this case?
A. Yes.
Q. Have you issued any reports outside of those particular handwritten yellow notes?
A. Written reports, no.
Q. Let me see those. [Witness handed them to counsel.]
Q. What is the average duration of pregnancy?

A.   Well, as a number, 40 weeks. The range for normals would be 37 to 42 weeks.

Q.   And one of your areas of concern in the obstetrical area is postdatism, is it not?

A.   Indeed, yes.

Q.   And would you explain to the jury what *postdatism* is?

A.   Well, *postdatism* means that the pregnancy has gone beyond 42 weeks.

Q.   And did this pregnancy go beyond 42 weeks?

A.   Yes.

Q.   Now doctor, we all know that you have authored a textbook and numerous articles in the medical literature on obstetrics. Have you published any papers regarding what steps physicians and hospitals caring for patients ought to take to determine fetal well-being after 42 weeks?

A.   Yes.

Q.   And would you explain to the jury what your article states what steps should be taken to determine how the child is doing in the intrauterine environment?

A.   There are various alternatives. Probably the most commonly used method to determine fetal well-being after that period of pregnancy would be antepartum fetal heart rate testing using the same fetal monitoring devices as were used on this patient, but applying them to the prelabor period. They could be used in one of two ways. Either watching the heart rate without contractions, and that's called the non-stress test. Or stressing the fetus by causing the uterus to contract and seeing the fetus' heart rate response to the contractions. That's called contraction stress testing.

Q.   Have you published a series of papers regarding your findings in that regard?

A.   Well, I've published more than one paper on contraction stress tests, and I have also published a specific paper with Dr. Jones on contraction stress tests on postdate patients.

Q.   Generally would it be correct to say that you favor the contraction stress test?

A.   Yes.

Q.   And the non-stress test you feel is somewhat a late indicator of distress if it's positive?

A.   Yes.

Q.   Did you find in this case that at 42 weeks or greater any type of testing was performed?

A.   No.

Q.   Is it generally your understanding that standards of good medical practice dictate that such a test be done in this day and age?

A.   Yes.

Q.   In terms of the fetus and the risk to the fetus, what does postmaturity carry with it?

A.   Well, there is an increased risk of death both prior to labor, in labor, and in the newborn period. There is an increased risk of damage to the baby from asphyxia, which can be to many organ systems, the most common and prominent of which is the brain. There is a risk of meconium aspiration syndrome which means that the baby passes a stool, feces, in the uterus and before, during, or after birth, breathes it into its lungs. And that causes a chemical irritation. There are several newborn complications that are associated with the fact that the baby is postmature, most of which if handled are not of any major consequence.

Q. Would it generally be correct to say that most individuals of your specialty today feel that significant brain damage to the child being delivered usually results from a combination of chronic lack of oxygen in association with some acute lack of oxygen?

A. Yes.

Q. And you and your group have resolved rather than to undertake excessive numbers of cesarean sections or inductions, to develop a method of determining beforehand whether or not that fetus has been affected, or the fetal-maternal unit has been affected, by the postdatism?

A. Yes.

Q. And that's because about 5 percent of postdate pregnancies will have some element of uteroplacental insufficiency?

A. Yes. Based on our data, that is correct.

Q. Would it be correct to say that one of the indications of postdatism is a diminished amount of amniotic fluid?

A. Yes, it would be.

Q. And you indicated in your textbook that that would be of some concern to you in terms of delivering a patient. Why is that?

A. Well, for several reasons. One is that it's an indicator of postmaturity. The postmaturity is how we describe the effects of being overdue on the baby. And about one out of five postdate pregnancies have a postmature baby.

Part of the complex is reduced amniotic fluid volume. So in one respect it's a—tells us which one out of five is postmature. Secondly, as the amount of the amniotic fluid disappears, the umbilical cord becomes more subject to compression. That can cause two problems. One, it can be so severe to actually kill the baby in the uterus before labor. Two, when the fetus rolls over on its cord and compresses it long enough, it often passes meconium. And so then it's a set up for meconium aspiration. So that I would—there is also probably a pretty good correlation though not as good as with other methods, between reduced amniotic fluid volumes and subsequently depressed babies.

Q. Doctor, I've handed you what I think is marked as Plaintiff's Exhibit No. 2 which I believe is a complete record of the prenatal visits to Moore Hospital. Do you find any indication in those records of an appreciation that this was a postmature patient?

A. Well, not—no. There is no direct evidence of that case. There are a couple of notes where the weeks of gestation are written. Forty plus, forty-one plus, on 8-7. There are pelvic exams documented on 8-7 and 8-12 and 8-9 which indicate to me that the physician is starting to think about when this lady is going to deliver. But other than that I see no appreciation, which is consistent with my recollection. Nor do I see, after having the opportunity to review these, any evidence of suspicion of ruptured membranes.

Q. Now, we can agree that the standard in August of 1979 would have been to do some tests to determine the ability of this fetus to withstand the rigors of labor?

A. I would agree.

Q. And that was not done here, was it?

A. That's correct.

Q. So the physicians who finally participated in the delivery did not have the availability of that information?

A. That's correct.

Q. When she came to the hospital, what was your understanding as regards whether she had oligohydramnios, or a diminished amount of amniotic fluid?

A. Well, I think there is evidence that she had diminished amounts of amniotic fluid because when—the patient had a history of possible ruptured membranes though it's not documented, when the, I believe it was a physician, who attempted to rupture membranes, found no fluid. And that could have indicated either that she had been leaking fluid or that there was oligohydramnios, and she had been tapped and there just was no fluid to come out.

Q. Well, the admitting physician at that point has reason to at least suspect that he or she may already be dealing with a fetus who might not tolerate labor as well as a full-term nonpostmature baby?

A. Yes, I believe that's correct.

Q. And certainly that should be kept in mind in the management of this patient?

A. Yes.

Q. Further, that particular physician would be aware that cord compression would be more likely to occur in this type of patient?

A. Yes.

Q. Now, she didn't have an oxytocin challenge test, though, did she?

A. No.

Q. Did she get oxytocin?

A. During labor.

Q. All right. And if that dose of oxytocin had been given prior to delivery and you got the same pattern that you got after oxytocin was started here, would you have said that that patient could withstand labor and delivery?

A. I would have given that patient a trial at labor. Yes.

Q. If that pattern had been reproduced that you see in the late—or early—late morning on August 30th, would you have persisted in trying to deliver this patient vaginally?

A. Well, I think if you were going to say that this patient's cervix was undilated with that pattern, no. But if her cervix was eight centimeters dilated with that pattern, I would have persisted until the point which I previously said I would have intervened, which I think there is a difference there which is— I mean, you can't stand—it's different to expect to stand two hours or three hours of such variable decelerations or fourteen or twenty-four hours.

Q. Since you mentioned prolongation of abnormal or the duration of abnormal fetal heart rate patterns, does the duration have anything to do with ultimate outcome in terms of brain damage?

A. Of the abnormal heart rate pattern?

Q. [Counsel nodded his head affirmatively.]

A. I believe it does. I'm not sure it's been adequately documented, but I believe it does.

Q. In terms of duration of abnormal fetal heart rate patterns, how long would you say that Mrs. Gorham demonstrated abnormal fetal heart rate patterns?

A. It depends what we mean by abnormal. Okay? If you're asking, how long did she have persistently abnormal heart rate pattern or how long since the first abnormality existed?

Q. Well, let's start first with how long since the first abnormality.

A. I believe it started at approximately 4:00 in the morning, and she delivered at 12:15. So eight and a quarter hours?

Q. Okay.

A. But that's since the first abnormality.

Q. Would you say that moderate to severe variables and severe variables would be considered ominous fetal heart rate patterns?

A. Severe variables which were persistent in and of themselves, yes.

When discussing the fetal monitor record, the entire strip, panel by panel, should be reviewed.

Q. I'd like to at this point go to the fetal monitoring pattern which has been previously marked as Defendant's Exhibit No. 1. At the first tracing that starts at 2:42 A.M. on August 29th, 1979, what do you see there—

A. I see a baseline fetal heart rate of approximately 160 beats per minute, some apparent long-term variability, no decelerations. Variability which would—I have previously described as somewhere which I would not describe as average but not absent. Somewhere in between. Decreased.

Q. This is an external monitor?

A. That's correct.

Q. Would variability be more pronounced on an external monitor or less pronounced?

A. Be artifactually increased, if anything. But long-term variability as seen here can be accurately assessed.

Q. And there are portions where the variability does not look good at all, does it?

A. Well, there—there are no portions where it's absent. There are certainly portions where it's decreased.

Q. Well, for an external monitor they are markedly decreased, aren't they?

A. No. I wouldn't describe it as such. There are—there is long-term variability there, and it's not markedly decreased.

Q. But it is decreased?

A. Yes.

Q. And then we have uterine contractions; do we not?

A. Yes.

Q. All right. And how long are those contractions lasting?

A. About a minute.

Q. Just to orient the jury, would you show them which markers—why don't you use red here—

A. Okay.

Q. —are a minute.

A. One minute is three centimeters, which is from here to here or from here to here.

Q. And that's how you're able to tell how long the contractions are—

A. Yes.

Q. —is that correct? With this second contraction, do you see a slight dip in the pulse rate?

A. Uh-huh.

Q. And where does that dip occur?

A. It's—it's a pretty nondescript dip. It occurs somewhere toward the latter half of the contraction.

Q. That's a late deceleration, but you don't think it's significant?

A. It's not a late deceleration.

Q. All right. It's a dip in fetal heart rate that occurs after the peak of the contraction?

A. Uh-huh.

Q. And you think it's a technical artifact?

A. No.

Q. What do you think it is?

A. It's a variation of the heart rate. It's not a late deceleration.

Q. All right.

A. You see normal fluctuations of the heart rate above and below the baseline. But you see here this thing is well over before the contraction even begins to be over. It's only of about 10 seconds duration, and late decelerations don't look like that. You can find other areas in the tracing which have decelerations like that, that are unrelated to contractions.

Q. On the second page, the dip at 422147, what is that dip there?

A. Small variable deceleration.

Q. How can you tell it's a variable?

A. Because of its shape.

Q. Well, is it in association with a uterine contraction?

A. Doesn't matter.

Q. 422148 and 422149, what do you see on that part of the tracing?

A. I see an apparently normal-looking heart rate. Baseline of 155 to 160 with accelerations present. Actually more normal appearing variability than appeared before.

Q. The fact that there is an intermittent tachycardia; that is, a pulse rate over 160, with diminished variability, would that have concerned you in this—

A. That is not an intermittent tachycardia. One must be very careful in describing monitor patterns to distinguish between accelerations and tachycardia. Tachycardia is a permanent change in the baseline, which could be bad. Accelerations or transient changes above the baseline are good so that those temporary rises of the heart rate above the baseline are reassuring signs.

Q. How do you account for the change in baseline that Mrs. Gorham had in this case from the baseline that had been the baseline throughout her entire pregnancy?

A. Oh, you mean during the prenatal care when they counted on 44—

Q. During the prenatal care and up until almost two or three days before she came into the hospital.

A. Well, I think that there are two possibilities. One is that counting heart rates is so notoriously inaccurate when physicians count heart rate in the office that Dr. Hon wrote a paper about it. He found in conclusion that even giving quite a number of professors the same exact tape of something to listen to, they tended to normalize the heart rate. People tend to do that. They—because of that I don't count heart rates in the prenatal office. I just say present or absent unless it's grossly abnormal. So that's one possibility.

   The other possibility is that perhaps this baby had some hypoxic insult, brain—some brain damage occurred. The oxygenation normalized, and then we arrived at the point where we are now.

Q. So the possibility is that assuming that the fetal pulse rates were done properly and recorded properly, that this child already had some decrease in the oxygen tension in the brain when the child came in?

A. No. That's not how I would word it.

Q. How would you?

A. The fetus had—had some reduction in the oxygen tension in the brain. If there was any persistent reduction in oxygen tension, it would be manifested in late decelerations.

Q. Would—okay. With Mrs. Gorham's status in terms of diminished amniotic fluid, postdatism and early loss on the initial tracing of diminished variability, would you have switched to an internal monitor?

A. I would have.

Q. Did they do that here?

A. Not till they started the oxytocin.

Q. Why would you have done that, Doctor?

A. Well, I just—I'm more comfortable looking at variability with an internal monitor directly. However, I would—I would say that if you have an adequate external monitor and you're comfortable that you're getting reasonably good tracing, that it's not absolutely essential to switch to an internal monitor. There is some concern that putting internal monitor may add to infections more, too. So there is a downside risk of using it. Given its long-term variability being reasonable, I think one can make a case for not doing it. I would have done it, I would have wanted to maximize my data, but I wouldn't be critical of someone not doing it.

Q. What is your opinion of these four panels of tracings?

A. There are these—which changes here which could either represent signal loss or small variable decelerations.

Q. Now, this early in the labor would those concern you any?

A. No.

Q. Even with postmaturity and diminished amniotic fluid?

A. No.

Q. And no prior testing to determine whether or not the fetus was susceptible to hypoxia?

A. There are no late decelerations occurring now.

Q. Are there any late decelerations anywhere in this record, Doctor?

A. No.

Q. Well, if the Defendant in this case thought they were late decelerations, was he wrong?

A. I don't see any. I see what—it may be a problem of semantics. I see what is—when later on as I've testified, when the fetus is having variable decelerations there is a late component to them. Some people call them late component. Others call them a slow return to baseline.

Q. All right. At panel between -75 and -76, that again you believe is interference?

A. Yes.

Q. And through -77, is that also—

A. Artifact.

Q. Artifact?

A. Yeah.

Q. During the artifact is the machine adequately—accurately recording the pulse pressure, pulse rate at the same time?

A. It's hard to be sure.

Q. Well, for instance at -77, the strip that shows the rapid squiggly lines, is that the fetal heart rate?

A. It's hard to know.

Q. Okay. You don't know what the fetal heart rate is there, do you?

A. That's correct.

Q. And then -78, what is that?

A. Small variable deceleration.

Q. And at -79 and -80?

A. Something's happening with the contractions. The probability is that the contraction monitor has slipped so that it's not recording correctly. And there is more of this artifact. There is the beginning at the end of -69 of a larger deceleration. It's hard to be sure because of the page change. It's probably a variable deceleration.

Q. Okay.

A. Because of the way it comes back up here, I'm wondering how much is artifact, how much is real.

Q. Okay. Could it also be a late deceleration?

A. It could be. Doesn't make any difference.

Q. If Dr. Moore called this a late deceleration, would you disagree with him?

A. See, the real issue is—and this is something that I don't mean to be difficult about. But, you know, worrying whether one deceleration is a late or not is really not worth any time at all.

Q. Okay.

A. Because if lates are present, they are reoccurring with most contractions. So it's hard. I mean, we could always sit here and argue with the tracing whether there is one deceleration on everybody's labor. And I try to teach the nurses and medical students to not do that because that isn't anything.

Q. If a late deceleration, if that is a recurring—or the physician thinks it's a recurring problem, say, in Mrs. Gorham's situation, would that be more significant than just variables?

A. Persistent decelerations are nonreassuring patterns, yes. And indeed they require some action.

Q. What type action do you suggest in your book?

A. Well, first you position the patient on her side and give her oxygen. Second, if she's on oxytocin you discontinue that. Third, if there is any precipitating event that you can treat, such as an epidural anesthetic with hypotension, give pressor agents, if necessary. And if you can't correct the Pitocin—and if Pitocin is on, you should turn that off. If you can't correct it, then you need to intervene.

Q. How about with moderate to severe variable decelerations? What steps do you usually take if they are repetitive?

A. Repositioning the patient and giving oxygen.

Q. How about in terms of oxytocin?

A. Well, if you have a pattern of persistently nonreassuring variable decelerations, you should probably not give oxytocin. It would vary with the individual tracing, and you have to make a decision on any individual whether it's safer to allow the nonprogress of labor and section at that point, or augment the patient. And that would depend on that pattern.

I hesitate to, you know—moderate to severe is a—is a real range, and it's hard to be specific. If they meet nonreassuring criteria, then I would not use oxytocin.

Q. Do you see any late or nonreassuring variable decelerations on this record?

A. Not—there are some that are nonreassuring, but they are not persistent until the point in the record where I said I would be willing to intervene.

Q. At 11:30?

A. 11:30. I think the big issue is, yes, you can find several of them that are in and of themselves nonreassuring, but they don't persist.

Q. At that point would Pitocin ordinarily be shut off?

A. Not if it were just one or two.

Q. Well, how about in this case? Would it be appropriate to shut it off at 11:30?

A. About then.

Q. If you continued running it, would that likely have made the hypoxia worse?

A. It depends how much the Pitocin was actually contributing to the contractions. I mean, if you start someone with Pitocin, say at six centimeters or seven centimeters and they get to nine centimeters, many times if you turn off the Pitocin at that point, you don't see any diminution in the uterine activity. So that—because there is a very good correlation between the stage of labor and the amount of uterine activity. Certainly people who are near delivery or near complete dilation have more uterine activity. So I don't know about turning it off at that time.

Q. In any case, you would have shut it off at 11:30?

A. Yeah.

Q. Okay. And I assume part of that is based on the fact that the pattern that you saw that was nonreassuring occurred after the onset of Pitocin therapy?

A. It was after. Yes.

Q. Did you see a place that documented the Pitocin was indeed stopped in this patient?

A. No. I did not.

Q. Let me ask you, do you give Pitocin that way at your university?

A. In which way?

Q. In terms of verbal commands for increasing it and decreasing it and stopping it?

A. Yes. We often do.

Q. Is it usually transmitted immediately into written form?

A. Yes, it is.

Q. Do you find that that was done here?

A. No. It was not.

Q. Is that in your opinion somewhat sloppy management of Pitocin therapy?

A. Certainly sloppy documentation.

Q. Why is it that at your particular university you make sure you have good documentation?

A. For several reasons. One is in case we come to a setting like this, it's always important to have adequate documentation. Two, is we do a lot of teaching off of our monitor strips, and the best way to be able to teach is to document events so you can relate events and happenings to the monitor. It's also good for patient care.

Q. For the safety of the patient?

A. Sure.

Q. And you weren't able to find any evidence that Pitocin was stopped up to the time the patient went to deliver, were you?

A. No evidence in the medical record.

Q. Would you agree that there are four decelerations in a row?

A. Yes.

Q. Variable decelerations?

A. Yes.

Q. An indication to you that at least for a period of time the cord is in some way compromised?

A. The cord is compressed.

Q. Compressed? You indicated earlier that those periods of compression could be best likened to periods of time in which you—an adult would hold their breath?

A. Yes.

Q. Could they also be likened to pulling someone under the water and holding them under the water for 30 or 60 seconds and then letting them up again?

A. Yes.

Q. And doing that three or four times in a row?

A. Yes.

Q. What do you see on this page of monitor strip?

A. There are two larger variable decelerations than before.

Q. Okay. Now, how low does the pulse rate get?

A. On one of them it gets to 50 to 60 beats per minute.

Q. And then the next one?

A. About 90.

Q. Okay. Now, why does the pulse rate go down as low as it goes here? What is the mechanism?

A. Well, the mechanism that causes the heart rate to go down is the heart senses an increase in resistance as it pumps against the cord. Most of the blood that comes out of the heart goes into the umbilical cord, or at least half of it.

Q. Talking about the fetal heart?

A. Fetal heart.

Q. Okay.

A. And when a heart is starting to pump against a closed system, it has a reflex that causes it to slow down, and that's why the heart rate goes down. The more closed it is and the longer that it's closed, the more profound the reflex. And that's as we understand variable decelerations, why the heart rate goes down. What controls the degree to which it goes down is anybody's guess, but it usually correlates with the completeness and duration of umbilical cord compression.

Q. How long does the variable last at -01?

A. One minute and 30 seconds, 20 seconds, in there.

Q. How long does the variable at -02 last?

A. The entire variable lasts about a minute and 10 seconds.

Q. Are those severe variables?

A. They would fall into the category of nonreassuring variables.

Q. Are they severe—

A. Or severe.

Q. Now, if you were concerned at your institution at this point about a child being postmature and the possibility that that cord compression superimposed on a child who might not be able to tolerate it well, that there was a problem, do you have a mechanism at your hospital for looking a little closer at that situation?

A. We put internal scalp electrodes on.

Q. And do you also have the ability to get any type of blood gas determination?

A. We do scalp pHs, but we rarely use them with variable decelerations.

Q. Well, what does a scalp pH tell you?

A. It tells us the degree with which either the hypoxia or carbon dioxide retention is causing the fetus to become acidotic. If the tissue is getting adequate oxygen, then tissue maintains a normal pH, or acid-base balance. And if the tissue is not getting enough oxygen, it changes the way it uses glucose and starts to use it without oxygen in which case you start to get a buildup of acid, and the pH goes down. That's what you're looking for when you use scalp pH.

Q. And that's an additional tool that you have that Moore doesn't have?

A. That's correct.

Q. And what you're telling the jury is that you have an additional piece of information that you can plug into your determination of whether or not the child is or is not getting sufficient oxygen?

A. We do have that. Yes.

Q. And indeed you are able to get a number and integrate it in and frequently determine whether in conjunction with the fetal heart rate changes, whether or not you are going to perform a C-section?

A. Yes.

Q. At -03, is there a slight variable?

A. Yes. Slight.

Q. At the next contraction?

A. Slight.

Q. At the next contraction.

A. Severe variable.

Q. How long does that variable last?

A. One and a half minutes. One and three-quarters minutes.

Q. How about the rate of return to the baseline?

A. It's a little confusing because there is a signal loss at this point. It looks slower than average, but then there is an abrupt point so—

Q. Okay. Now, that's one, two—this one you can't say because there is artifact.

A. Uh-huh.

Q. Three, four—the next five contractions that can be recorded have variables, do they not?

A. Variables.

Q. Okay. Is that by your definition repetitive?

A. Yes. But not repetitively severe.

Q. All right. Let's assume that at -04 you had the discretion to think about cesarean section. At your hospital how long does it take after you make the decision to perform a cesarean section and the time that everything is usually together to do that?

A. We can do them as soon as five or ten minutes, if necessary.

Q. Tell me how, the procedure that you do that. How do you manage to do that at your hospital?

A. We rush the patient across the hall to the cesarean section room. And we have an operating crew in the house and an anesthesiologist in the house, and we just do it.

Q. Now, is that an appropriate standard of good medical practice?

A. It's unfortunately well above the standard that most hospitals meet.

Q. Now, if you have variability intact, does that suggest to the practitioner that irreversible and permanent brain damage has not occurred?

A. Not necessarily.

Q. It is at least some indication that that may be true?

A. Not necessarily.

Q. Well, if you have a dead brain, are you able to get variability?

A. If the—if the cortex is not functioning but your midbrain and lower brain are functioning, you probably still have normal variability. So it depends, you know, what we're talking about. I don't know, you know, how well that's been documented.

We have a sense that severely brain damaged babies don't have normal variability. However, for example, you can take an anencephalic baby, and if

the cortex—baby with essentially no head, but they have lower brain struc-
tions intact. Some of those have normal variability. They don't have any cortex to speak of.

Q. And some don't have?

A. And some don't.

Q. Okay.

A. So it just depends how much of the brain has been damaged.

Q. All right.

A. It's not an all or not phenomenon.

Q. But the general theory is that if you have good variability, that it's at least a
good suggestion that you have a brain that's intact?

A. If we're dealing—if we're talking about acute situations—okay? I think that
that would be a fair statement. But I don't think it's fair to extrapolate that
statement to the chronic effects and the acute effects.

Q. What kind of deceleration is this [counsel pointed]?

A. An unusually shaped deceleration. Looking at it of itself, I can't be sure what
kind of deceleration it is. Based on the company it's been keeping, it's probably variable.

Q. Except it appears to start—

A. Yeah. That's why I said—

Q. —late?

A. It's late, but it has these jagged things in it like a variable. So that's why I said
it's unusual. But then there are no more.

Q. And at that point the Pitocin is started?

A. Yes.

Q. Now, you feel that Pitocin is appropriate for protracted labor—

A. Yes.

Q. —is that correct? All right. Are there some who would disagree with you on
that?

A. Yes.

Q. How—how would you characterize Mrs. Gorham's labor up to that point?

A. Protracted.

Q. What does that mean?

A. It means it's not following a normal labor curve. The accepted lower limits of
normal would be—in the active phase of labor would be one centimeter per
hour.

Q. What are the causes of that?

A. Well, it can be uterine inertia, whatever causes insufficient contractions. Can
be cephalopelvic disproportion. Can be a head that's in the wrong attitude
creating a functional disproportion. It can be something—some tumors or
other mass effects that obstruct the progress of the labor through the birth
canal.

Q. Do you ever see any indication that anybody has determined the position of
the fetal head?

A. Not that I can see. No.

Q. Is that good obstetrical practice to go forward with starting Pitocin without
determining the position?

A.   I wouldn't say it's good obstetrical practice. No.

Q.   At -71 and -72, 422371 and -72, an internal lead has been put on finally.

A.   Indeed.

Q.   Something you would have done probably much earlier in the evening?

A.   Yes.

Q.   And Pitocin is started?

A.   Yes.

Q.   All right. The patient is eight or nine centimeters dilated?

A.   According to that notation, yes.

Q.   Okay. You would have started Pitocin with eight or nine centimeters dilatation?

A.   Yes.

Q.   How were the contractions throughout the night according to the monitor?

A.   Well, the limitations of the external monitor are many. But given the amount of limitations, they were—you can't tell anything about strength, and the frequency prior to starting oxytocin is every four minutes there, three and a half there. I don't know how long there. Here I can't tell because of the artifact. Here we go a long period of time, about five or six minutes without a contraction. Here we have a contraction that only lasts about 40 seconds. They appear to be inconsistent and somewhat irregular at the time the Pitocin is started.

Q.   Now, what was the pattern through the night and through the early hours? Labor look pretty good?

A.   You really can't say on an external monitor. In terms of frequency it looked frequent enough. But in terms of strength, I couldn't say.

Q.   Is there any notation in the record through the night or through the early morning that the strength was not adequate?

A.   No, there isn't.

Q.   Would you have started the Pitocin if clinically the contractions seemed normal?

A.   Not if I thought the contractions were adequate.

Q.   Immediately after the Pitocin was started at -71, the second contraction after the Pitocin was started, what do we see there?

A.   See a deep variable deceleration.

Q.   How low does it get?

A.   Fifty beats per minute. Well, excuse me. Sixty—70 beats per minute.

Q.   How long does it last?

A.   Total duration of that deceleration is 50 seconds.

Q.   And then at—the contraction at -73, is there any type of deceleration there?

A.   There is a deceleration. It's probably a variable. Could be something else.

Q.   What else could it be?

A.   Could be a late.

This expert has finally admitted there could have been late deceleration with this patient.

Q.   And then at -74, what's occurred with that contraction?

A. Very long variable deceleration.

Q. How long does that last?

A. A minute and 40 seconds.

Q. And how low does the pulse rate get?

A. Seventy—60 to 70, in there.

Q. Okay. And let's see. There are four contractions on this page; is that right?

A. I'm not sure if there are three or four.

Q. Three or four. Okay. At least with the three you can identify, there are decelerations, are there not?

A. Uh-huh.

Q. And two of them last longer than 45 seconds?

A. That's correct.

Q. Let's see. That's at 8:06—8:06 A.M. At 8:12 someone places oxygen on.

A. Uh-huh.

Q. What is the purpose for giving the mother oxygen?

A. It's to supplement oxygen transfer to the baby between the variable decelerations so it is better able to compensate for its cord compression.

Q. Okay. You're raising the amount of oxygen in the—

A. Mother's blood.

Q. —mother's blood and hoping that that will get across to the child?

A. That's correct.

Q. On the next contraction after the oxygen or, I guess, with the oxygen at -76, do we see anything there in terms of fetal heart rate?

A. Yeah. It could be a late deceleration. I can't be sure at this point.

Q. Okay. And then at the next contraction at -77, contraction—

A. It is a variable deceleration, and that one has a slow return to baseline.

Q. How long does it last?

A. About 45 seconds.

Q. And the pulse rate gets down to what, 90?

A. Yes.

Q. Now, this is with an internal lead at this point?

A. Yes.

Q. In response to these fairly repetitive and deep decelerations, would you have increased the Pitocin?

A. Given the overall pattern, at this point I might have waited a little bit. But I don't—I don't object to it. They are no longer present in any significant quantities when that Pitocin is increased.

Q. Is it possible for the fetus to reach a stage where it can no longer develop late decelerations?

A. Some people believe it is.

Q. Okay. Out of the last five contractions, how many are associated with variable decelerations?

A. All of them probably.

Q. And at -95 is there also another to the right of that one you just looked at, is there a variable?

A. Yes, sir.

Q. How long does it last?

A. Sixty seconds.

Q. Okay. And how deep does it get? How slow does the fetal heart rate go?

A. Eighty.

Q. And how about the return to baseline?

A. It's slower than before. It's now becoming a slow return to baseline, or a late component.

Q. Okay. Now, based on the last three pages and assuming you had available the ability to get blood gases and resources to perform a cesarean section as quickly as you needed to, within five or ten minutes, in this strip would you have gotten pHs?

A. No.

Q. Would you have done a C-section?

A. Yes.

Q. And that's at 42295?

A. Yes.

Q. That would be based on your evaluation of the entire record including her postmaturity and the fetal monitoring records through the night?

A. Yes.

Q. And what time is it, the 42295—

A. My best estimate of going over the monitor records, at 9:20.

Q. Now, at 9:20 at your institution you could have done your cesarean section within five minutes?

A. Had I wanted to, yes.

Q. Would you have wanted to do it as quickly as possible in this case?

A. Yeah. But not—I wouldn't crash her.

Q. Okay. But you wouldn't drag your feet either, would you?

A. No.

Q. And if you had everything ready to go, you could do it in five to ten minutes?

A. In this situation I wouldn't. You're compromising the mother so much if you go in five to ten minutes. Then if you go in five to ten minutes, you can't prep her abdomen, can't get the Foley catheter in. You can't take every precaution and make sure that her blood pressure is stabilized and the anesthesiologist has everything. That's a crash cesarean section where you're throwing maternal safety to the wind for the baby's benefit.

This is a gradually progressive pattern which doesn't indicate the necessity for a five-minute cesarean section.

Q. Could you do it in 15 minutes and still do the prep?

A. From there? Probably not. Take you 20 or 30 minutes.

Q. What's the prep time for skin?

A. Six or eight minutes. But you got to get the Foley in. Got to get the anesthesiologist set up.

Q. And the next contraction, are you able to make anything of that?

A. Yeah. It looks like there is a variable with a late component.

Q. What does *late component* mean?

A. That the baby is developing residual hypoxia between contractions.

Q. What does that mean to the jury? What does *hypoxia* mean?

A. My interpretation of this is that the cord compression has occurred recurrently enough that the baby is beginning to have an oxygen debt so that it's not able to recover its oxygenation between contractions.

Q. Okay. So that now pulling the baby under the water has resulted in less oxygen in the child's brain clearly?

A. Yes. And we're having a beginning in a rise of baseline at this point which is different from accelerations and a loss of variability.

Q. Okay. What does that mean?

A. Means that the baby's brain is starting to reflect a depression from a lack of oxygen.

Q. And then the next contraction, is that also—

A. Same thing.

Q. At—at any point here are there any examinations you can do to determine where the cord is?

A. A pelvic examination would reveal a prolapsed umbilical cord.

Q. When were you first contacted regarding testifying in this matter?

A. I'd have to check my briefcase.

Q. All right.

A. Want me to do that?

Q. Sure. And why don't you bring all the correspondence and everything.

A. Certainly.

Q. Doctor, let me show you what has been marked as Plaintiff's Exhibit No. 7. Is that a—the notes which were compiled during your review of this matter?

A. Yes.

Q. I didn't notice in the correspondence any set of billing. Have you submitted any bills to the firm of Jones & Smith?

A. I believe I have.

Q. What is the amount of that bill to date?

A. My best guess is $750.

Q. That's for your initial review?

A. There may be—there may have been an additional bill sent after subsequent depositions were received.

Q. What is—what is your bill per hour for reviewing them?

A. I bill a minimum of $750 to review a case and give a verbal report. If the bill goes beyond $150 an hour, I bill $150 an hour over that.

Q. And how about your trip here today? How much are you billing for?

A. I don't know. This is my first time I've done this. I'll have to consult.

Q. What do you think it's going to be per hour?

A. At least $200.

Q. Is this the first case you have ever reviewed medically?

A. It's not the first case I've ever reviewed. No.

Q. How many cases have you reviewed in the past?

A. I could give you an approximation. Nine.

Q. How many on behalf of defendant and how many on behalf of plaintiff?

A. All on behalf of the doctor.

Q. Which journals do you recognize as standard references in the area of obstetrics?

A. Well, the peer review journals that I recognize are the *American Journal of Obstetrics and Gynecology* and *Obstetrics and Gynecology.* To a lesser extent others would include *Journal of Reproductive Medicine, British Medical Journal,* and occasionally I'll read a few other peer review journals. I do review the *New England Journal of Medicine* so that I don't miss anything that I want to see.

Q. When you read Dr. Moore's deposition, you were aware that he called many of the decelerations that you called variable, late decelerations?

A. Yes, I did. I'm aware.

Q. Assuming that he was correct for the purposes of the next question and assuming indeed that he was under the impression that those were late decelerations, which apparently he was at the time he was handling the case, at that time would a cesarean section have been ordered by you in light of —

A. Well, that —

Q. —that suspicion?

A. It's sort of hard to know what was going through his mind. But you see, late decelerations are not typically isolated. They are present with the majority of contractions or all the contractions, or they're not. So I can't say, you know, a late here and a late there, that I've ever sectioned a patient.

Q. Well, assuming that Dr. Moore—

A. But all the variables that I saw were late?

Q. That's right. And assuming Dr. Moore thought they were late.

A. Okay. But let's say that each—for the purposes of your question, that each deceleration was a late?

Q. Right.

A. Well, then we'd have to go back to somewhere around the point where the decelerations become persistent.

Q. Around—

A. Which is—

Q. —8:06 A.M.?

A. Yeah. About that. 8:36 A.M., 8:06 A.M. In there. Or become present with most of the contractions.

Q. Okay. If Dr. Moore was laboring under the impression—and apparently in his deposition he indicated that he was—that these were late decelerations from 8:06 A.M. on.

A. My impressions were that he was under the impression that some were late and some were variables. But that's my recollection of his deposition.

Q. Well, assuming he thought most of them were late decelerations, what significance does that have if, indeed, he was right, and you're incorrect?

A. Well, it would be more likely to be associated with a depressed baby.

Q. And your opinion regarding at what time cesarean section intervention should have been performed would be different if those are late decelerations, assuming that they are?

A. I can't answer that because I can't assume that they are.

Q. Well, for the purposes of the question you're allowed to assume that those are late decelerations as Dr. Moore thought. If that is correct, you would have intervened with cesarean section around 8:25 or 8:40, wouldn't you?

A. If they were all late decelerations?

Q. If the majority of them were.

A. Okay. Not—not at that point, no. I would have repositioned the patient, given her oxytocin as they did, and maybe at—okay. Somewhere around 8:40.

Q. The question I asked you is—did you have an opportunity to read Dr. Robin's deposition?

A. I doubt whether I read it. Would you refresh my memory?

Q. He was the neonatologist who attended the child.

A. I believe that I did scan it, sir. Yes.

Q. And you disagree with his opinion that the child was asphyxiated at birth?

A. I think this baby could have been—was asphyxiated to a degree at birth. But asphyxiated to a sufficient degree to cause damage, I don't know that. We don't know what happened to the baby after birth before it got to Dr. Robin.

Q. Would the neonatologist who actually attended this child, be in a better position to render an opinion on that?

A. Not unless he was there from the time of birth till he took care of it.

Q. Well, assuming that he was there from the time of birth virtually.

A. Well, then I would think he would be in an excellent position.

Q. Have you read his deposition?

A. I believe I scanned it, sir. I don't—I don't remember it in depth.

Q. So basically you would have to rely on his testimony as to how this asphyxia occurred and when it occurred?

A. From my review of the chart, I would say not necessarily. Okay? Because the baby was born at Glendale, was transferred to Newton Hospital and that, I believe—and please correct me if I'm wrong—was where Dr. Robin got involved. And there was a period of time during which that baby may have not been getting oxygen in the newborn period between birth and transfer, that he had no more knowledge of than I had knowledge of.

Now, based on my ability to interpret the heart rate pattern, I'm a little surprised that this baby is this bad from this intrapartum event. So that my opinion might be that I'd be—my guess would be maybe something happened in the newborn period.

Q. Did you look at the record to determine whether that happened?

A. Yes, I did.

Q. Did you find anything?

A. Well, there is a—there is a blood gas that was determined probably an hour or two or more after birth—I'd have to refer to the Newton Hospital record to be precise—that showed a significant base excess, significant acidosis. And how—who knows how that fluctuated between birth and arrival there.

Q. Well, a base excess would indicate that an acidosis had been present for a period of time?

A. Could have developed afterwards.

Q. How long does it take to develop a base excess?

A. Depends on how severe the hypoxia is.

Q. After you've discontinued electronic fetal monitoring, do you continue to monitor the baby by auscultation?

A.   No. We usually take the fetal monitor to the delivery room.

Q.   Was that done here?

A.   No.

Q.   Do you know why it wasn't?

A.   Probably because there was a fairly short interval between discontinuance and delivery.

Q.   Forty-five minutes?

DEFENDANT'S ATTORNEY: The record doesn't indicate that.

Q.   How long is your recollection of how long it was?

A.   Well, from the time it's discontinued until the institution of anesthesia, in my best estimation, was about 20 minutes.

Q.   Does the continuing monitoring during that period of time give you a better idea what's going on in terms of whether the situation is worsening and you need to hurry even more than you might ordinarily?

A.   Yes. It has that potential.

Q.   And that's why you do that?

A.   Yeah.

Q.   And that's in keeping with good standards of obstetrical practice, is it now, and hospital obstetrical practice?

A.   I think that's optimal.[9]

§ 16.12   Scope of Expert's Testimony

In *Bank of Illinois v. Thweatt,*[10] the plaintiff parents had brought a medical malpractice action against the defendant obstetrician/gynecologist alleging that as a result of the defendant's negligence, their son Nicholas was born prematurely and suffered multiple injuries and disabilities; judgment was for the defendant. On appeal, the plaintiffs argued that the trial court erred in allowing an expert called by defendant to testify regarding Nicholas's condition had the pregnancy been prolonged, because such testimony exceeded the scope of his Supreme Court Rule 220 disclosure during discovery. The appellate court held that the intended solicited opinion from the expert did not exceed the scope of pretrial disclosure based on the following discovery:

In response to plaintiffs' interrogatories, the defense stated that Dr. Lawson [defense expert] is expected to testify regarding the subject matter of the causation of the conditions of ill-being sustained by Nicholas. . . . Dr. Lawson is of

---

[9] Note that in Mundell v. La Pata, 635 N.E.2d 933 (Ill. App. Ct. 1994), the court explained that in order to be certified as an expert witness, a physician "must be (1) a licensed member of the area of medicine about which [the physician] is to testify; and (2) must show [familiarity] with the methods, procedures and treatments ordinarily observed by other physicians in either the defendant's community or in a similar community." *Id.* at 938. The court went on to state that if "testimony establishes that a standard of care is one followed by all doctors in the country, then a witness may testify as an expert even if he has not practiced in the community because [the witness] is thus aware of the standard in a similar community." *Id.*

[10] 630 N.E.2d 121 (Ill. App. Ct. 1994).

the opinion that [defendant] appropriately initiated the administration of Rito-drine [a tocolytic medication given to arrest preterm labor contractions] in a timely fashion. He is of the opinion that the same outcome would have resulted, even if [defendant] had initiated the administration of the Ritodrine prior to the time he did. Dr. Lawson has concluded and it is his opinion that the premature birth of the [infant] is the cause of the conditions of ill-being sustained by Nicholas.[11]

Attached to the response was a letter from Dr. Lawson to the defendant's attorneys which stated in part: "You have asked me to be an expert witness regarding survivability and outcome of [infant] born at this gestation and at later gestation."[12] Finally, there was a letter from the defendant's attorneys to Dr. Lawson which stated in part:

> Specifically, we would like to know in your experience would earlier tocolysis have made a difference in the outcome. . . ? Assuming [plaintiffs' expert's] opin-ion that early tocolysis would have prolonged the pregnancy two weeks, would it be your opinion to a reasonable degree of medical certainty that it is more prob-ably true than not that the morbidity . . . in this case would have been substantially the same?[13]

The testimony of plaintiffs' expert Dr. Dattel regarding the amount of morbid-ity suffered by fetuses delivered at different gestational ages was found by the appellate court to be beyond the scope of Supreme Court Rule 220 disclosure and properly stricken by the trial court. Dr. Dattel had been disclosed as an expert concerning negligence, and the plaintiffs had disclosed that she had con-cluded that the defendant had been negligent in several matters, including not starting tocolysis sooner. The disclosure also indicated that it was her opinion that if tocolysis had started earlier the preterm labor would have been prevented. Testifying about morbidity at different gestational ages was beyond the scope of this disclosure.[14]

---

[11] *Id.* at 127.

[12] *Id.*

[13] *Id.* at 128.

[14] *Id.*

CHAPTER 17

EXAMINATION OF THE EXPERTS IN A MERITORIOUS LABOR AND DELIVERY CASE WITH RESULTING DEATH OF MOTHER AND CHILD

Michael D. Volk

§ 17.1   Introduction

This chapter deals with the testimony in a medical malpractice case involving the death of a mother and child during labor and delivery. The mother had a condition known as congestive heart failure. The fetus predeceased the mother by approximately five hours. After admission to the hospital, the child's fetal heart rate pattern was abnormal from the beginning of the electronic fetal monitoring. The child was pronounced dead in utero and the mother was given Pitocin to establish a contraction pattern sufficient to expel the dead fetus. Five hours later, while in a birthing chair, the mother collapsed and died.

The physicians who were sued were the obstetrician/gynecologist and the two family practitioners who took care of the mother approximately six weeks before her labor for a condition they diagnosed as pneumonia, which was in reality probably a combination of congestive heart failure and pneumonia.

§ 17.2 Cross-Examination of Treating General Practitioner

The following transcript shows the cross-examination of one of the two general practitioners who cared for the mother during her hospitalization about six weeks before her labor and resulting death. Her condition was diagnosed as pneumonia. The preliminary portions of all the depositions in this chapter have been omitted.

Q. In your medical school training did you come to learn some of the symptoms of heart disease?

A. Yes, I did.

Q. And could you tell the jury what some of those symptoms can be?

A. Symptoms of heart disease? Well, they could be numerous things, they would be chest pain, they could be shortness of breath, they could be blueness of the lips or fingernails.

Q. How about edema?

A. Swelling of the legs, yes.

Q. Palpitations?

A. Palpitations would be one, yes.

Q. Explain to the jury what a palpitation would be.

A. Palpitation is a sensation that a person feels, feels as if his heart is skipping or jumping.

Q. Easy fatigability?

A. This could be a symptom, yes.

Q. Any other symptoms that you can think of that are generally associated by you with heart disease?

A. Not any that I can think of at the moment.

Q. Some of those same symptoms can be seen with lung disease, is that right?

A. Some of them can, yes, that's right.

Q. Which ones would be the ones that you would associate with lung disease?

A. Chest pain would be one, and also shortness of breath, and the blue fingernails and blue lips, cyanosis, in other words. I can't think of any others off-hand.

Q. What happens to the heart if it becomes diseased in terms of its capabilities to push blood around to the organs of the body?

A. If it becomes diseased, the heart loses its ability to push blood around through the heart—through the body, excuse me.

Q. When the heart fails, is there a term we use?

A. It's called heart failure, cardiac failure.

Q. And explain to the jury what you mean by the term *cardiac failure*.

A. *Cardiac failure* is a situation where the blood loses its ability to pump, the heart loses its ability to pump blood through the heart—excuse me, through the body rather, and as a consequence the—frequently the lungs fill up with fluid and also the ankles and the feet swell as a result of this fluid being able—being forced out into the tissues.

Q. And this condition of heart failure, if it progresses, can result in the patient being short of breath?

A. That's true

Q. A term that will come up, I think, in the course of this matter is *dyspnea*. Would you explain to the jury what that term means?

A. *Dyspnea* is a sensation that a person feels when they are short of breath, they feel as if they're not able to get enough breath.

Q. And what is the mechanism of that, why is the patient sensing that, would air hunger be a proper term for it?

A. Air hunger is another way of describing it, I think rather than a—it's just another term for dyspnea.

Q. Now, the worst degree of dyspnea in the functional classification, and correct me if I'm wrong, would be a patient who had dyspnea at rest? In bed?

A. Yes.

Q. In the course of evaluating a patient, a careful physician will take a history, will he not?

A. Yes.

Q. And a physician will also, in the course of evaluating that patient and being careful, do a physical examination?

A. Yes, that's right.

Q. And some of the things you listed earlier, in terms of things that one would see either historically or on physical exam as indicative of possible cardiac disease, were things that you would obtain in the history and part of them by physical exam?

A. That's correct, yes

Q. Have you done any research to determine what happens to mid and late systolic click during pregnancy?

A. I have not.

Q. Did you know that they tend to disappear?

A. I did not know that.

Mid and late systolic clicks do tend to disappear during pregnancy. The mortality rate for women who have recognized congestive heart failure is very small. Death usually results only when the congestive heart failure is not diagnosed.

Q. Now, Mrs. Lawton's EKG during her September admission was abnormal, was it not?

A. That's true, yes.

Q. And it was read as nonspecific, T wave abnormalities?

A. That's correct.

Q. And by that, we mean that the recording of the electricity from her heart seemed not to be exactly what it ought to have been, at least electrically?

A. That's correct, yes.

Q. Now that, in itself, might not be too significant. On the other hand, it might be significant. Would that be a fair statement?

A. That's correct, yes.

Q. Would it be more significant if those were changes on her electrocardiogram that hadn't been present before?

A. Yes, that's true.

Q. And as a matter of fact that's why someone specifically stamped *old EKG* not available for comparison?

A. That's true.

Q. So someone looking at this electrocardiogram would tend to be more alerted to the possibility of heart disease with this nonspecific T wave abnormality if a prior tracing, electrocardiogram had been essentially normal?

A. It would have to be put together with the patient's clinical symptoms at that point.

Q. All I'm saying is one would be more inclined to be concerned if a prior EKG was normal?

A. Was normal, that's true, yes.

Q. And did Joan have a prior EKG that was normal?

A. I'm not aware of any.

This physician had in the office records of this patient a prior EKG that was in fact normal. The physician had failed to review his medical record with his lawyer before the deposition.

Q. If you had been aware that she had a change in her electrocardiogram from a prior tracing, would you perhaps have had a cardiologist see Mrs. Lawton when she was in the hospital in September?

A. Not necessarily.

Q. Would it have pushed you towards tending to do that?

A. If I couldn't account for the—for the changes myself, I would probably have gotten a consultation, yes.

Q. Were you able to determine whether these were changes that Joan had had in her heart for many years or were you able to determine whether these were new changes on her electrocardiogram?

A. I was not able to tell.

Q. And I guess that's basically because you had no old EKG to compare it to?

A. That's correct, yes.

Q. Had you had an old EKG you would have been able to compare them?

A. That's true.

Q. And if the old EKG had been normal, that would have led you to question maybe something had changed in Joan's heart at that time?

A. That's true, yes

Q. Let me show you what has been marked as Plaintiff's Exhibit No. 2, which I believe is in your office records, and ask if you can identify that for me?

A. Joan Barrett. Yes, I—

Q. Is that Joan Barrett also Joan Lawton?

A. I don't know.

Q. Well, it is to be found in the file which was provided me as being representative of your office records on Mrs. Lawton.

A. I see. I don't recall seeing this before.

Q. Okay. Could you review it and indicate whether or not there are any abnormalities on it in terms of T waves?

DEFENSE ATTORNEY: I take it that's a prior EKG?

PLAINTIFF ATTORNEY: Yes.

DEFENSE ATTORNEY: What is the date of it?

PLAINTIFF ATTORNEY: The date is 8/5/73, I believe.

A. Yes, there are no T wave abnormalities on this tracing.

Q. And this, I want you to assume that this indeed comes from your records since it was provided to us as from your records. Perhaps we can look through your originals this afternoon to determine if there's been an error made.

But if this is correct, this electrocardiogram was in Mrs. Lawton's file when she was in the hospital in January of 1981?

A. It was in our office file? Is that what you're saying?

Q. Yes.

A. Yes, I believe so.

Q. And if you wanted to answer the question when or whether or not the T wave changes had been present on a prior EKG, you could have compared the two EKGs, could you have not?

A. That's true, yes.

Q. And in this instance, as far as you know, you did not do that?

A. I did not, that's right.

Q. In the course of your care of Mrs. Lawton, had she demonstrated any symptoms in the past suggestive of heart disease?

A. I'd have to refer to my record. I don't recall any off-hand.

Q. If that EKG from 8/5/73 is correct, do you know for what reason you performed the electrocardiogram?

A. I have no idea.

Q. Is it likely, in the course of your practice, in a young lady that you would do an EKG to investigate symptoms that the patient might be having?

A. That's correct, yes.

Q. Do you know whether in Joan's case that was indeed the reason that it was done?

A. I don't know why I did it at that time.

Q. You would have to review your records to determine that?

A. That's correct, uh-huh.

Q. Is there a reason why you were not aware of the prior EKG?

A. There was no—there was no reason to suspect that there had been a previous one.

Q. Okay. You really didn't go back and look in your records to determine it?

A. That's correct, I didn't.

Q. In the course of your medical education and experience, have you determined that patients with pregnancy and heart disease should be managed differently and more carefully than patients without heart disease?

A. That's true.

Q. And would you explain to the jury why that is so?

A. A person with heart disease in pregnancy puts a great stress on the heart, and can go into heart failure unless the individual is watched very carefully, and the symptoms and signs are observed, so that they can be treated at the first sign of problems.

Q. And would it be correct to say that a patient might have a heart that was able to tolerate the nonpregnant state, but would not tolerate the pregnant state?

A. That's true, yes.

Q. And that is the type of patient who may have subtle symptoms of heart disease for a long period of time but not have any signs of heart failure until pregnancy?

A. That's true.

Q. When did you next have the opportunity to see Mrs. Lawton relative to her hospitalizations?

A. The next time I saw her was at the hospital emergency room when she was admitted in September of 1981.

Q. And do you recall the circumstances that led you to be called? I think that's the pink sheet in the front there.

A. Yes. Mrs. Lawton presented at the emergency room with a complaint of cough and congestion for three days and severe pain in the left chest which was aggravated by deep breathing.

Q. Now, concerning the X-ray of her chest, can you definitively call that pneumonia versus fluid from something else?

A. No, you cannot.

Q. Do you know that that film is not heart failure?

A. I can't say that it is not heart failure.

Q. That is one of the possibilities, is it not?

A. That's one possibility, that's right.

Q. She was severely short of breath to the point that she needed oxygen, is that right?

A. I think I gave this to her more for the idea that she was pregnant, than—to assist the pregnancy.

Q. You didn't give it to her to relieve her shortness of breath?

A. I don't really know the reasons.

Q. Okay. Would it have been logical for you to start it to relieve her shortness of breath?

A. Yes, it would have, yes.

Q. That shortness of breath could either have been due to heart failure, cardiac disease, or lung disease at that point? Or a combination?

A. Shortness of—as we've covered, shortness of breath can be a symptom of any of those things you've mentioned.

Q. With a patient who has had mild heart disease before pregnancy, when is she most likely to go into heart failure?

A. If she was going into failure she would when some stress came along. The time of labor and delivery.

Q. How about when her blood volume reached the maximum? During the pregnancy?

A. This would seem logical, yes.

Q. Do you know when the blood volume of a pregnant patient reaches the maximum?

A. I do not, no.

Q. In your differential diagnosis, based on everything you knew on September 9, 1981, after you had reviewed the chest X-ray and admitted Mrs. Lawton to the hospital and started her on oxygen, was part of your differential diagnosis an inclusion of possible heart disease worsened by pregnancy?

A. No, it was not.

Q. Did you ever entertain the possibility of cardiac disease?

A. No, I did not.

Q. Why the EKG then?

A. I didn't order the EKG, my partner did.

Q. So the consideration of whether or not there was heart disease would have been Dr. Parker's?

A. I presume there must have been some reason why he ordered it.

Q. Well, the electrocardiogram looks at the heart, does it not?

A. That's correct, yes.

Q. So that you would expect ordinarily that someone ordering an EKG would indeed be looking for the possibility of heart disease?

A. Of heart disease, that's correct, yes.

This physician's partner was called in to consult and review the case. The partner was no more qualified to diagnose heart disease because they were both general practitioners. However, the second physician did order the electrocardiogram but also failed to review the prior tracing.

Q. When a patient has heart failure, and you put them to bed and start them on oxygen and they respond, do their hearts get smaller, commonly?

A. When their heart failure resolves, yes, it does get smaller.

Q. And the infiltrate that you see on X-ray clears somewhat?

A. It could, yes.

Q. And that's not an uncommon thing to see in a patient with heart failure?

A. That's true.

There were two chest films taken during the hospitalization. The second one showed a clearing of the infiltrate, which the defendants claimed was because the patient's pneumonia was clearing with the use of the antibiotic Erythromicin. The plaintiff contended that the reason the patient's chest was clearing was that she was on bed rest with no stress and getting supplemental oxygen.

Q. Did she have any other complaints on September 20th other than what you have recorded in your chart?

A. Not that I'm aware of.

Q. Did you inquire of her on September 20th how far she could walk before she got short of breath?

A. No, I did not.

Q. If she told you that she was unable to walk more than 20 feet without getting shortness of breath, would you have repeated her chest X-ray?

A. I probably would have, yes.

Q. Okay. The left chest pain, what did you attribute that to on September 20th?

A. I felt this was just the residuals of her pleurisy.

Q. Did you do a physical exam on September 20th?

A. I have no record of it.

Q. And do you have any recollection of having done one?

A. I don't recall having done one.

Q. If she still had complaints about having to sit up to breathe, would you have repeated her chest X-ray?

A. Not necessarily, because most pregnant woman have trouble—excuse me. Did you say she was having trouble—what was your question?

Q. If she had paroxysm, nocturnal dyspnea, shortness of breath that caused her to have to sit up to breathe, would you have repeated her chest X-ray?

A. Have we established that she had nocturnal dyspnea?

Q. I'm asking you to assume she did.

A. Oh, assuming she did. I might have repeated her X-ray, yes.

Q. Did she complain to you of any swelling of her extremities?

A. Not that I recall.

Q. Did you ever see any swelling of her extremities?

A. Not that I recall.

Q. Did you look for it?

A. I don't recall.

Q. Did she complain to you of any swelling of her extremities?

A. I don't recall her doing that.

Q. And when did you—and just to have it clear, you don't remember what you told Dr. Wesley?

A. I don't remember, no.

Q. When next did you have an opportunity to learn about Joan's case? Either by telephone call or conversation or actual knowledge?

A. I didn't see her, the only thing that I recall hearing was that she had died in labor. There was talk around the hospital, quite a shock that a maternity case would die, a maternity patient would die.

This last statement brings home the fact that it is rare for a maternity patient to die during labor and delivery.

Q. I want to assume that you had made a diagnosis of Joan having some type of heart disease in—on either the admission in September 9, 1981, or on her visit on September 20, 1981, would you have referred her to a cardiologist?

A. If I thought she had heart disease I would have referred her, yes.

Q. And that's because the management is very specialized for patients with heart disease, is that right?

A. That's correct

§ 17.3 Cross-Examination of Defendant Obstetrician

The next testimony is of the obstetrician/gynecologist who cared for the patient during the pregnancy and during labor and delivery. This physician also directed the attempt at resuscitation when the patient collapsed and died. Throughout the prenatal course, his records, for the most part, reflected minimal problems with the patient. Contrary to this was the testimony of the husband and two independent persons who knew the decedent. The first person was a co-worker who stated the patient could not even walk a few feet to a water cooler without getting extremely short of breath towards the end of the pregnancy. The second person was a close friend who testified to essentially the same thing. The husband and the two lay witnesses testified that the patient and husband reported to this physician the symptoms of shortness of breath, inability to sleep without sitting up, swelling, and the like, but that the physician told the patient that that was normal for a pregnant lady. This patient died from mitral valve prolapse which led to congestive heart failure.

Q. What did you do next professionally after your internship was completed?

A. Went into the OB-GYN residency program, the same medical school.

Q. And that would be in 1965, approximately?

A. From '65 to '69.

Q. During that period of time did you have an opportunity to handle pregnant ladies with lung disease and heart disease?

A. Yes.

Q. And did you become familiar, actually even before your obstetrics and gynecology experience, with signs and symptoms of heart disease?

A. Yes.

Q. That's something that you would have seen throughout your entire education, would you not, that is heart disease and lung disease?

A. Yes, I had experience during that time period.

Q. And did you actually see patients present with heart failure?

A. Yes.

Q. And did you participate in the treatment of heart failure?

A. Yes.

Q. And what was the type of standard treatment that you would give for acute pulmonary edema during the course of your internship and residency?

A. Well, depending on the findings, we might use diuretics.

Q. A diuretic?

A. Yes.

Q. Something to get the excessive fluid off the patient?

A. Yes.

Q. A quick-acting form of digitalis?

A. Lasix yes, digitalis for heart problems.

Q. Cedilanid, quick-acting form.

A. Yes.

Q. Of digitalis?

A. Yes.

Q. During the course of your medical education, did you come to understand that there was a group of pregnant women who were at higher risk to develop problems of morbidity and mortality during the course of their pregnancy?

A. Yes.

Because this was a foreign-trained physician who did not understand English very well, counsel for the plaintiff wanted to make sure that there was no question that he was familiar with pregnant women who had heart disease. This was an attempt to avoid the claim that he did not understand the question.

Q. Are patients with heart disease managed the same way as patients with pregnancy and no heart disease?
A. You have to manage them differently.
Q. Why?
A. Because they can die of their heart disease.
Q. And obviously the first thing that an obstetrician needs to do in management of a pregnant patient is ascertain, of course, first whether that patient has heart disease?
A. Yes.
Q. And then he would take steps to manage that heart disease as well as the pregnancy?
A. Yes.
Q. And would you tell the jury what type of symptoms might alert you to the possibility of some type of heart disease with the pregnancy?
A. A mild case shows swollen legs and shortness of breath, and if it progresses, then chest pain and exertion from physical activity.

The physician has admitted that this patient, if the co-worker, friend, and husband can be believed, had signs and symptoms of heart disease which were ignored by the obstetrician.

Q. And then I guess a very late symptom would be blueness, cyanosis?
A. Yes.
Q. An almost terminal event in most cardiac patients?
A. Yes.
Q. Now, is there anywhere in your prenatal records, or do you have any recollection of either Joan or Roger Lawton telling you that Joan was having shortness of breath?
A. I don't recall anyone ever complaining to me about shortness of breath.
Q. Do you ever recall Joan or Roger complaining to you of swelling of the ankles, hands, or face?
A. No, sir.
Q. Who in your office checks for swelling of the ankles?
A. I do.
Q. The nurse doesn't check those things?
A. No, sir.
Q. And you never found any swelling of her ankles, did you?
A. That's correct.

The patient was admitted to the hospital with pitting edema and on autopsy she had three-plus pitting edema which was a finding of significant swelling. This edema was not only of her lower extremities but also her upper extremities and face.

Q. Had you found swelling of Joan's ankles and had Joan indicated to you that she was having shortness of breath on walking as little as 10 or 20 feet, would you have referred her to a cardiologist for evaluation?

A. If I hear either heart murmur or lung sounds compatible with pneumonia or heart failure, I would do it. But since pregnancy itself may increase pitting edema, I wouldn't refer her simply on some minor pitting edema.

Q. Well, how about pitting edema as much as a half-inch or three-quarters of an inch? Is that normal in pregnancy?

A. I think that's abnormal.

Q. Oh, all right.

A. And I would have to investigate further at that time.

Q. In terms of when a woman gets into her seventh and eighth month, I assume some women do have some shortness of breath, is that right?

A. Right.

Q. Do all of them have shortness of breath at that time or just some of them?

A. Some of them.

Q. How about having to wake up in the middle of the night and sit up to catch your breath, is that something you've seen with cardiac patients?

A. I think if that's happening every night, this is a matter of concern.

Q. And that's because that's called paroxysmal nocturnal dyspnea, isn't it?

A. Yes.

Q. And what it means is the lungs are filling up with fluid when the patient lies down at night so that they have to sit up to catch their breath, get enough oxygen at night?

A. That's one type of problem. But in the last one or two months of pregnancy, some of the patients have orthopnea because of pregnancy.

Q. In late November and December you do not recall any complaints from the Lawtons, then, regarding shortness of breath on exertion or swelling of the ankles or chest pain until the entry of September 9, 1981, when she was hospitalized?

A. That's correct.

Q. And did you come to realize that after your visit with Joan on September 8, 1981, that she was subsequently admitted to Rockland Memorial Hospital?

A. Yes.

Q. And how did you come to find that out?

A. I think that was September 9th, in the morning, I found her in her room. First I met with Roger Lawton and then I asked him why he was here, and he said that his wife was in the hospital.

Q. Well it must have been somewhat of a surprise since you had just seen Roger and Joan the day before, at which time all you found was a little bronchial congestion?

A. Yes.

Q. So you did, then, I guess, undertake an investigation of what had happened between the time you had seen her and when she got into the hospital?

A. Yes.

Q. And what did you determine had happened to Joan?

A. I—shortly after that I met Dr. Johnson, around—at the nursing station, and he gave me the impression that she had pleural effusion.

Q. And by pleural effusion we mean fluid in the space between the visceral and parietal pleura in the lung?

A. Yes.

Q. Before the death of Joan Lawton at Rockland Memorial Hospital, were you ever apprised, did you ever come to know the results of the electrocardiogram performed on the night of September 9, 1981, at Rockland?

A. I didn't know about any EKG.

Q. What was Joan's weight on October 11, 1981?

A. 206 and a half pounds.

Q. How much?

A. 206 and a half.

Q. Had she gained an inordinate amount of weight during her pregnancy?

A. Yes.

Q. How much had she gained over the course of her entire pregnancy?

A. From 148 to 206, makes 58 pounds.

Q. When did you next have any contact with Joan, Roger, Dr. Parker, or Dr. Johnson with regards to Joan?

A. On her next regularly scheduled visit.

Q. On September 25th or thereabouts, did Dr. Johnson call you to discuss the case with you at all?

A. September 25th? I don't recall that.

On part of the medical record was a handwritten note that this physician had been called by the admitting physicians for Joan's hospitalization for pneumonia. Neither physician could remember it, but the only logical assumption was that a discussion of her problem had occurred.

Q. And you didn't call Dr. Johnson to discuss Joan's status after she was discharged from the hospital?

A. That's right.

Q. The next contact you had with Joan was when she was admitted to the hospital?

A. Yes.

Q. When you were first called at home and told she was at the hospital in labor, were you apprised of any swelling of Joan's hands or feet or face?

A. No, sir.

Q. Were you apprised of any swelling of Joan's hands and feet at any time during that day?

A. No, sir.

Q. In light of the prior history of pleural effusion and abnormalities and EKG, if she was admitted to the hospital and was found to have, or someone told you that she was having swelling of her hands and feet, would that have concerned you since she was going into labor?

A. If significant swelling, yes, I would.

Q. What type of effect does active labor have on the heart, does it place an extra burden on the heart?

A. There are many studies, but unless there is evidence of heart failure, it shouldn't affect the heart very much, from what I understand.

Q. Well, does it increase cardiac output any, for instance?

A. Yes, increased cardiac output and stroke volumes.

Q. Would by 30 or 40 percent be an accurate reflection of what you've read in the literature?

A. About 20 percent increased.

Q. It's the type of work load that a normal heart can withstand?

A. Yes.

Q. But a heart that is abnormal might not be able to stand it?

A. Valvular heart problems should be the most critical type of heart problems affected.

Q. And by that we mean problems of the mitral, aortic, pulmonic, or tricuspid valves?

A. Yes.

Q. And when the kind of difficulties arise with a lady in labor with preexisting heart disease do arise, they present the doctor usually with the picture of acute pulmonary edema?

A. Yes.

Q. The treatment of which we discussed earlier in your deposition, did we not?

A. Yes.

Q. Well, did you see any swelling yourself of her extremities or face?

A. No, sir.

Q. I ask it only because the nurses did note swelling of her hands and feet that you didn't note then.

A. That's correct.

Q. Okay. And how is it that the nurses noted swelling of her hands and feet and you didn't?

A. Would you show me the nurse's note?

Q. You've never seen a nurse's note that indicates that on the day of admission at 6:20, the nurses did see that there was swelling of Mrs. Lawton's hands and feet? Did you never see that entry in this chart?

A. I don't remember now.

Although not set out in this section, this hospital had only two fetal monitors. One of them did not work at the time of the death of the patient. Of course, the hospital was sued for failure to have adequate equipment that was working, as well as the fact that the nurses were negligent in failing to recognize a significant number of late decelerations, from the beginning of labor.

Q. And what time did they begin the external monitor on Joan, do you know?

A. As soon as she arrived.

Q. Did the nursing staff ever apprise you of any abnormalities or problems with the external monitor?

A. No, sir.

Q. Have you had an opportunity to review the fetal monitoring records between 6:20 and 11:30 A.M.?

A. At 1:15 P.M. that was the first time I looked at it.

Q. And were you able to determine whether the monitoring records between 6:20 and 11:30 A.M. showed any abnormalities or any areas that concerned you?

A. I didn't have a chance to look all through the fetal monitor papers, but at the last portion of the fetal monitor I looked at it.

Q. And have you been able to determine whether there were any fetal monitor patterns that were suggestive of fetal distress during the night that you were not apprised of by the nursing staff?

A. Yes.

Q. Would you ordinarily expect nurses to apprise you of those changes by telephone?

A. Yes.

Q. All right. Did you order the monitor to be taken off at 11:30?

A. No, sir.

Q. Do you feel that the monitoring should have been discontinued by the nurses at that time, at 11:30, without your being apprised of the prior difficulties with the tracing?

A. I don't think so.

Q. However, in this case, the nurses took the monitor off even though the earlier monitor pattern was not normal. Is that correct?

A. Yes.

The hospital had a policy to monitor a patient for a short period of time and if there were no abnormalities to take the monitor off. The nurses failed to recognize the abnormalities and discontinued the fetal monitor on this patient. The physician looked at a short portion of the strip early in the morning but did not look at the entire strip.

Q. At what time did you make a decision to intervene in this matter, in some way other than what you had been doing?

A. Around 1:15—1:45 to 2:00, I saw the nurse was having a very difficult time in locating the fetal heartbeat on Joan Lawton. Finally she asked me to help her check. So I checked, I couldn't hear the heartbeat. I ruptured the bag of water right away. There was dark meconium stained fluid and I applied the internal fetal monitor and there was no fetal heartbeat.

Q. Now, was there no tracing or was the machine not working?

A. Well, that's always an obstetrician's problem to determine whether the electronics device is working. But there was no heartbeat, so we waited for a while and tried another conventional fetoscope and we still couldn't hear a heartbeat. So about 10 or 15 minutes later we decided the infant was dead.

Q. And at what point were there more than one alternative on how to handle Joan's care from that point, that is Pitocin augmentation of labor and expulsion versus cesarean section?

A. Once the fetus is dead, we don't do a cesarean section.

Q. If you had been aware that Joan had any type of heart disease, would you have elected not to put her through Pitocin augmentation and full labor and instead perform a cesarean section even though the child was dead?

A. Depending on how bad, how severe a heart problem the patient has I might not.

Q. In light of everything you know about the case, Joan's case, do you believe that Joan more probably than not would have survived and her child would have survived, if you had performed a cesarean section before her fetus died on the 28th of October, 1981?

A. That's correct.

Q. Now, when did you first become aware that Joan's condition was changing and something was happening?

A. It was after we transferred her to the delivery room.

Q. And I would appreciate if you would look at your records on this so we can get the times.

A. It was about 3:20 A.M.

Q. Okay.

A. And as usual, she was put in a birthing chair.

Q. Can we use the times that are in the chart so that, I think its 3:20, is that correct?

A. Yes.

Q. Did the nurses at 3:00 apprise you that Joan's pulse was up to 120, did they tell you that?

A. About 118.

Q. Well, at 3:00 it was 120?

A. Right.

Q. Did they tell you about that?

A. Yes.

Q. Okay. Had it been slower than that before?

A. Around 80 was her pulse.

Q. Do you know why it is that her pulse went from the baseline of 80 that you talked about to 120 at 3:00?

A. I've seen many active labor patients at the last stage of labor going up to 100, 120.

Q. Okay.

A. Without any significant problems.

Q. If, at 3:00, Joan was complaining of shortness of breath, would that have concerned you at all?

A. That—yes or no, because she was practicing Lamaze breathing technique. So it's—it was very difficult whether it was from the Lamaze breathing technique or truly shortness of breath.

Q. And so at 3:20, Joan was transferred to the birthing chair and what occurred at that time?

A. The nurse did a prep on the perineum, and I got the drape on her, as usual, and then had her push. Right after a few times of pushing, she experienced marked shortness of breath suddenly.

Q. And what, that would have been around 3:25?

A. 3:25 or 3:30.

Q. Okay. Well, it looks like the oxygen was started around 3:25, according to the nurse's notes.

A. Yes. That should be correct.

Q. And what did you do at that time to determine why this sudden need for oxygen was occurring?

A. I thought she was practicing Lamaze breathing, and she had experienced shortness of breath from that breathing technique first.

Q. All right. And how long did you continue to think that that was the cause of her shortness of breath?

A. About, for 10 minutes.

Q. Okay. Did—was Joan able to keep her oxygen mask on?

A. About 10 minutes later, she was getting excited and throwing away the oxygen tubes, and her husband was trying to help her.

Q. Have you seen air hunger in patients?

A. Yes.

Q. And does that occur in pulmonary edema?

A. Yes.

Q. Kind of like a fish out of water?

A. Yes.

Q. Patient jumps around a lot and tries to get air?

A. Yes.

Q. And at that point what did you do to determine what was causing this change in Joan's condition?

A. At that time, since she was very excited and the infant's head was pretty much down, I could apply the forceps. But since she was so uncooperative, I decided to give her a general anesthesia and then use the forceps. So I called an anesthetist.

Q. Did you do anything more to determine why this sudden change of events in Joan's condition?

A. That time, I didn't think anything else. Ten minutes before was fine and then suddenly that happened, so I thought she was a little bit excited because of some medication she had, she had a mild sedation with Demoral, 25 milligrams, IV, and Largon, 20 milligrams, about 40 minutes prior to that.

Q. Was she telling you at that time that she couldn't breathe. She couldn't get any oxygen?

A. She didn't talk much, she just kept pushing the oxygen away.

Q. And what happened next?

A. And at that time the anesthetist came.

Q. No, what did you do between the time all this started and the time the anesthetist came?

A. We still kept the oxygen on and then tried to let her calm down.

Q. Did you administer any medications to her?

A. Just before the anesthestist came, the nurse checked the blood pressure again, and it had dropped down to 60 systole, so we gave her Ephedrine, 25 milligrams, IV.

Q. And what were you treating?

A. That time I was just blocking because she was so good 10 minutes before, and just suddenly her blood pressure dropped, so I tried to raise the blood pressure up first and then at the moment the anesthetist came in. We decided to forget about the forceps delivery, and since she had shortness of breath, we better take her to the X-ray and her lungs to find any problem. But when we tried to move the patient to the stretcher right away, and she just went into convulsions and a coma and died.

Q. What steps did you take, other than transferring her to X-ray, to handle the situation?

A. Since I suspected she had pulmonary edema, we gave Lasix, 20 milligrams IV, and then kept checking her blood pressure. We moved the patient to the stretcher; meanwhile I asked the anesthetist whether it would benefit her to intubate her, but there was a very short time. She just went into the coma in a few seconds. So we didn't quite have time enough.

Q. What time did you administer the Lasix to Joan?

A. I don't have the anesthetist notes on my—

Q. Looks like 4:10, would that be right? It's in the nurse's notes at 4:10?

A. Yes, around 4:10.

Q. At—is that the first time you suspected that Joan had pulmonary edema?

A. Yes.

Q. At—between 3:20 and 4:10, you didn't suspect that Joan had pulmonary edema?

A. First I didn't suspect that she had pulmonary edema. I simply was going to find out why she had hypotension. And then after Mr. Cook came in and then she showed progressive cyanosis on the lips, so at that time, it's around 4:00, then we decided to try with the Lasix and then I think it was given around that, 4:10.

Q. Well, in our earlier discussion we touched upon some of the ways to treat acute pulmonary edema and Lasix is only one of those ways, isn't it?

A. Right.

Q. The other way is to give Cedilanid, a quick-acting digitalis preparation, is that right? Do you remember your earlier testimony?

A. If we suspected congestive heart failure. But I thought it was just simple pulmonary edema, not from cardiac origin.

Q. Well, from what origin would you have suspected it to be from?

A. Well, she had a history of bronchopneumonia, so I first in my head thought, it's a pulmonary problem rather than a cardiac problem.

Q. When was the decision made to try to pass an endotracheal tube, at what time, to give Joan additional oxygen?

A. As soon as Mr. Cook came in and we discussed the possibility of a general anesthesia, of an intubation, since then her blood pressure dropped and I didn't think it's appropriate to put her to sleep. First I wanted to find out what's the problem and then I gave her Ephedrine and her blood pressure went up a little bit. We then tried to go to X-ray to check chest. And then suddenly she just became cyanotic when we moved her to the stretcher. She just went into a seizure and died.

Q. Well, the period of time from the nurse's notes from starting of oxygen at 3:40 to 4:10, when the first dose of Lasix was given, you did not, at any time, consider passing an endotracheal tube so that she could get an adequate amount of oxygen?

A. If her blood pressure was fine, then of course, no doubt, we go ahead to have induction of anesthesia and intubate.

Q. I'm not talking about anesthesia, for anesthesia. Have you taken a course in cardiopulmonary resuscitation, Doctor?

A. Yes.

Q. And do you have any type of certificate showing that you have taken this CPR course?

A. Yes.

Q. Okay. And do you understand the basic fundamentals of cardiopulmonary resuscitation?

A. Yes.

Q. And do you understand that if a patient demonstrates signs of oxygen deficit that the first thing that has to be done is to give that patient oxygen?

A. Yes.

Q. Do you understand that on some patients, because they are agitated because they have air hunger, that the only way to give them an adequate amount of oxygen is to intubate them first to give them an adequate amount of oxygen?

A. Most of the time yes, it was very difficult to decide. The airway was not an obstructive type of problem, apparently, but I thought the lung bed was the problem.

Q. In the course of your experience in cardiopulmonary resuscitation, you have not been instructed that no matter what the pulmonary disease is, if the patient lacks oxygen and is combative, that the way to handle that is to pass a tube and put in oxygen under positive pressure? No matter what the cause of the cyanosis is?

A. The cyanosis was appearing at the very last minutes, about 4:00.

Q. Where did you take your course in cardiopulmonary resuscitation, Doctor?

A. We had a course in town, about two years ago.

Q. Did you get a certificate?

A. Yes.

Q. And was it the advanced life support, advanced cardiac life support course? Or the basic life support system?

A. Just basic.

Q. Just basic?

A. Yes.

Q. Have you been trained more extensively than that?

A. I didn't have any more formal training.

Q. Have you ever passed an endotracheal tube?

A. Yes.

Q. Do you know how to do it?

A. Yes.

Q. Have you passed endotracheal tubes on patients who require oxygenation?

A. Yes.

Q. You know how to do that, don't you?

A. Yes.

Q. Have you given bicarbonate to patients who have problems with acidosis from lack of oxygen?

A. Not by myself. But I have seen that done.

Q. And you know that it's part and parcel of the resuscitation process?

A. Yes.

Q. Doctor, does a last blood pressure shown on the record show that Mrs. Lawton was shocky? Before you tried to transfer her for an X-ray?

A. That time she was not really shocky. Her blood pressure was fluctuating, once 60 systole and then it would go up to 90. And she was breathing all right. But she had shortness of breath. And then progressively, about 4:00, she became cyanotic.

Q. Was it proper for you to attempt to transfer a patient who was unstable to the X-ray department for a chest X-ray?

A. Another reason why I decided that was she was sitting on the birthing chair. It was not helpful for the hypotension, the birthing chair was upright. Since I was wondering whether she had amniotic fluid embolism or pulmonary embolism or just simple hypotension, I wanted a chest X-ray.

Plus there was another problem; she was having active contraction of labor and the baby's head was way down in the pelvis. The decision was very difficult, whether we go ahead, give her sedation and take baby out or just forget about the delivery and then go to X-ray or some other diagnostic procedure. Then the time was passing.

Q. A very simple question, it's the last question I'm going to ask you. Simply, what did you do during that period of time to treat the cyanosis? Or to treat Mrs. Lawton?

A. We tried to elevate the blood pressure first, and—

Q. I'm just—just tell me what drugs you gave and what maneuvers you went through and we'll be finished.

A. We gave first the Ephedrine 25 milligrams IV and blood pressure went up to—

Q. You don't have to tell me the results, just tell me what you did.

A. And then another 25 milligrams of Ephedrine again, and then Lasix, Lasix, 20.

Q. So basically what you did for Joan between 3:50 to 4:10 was to give two doses of Ephedrine and one dose of Lasix.

A. Yes.

Q. And you did not intubate her?

A. No.

Q. And you did not give her positive pressure oxygen?

A. No.

Q. You did not give her morphine?

A. No.

Q. You didn't give her Cedilanid?

A. No.

Q. You didn't use rotating tourniquets?

A. No.

Q. You didn't do a phlebotomy?

A. No.

§ 17.4 Direct Examination of Plaintiff's Anesthesiologist Expert

The following transcript is of the examination of an anesthesiologist who testified as an expert for the plaintiff concerning the standard of care of a physician faced with a respiratory emergency.

Q. Doctor, would you tell the jury whether or not there is a national standard of care that applies to the management of cardiorespiratory problems in patients?

A. There—it depends on what the problem is obviously. I think there are baseline standards of care that would apply throughout the country in terms of preventing the cardiac arrest, respiratory arrest, or responding to a cardiac or respiratory arrest. We're talking about fairly gross events and I think that the baseline—there are baseline standards that would apply throughout the country at large and small hospitals.

Q. Do these baseline standards, in your opinion, apply to the medical conduct that you examined in this case?

A. Yes. I think so.

Q. Why are there such things as baseline fundamental standards of care through-out the United States, in your opinion?

A. Well, I think the dissemination of knowledge in this country is such that it is reasonable to expect a level of care by practitioners that it reasonably—that meets at least some floor of a standard. There is access to continuing educa-tion, to journals, to books, to videocassette tapes. There are meetings. People have trained at many different parts of the country. Various specialties have board certification that are nationalized. The state societies in general tend to follow AMA guidelines.

   The AMA is a national organization. I mean I could go on. I think it's not necessary, but the point is I don't think any of us practice in a vacuum anymore.

Q. And Doctor, do you have a working knowledge of these fundamental and baseline standards of care as they apply to this case?

A. I think so, yes.

Q. And do these baseline fundamental standards of care apply in your opinion to Dr. Wesley?

A. Yes.

Q. Do they also apply—

DEFENSE ATTORNEY: Excuse me. Note my objection for lack of foundation.

Q. Do they apply to Dr. Johnson?

DEFENSE ATTORNEY: Same objection.

A. Yes.

Q. Dr. Parker?

A. Yes.

DEFENSE ATTORNEY: Same objection.

Q. And Mr. Cook, the nurse anesthetist?

DEFENSE ATTORNEY: Object on the basis of foundation.

A. Yes.

Q. And Doctor, can we agree here today that you will base your testimony that you give here today on those minimal fundamental standards of care as they apply to Dr. Wesley, Dr. Johnson, Dr. Parker, and Mr. Cook?

A. Yes.

The above exchange gets around the problem of a locality rule when the physician testifies that there is a minimal, fundamental standard of care that is to be followed everywhere.

Q. And I would ask you, based on your education, training, experience, knowl-edge of the standard of care, and reasonable medical probability, as to whether or not Drs. Johnson and Parker adhered to acceptable standards of medical practice?

A. Just in a general sense, my criticism of them has to do with prior to her hospitalization, what I considered to be not very thorough evaluation of her medical condition, the evaluation having started around 1973. And the followup was not very, I think, carefully done and certainly in terms of following through on the cardiac type complaints that she had even started mentioning in 1973, but were much more up to date in 1981 or—I guess, '80 and '83. But my major criticism has to do with her hospitalization in 1981.

Q.   And if you would explain to the jury what steps you feel should have been taken to adhere to good standards of practice?

A.   Okay. She is in her eighth month, end of her seventh month, early eighth month of pregnancy and comes in with a supposed pulmonary problem, shortness of breath, coughing.

Dr. Wesley had thought she had some sort of pneumonia and started her on antibiotics. And the next day, I guess that was September 8th, if I recall correctly, and the next day she takes herself to the hospital because she's doing so poorly.

And I think from that point on, they just assumed or took for granted more than they should have. I think their care was below the standard. There was no attempt to evaluate what else might be going on besides their consideration of bronchial pneumonia.

And this lady was giving off clues that she had some serious problems. Bronchial pneumonia would have been very low, very low on my differential diagnosis list and it should have been low on anyone's list.

She did not have a fever. Her white count was somewhat elevated, but that's not specific. It can certainly happen in stress response.

Their failure to do a gram stain on her sputum, to look for the kind of sputum that she was producing—was it an infected sputum? Did it have an organism in it that would be causing her pneumonia?

She was started on antibiotics without any basis for the antibiotics. A later sputum culture turned out to be negative.

They didn't communicate at all with the radiologist, which I think is a major error, and this is why I say it's more in the realm of common sense than in the realm of specific attention to medical detail.

They have a patient in the hospital who has some serious problems and is pregnant and the radiologist knows nothing about this patient. He's just asked to look at a chest X-ray and nobody communicates with the radiologist as to what the clinical problem is. The radiologist doesn't know the clinical situation, yet they're depending on the radiologist for an interpretation of a chest X-ray.

I haven't seen the X-ray. My guess would be that—and based on what I read of the reports, it's kind of a nonspecific problem. He describes it as bilateral infiltrates which one can get with congestive failure; one can get with a pneumonia; one can get with a viral inflammation, a variety of causes.

You can't expect the radiologist to know what the problem is in the absence of any clinical information and I don't get any inference that there was any communication. If I am wrong, if there was a communication between them, that's fine, but I didn't get any impression from reading their depositions that they did communicate.

So the radiologist is left in the dark and yet they use that X-ray as an important piece of evidence that this lady did, in fact, have pneumonia.

I think the other pieces of evidence don't support pneumonia, yet they treat her for it and don't go into any other possibilities that might have caused her to become short of breath, coughing, dyspneic, et cetera. If those things had been looked into or if the questions had been raised in their minds, if they had gotten appropriate consultations, if they had informed the radiologist that this lady is in her eighth month of pregnancy; she's had some symptoms in the past of cardiac problems; she has an EKG that's different now than it was a few years ago; she really doesn't have the classical picture of bronchial pneumonia; what do you think is going on? The radiologist might have been able to search his mind and review the X-ray. But these things were never brought in and that is not basic good medical care.

Any time somebody in their last third of pregnancy gets into this kind of difficulty, you have to wonder seriously about cardiac problems because this is a well-known precursor for the third trimester of pregnancy for reasons we can get into physiologically later. It sets up a situation where patients do get into the respiratory difficulties on the basis of heart disease and it ought to be something that is in the front of a practitioner's mind.

In addition to that, she had some other things we have already mentioned, such as an abnormal electrocardiogram. The opportunity was there to see that the cardiogram was quite different than the one obtained in 1973, although that wasn't done. But the opportunity to do it was there.

Q.   What are the changes that occur in pregnancy that affect the heart?

A.   Assuming that we're dealing with a normal situation, the normal changes of pregnancy primarily involve the dramatic increase in blood volume, so that by the third trimester, the patient's blood volume is greatly increased, about 50 percent increased above normal. And this is in anticipation of the labor and delivery process which is going to put an additional strain on the cardio-vascular function.

In addition to that, the geometry of the heart changes because the uterus enlarges, the diaphragm pushes up against the heart and the heart configuration changes. There is less room for the lungs to expand.

The left ventricle changes its configuration and, therefore, changes the way it contracts.

In a normal situation, there is no problem with this and it handles these changes perfectly well.

The pulmonary arteries increase their vascularity as more and more blood flows into them. The pulmonary arteries become more congested and more of the pulmonary vessels open up and start accepting blood flow per given unit of time. So it becomes just a richer circulation in the pulmonary vasculature as well.

Breathing becomes more difficult because the sensation of breathlessness, which is caused by the enlarged uterus and the high diaphragm, bothers people, particularly when they lie down. So they will feel like they're not able to breathe as deeply as they would like to. And they start feeling some degree of breathlessness anyway.

These are the major changes that we can talk about.

Q.   Assuming in September of 1981 that Mrs. Lawton was unable to walk more than 10 to 15 feet without severe shortness of breath, would that indicate to you that she was decompensated at that point?

A.   Yes.

Q. Now, further assuming that in January that a diagnosis of heart disease had been made, in your medical opinion what did the fundamental standards of care in 1981 dictate with regard to management of that patient from that point on?

A. I think that at a very basic level this lady would have been informed about what her problem was, educated about it, put on bed rest, her diet significantly restricted, sodium restricted, fluid intake restricted, and plans would have been made for a controlled labor and delivery.

 Whether she would have been given diuretics in addition, whether she would have been given digitalis or other cardioactive drugs, I can't say, and may be beyond the expertise, my expertise and perhaps those of the primary caretakers in this situation. But at least some very basic standard medical approaches would have been initiated.

Q. Would it be generally true, that swelling of the upper extremities and face during pregnancy is something that should be evaluated as being abnormal?

A. Yes.

Q. I want to direct your attention to the second or the November 3rd admission to Rockland Memorial Hospital. Have you reviewed those records?

A. Yes.

Q. And have you been able to reach any opinions regarding the conduct of Dr. Wesley?

A. Yes.

Q. And I would appreciate it if you would tell the jury based on your education, experience, and reasonable medical probability, as well as your knowledge of the national standards of care as they apply to this patient, what your opinions are?

A. First, my opinion with regard to Dr. Wesley is that he deviated from the basic fundamental standard of care in a variety of ways.

 First, let me backtrack and say that I think, again based on common sense rather than on a specific medical standard, I think Dr. Wesley, knowing that his patient was in the hospital in September, essentially did nothing to take care of her or participate in her care when she was hospitalized in September with "pneumonia," and I think this is an indication of a very—an attitude which takes a great deal for granted that is not acceptable.

 He was supposed to know this patient and her problems and the kinds of problems that occur during pregnancy. And it seemed, from his own deposition and the other material that I read, that he really wasn't at all involved in her care in September.

 I think that is really unacceptable right from the start. From the time she was admitted to the hospital—I believe it was around 2:15 in the morning on March 3rd—Dr. Wesley was notified at 2:15 that she was admitted, but he did not come to see her until morning. Now, since he didn't know that she had a cardiac problem, and it never entered his mind that she had anything wrong with her, she was just a normal term pregnant patient. I really can't fault him for not coming in at 2:15 in the morning to see her. The fault lies in the fact that—he didn't know what was wrong with her right from the start.

 My next criticism of him, I guess, occurs at 7:00 in the morning when he does come to see her and the tracings that are available on the intrauterine pressures, the monitoring devices, indicate many, many patterns of fetal distress.

Although this was an anesthesiologist, he can testify about certain things that are in the realm of medicine not particularly related to his own specialty. For instance, any physician can testify that medical records have to be reviewed. Also, any physician can testify about standard and authoritative works in the medical field.

A.   The tracings which were available to him and which indicated a number of times that there were patterns of late deceleration which represent fetal distress, he either didn't see those tracings or didn't respond to the fact that he did see them. So that at 7:00, when he saw this patient, regardless of what her condition was, the fetus was in distress. And he was not responsive to that or didn't even know that the fetus was in distress because he didn't review the records carefully.

Then we get into the situation where this lady becomes acutely stressed and she's acutely stressed because he has her sitting in a birthing chair and pushing. She's now had five hours of Pitocin-induced labor which creates a number of stresses to her.

First of all, there is a—with the Pitocin, she will increase any salt and water retention that she might have, although in the five hours she didn't get that much fluid. I don't think that's really an important issue.

Pitocin is a pretty good vasopressor and will vasoconstrict blood vessels and increase resistance to outflow from the heart. So that will worsen any congestive failure and mitral regurgitation that she might have.

He puts her on several hours of Pitocin to induce her labor, to get the baby expelled, and this is only going to worsen her cardiac function.

When she gets acutely stressed by going into the birthing chair and pushing, that's going to produce a maximum increase in venous return and that's going to acutely—whatever she was able to compensate for up until now is just going to dramatically worsen her condition.

At that point, he has no idea what's going on and I think his response to this acutely stressed and severely ill patient—and she is truly a critically ill patient by this time—his response is very inadequate.

Q.   Based on your education, training, experience, and reasonable medical probability, and based on the fundamental standards of care for any physician in the United States treating patients medically and surgically, what steps should Dr. Wesley have taken when Mrs. Lawton began to deteriorate?

A.   First thing I think he should have done when this lady started, assuming he knew nothing about a cardiac problem beforehand, he should have examined her. She's short of breath and all he's concerned about is getting the dead baby out. And instead, he should have been concerned with her medical condition and why she is short of breath. Take a stethoscope and listen to what her lungs sound like; get her into a position that would be more comfortable for her; stop pushing, if that's what started the problem.

He thinks the solution to the problem is to have her push more and get the baby out. If that made her worse, then he should have stopped and said,

"What's going on here? This lady is in severe medical straits. What have we done or what can I do to improve the situation?"

And that's based on: Number one, knowing what her diagnosis is, but he doesn't know that. At least he could examine her and find out what her lungs sound like, how she's breathing, what the pattern of her breathing is and is there something he can do to help this out.

Instead, as I understand the medical record and his deposition and Mr. Cook's testimony, he merely assumes she had asthma, that she was wheezing and he gives her some oxygen to breathe or maybe she was already on oxygen by this time. I don't recall exactly the time sequence.

And this lady is too agitated and too distressed to breathe adequately with a face mask with oxygen because: Number one, it feels confining to patients when they are in this kind of distressed state; and number two, breathing oxygen is not the solution to the problem. She's got to get the oxygen into her bloodstream and she's got to mainly get her heart decompressed. So giving oxygen is not going to be very useful in this situation. Diagnosing the problem is going to be useful.

The only other action that he then takes, as I recall, is to then call for Mr. Cook to give her a general anesthetic so he can deliver the baby. In other words, this patient is moving around too much, making it difficult for him to deliver the baby. His concern should not be with delivering the baby, it should be with her medical condition. And instead of trying to knock her out for delivery, his concern should be how can he improve her medical condition so she doesn't die.

The question of moving her down to an X-ray area to get an X-ray is absurd under these conditions. I'm sure if she hadn't arrested in the delivery room before she got moved to X-ray, she would have arrested on her way to X-ray or in X-ray. A chest X-ray is not ordered to know what to do.

So therefore, he then needs to take the steps to say regardless of the cause, assuming he doesn't know that she has a cardiac problem, assuming all he knows is that he's got this lady who's suddenly decompensated, is cyanotic, is dyspneic, is confused, agitated, et cetera; we've got to get this lady oxygenated and we've got to get her ventilated. And he should be directing his efforts towards that.

If he can't do it, getting somebody there who can do it, not to administer a general anesthetic, but to get her intubated, oxygenated, and ventilated and that's got to be his thrust.

There are other medical things he can do which might also alleviate the situation if he can figure out what the cause of the problem is. But if he thinks it's asthma without even examining her, then he's not going to take these steps. He's not going to give her Lasix or a diuretic. He's not going to give her digitalis. He's not going to give her morphine because those wouldn't be appropriate first steps to treat asthma.

They are appropriate to treat congestive failure, but a major criticism is that he never makes a diagnosis because he never examines the patient. And something that can be done at Rockland Memorial Hospital as well as the Massachusetts General Hospital—is to listen to her chest with a stethoscope.

And that's why I talk about common-sense-type, basic standards of care. We're not talking about Ivory Tower medicine.

Finally, his actions, after Mr. Cook arrives and tells him that the blood pressure is 60 makes me think, first of all, was this patient being monitored in the delivery room even by the delivery room nurses? Was anybody checking her cardiovascular function, routine vital signs, checking them periodically in the delivery room, frequently enough?

And number two, his response to that is to give her Ephedrine, which is, under the conditions, about the worse thing he could have done. But it doesn't really do anything anyway. It doesn't make her any better, that's for sure. But it would only increase this vasoconstriction that I have talked about and make her heart back up even more because it would make it harder for the heart to eject blood against the aorta and more of it would back up. And it's precisely the wrong kind of therapy. She needs control of her airway and oxygenation and ventilation. She does not need this kind of drug therapy.

Q. Would it generally be correct that a physician such as Dr. Wesley, although he's an obstetrician, should be well enough versed in the fundamental standards of resuscitation of a patient to have taken care of Mrs. Lawton properly?

A. Yes.

Many attorneys make the mistake of controlling the direct examination too tightly by asking long questions and letting the expert answer yes and no. The more preferable route is to let the doctor or other expert talk, since the jury probably cares little about the lawyer's opinion but wants to hear the expert's opinion.

Q. Why is that?

A. Again, this is basic. Any physician who takes care of a patient, particularly any physician who works in an operating room or who deals with changes in cardiac and respiratory function as part and parcel of disease processes, needs to know how to handle the basic resuscitative measures that patients will undergo in an operating room environment or in a delivery room environment. And there is no question that problems of labor and delivery spread out into all kinds of cardiorespiratory disasters. The obstetrician, as part of his basic training, if he is going to take care of pregnant women, needs to be able to manage disasters when they get into the cardiac or respiratory area acutely because there won't be time to call for sophisticated experts in all kinds of fields.

And we're talking about basic stuff here. We are not talking about open heart surgery type problems. This is very basic nationwide, if not worldwide, but certainly basic medical practice for any practitioner who deals with surgical patients or obstetrical patients.

Q. And in summarizing your opinion, would it be correct then that an obstetrician such as Dr. Wesley practicing anywhere in the United States should have knowledge of the standards of basic resuscitation?

A. Yes.

Q. Now, I would ask you at this point, assuming that Dr. Wesley had adhered to these fundamental basic standards for resuscitation for a patient such as Mrs. Lawton, what steps should he have undertaken when the problems arose in the delivery room?

A. I think he should have examined her to try and figure out what the problem was. And I think the problem was not subtle in the slightest, that if he had listened to her, he would have heard that she wasn't wheezing and, therefore, that would have made life very easy for him. He should have been able to immediately determine that this wasn't asthma and if it isn't asthma and she's this badly off, it can really—there aren't too many other treatable possibilities it could be and the most important one is that she has acutely gone into heart failure.

Given that, he then would have been able to take some drug-related steps to improve her condition before she got this far. Number one, he would have stopped having her try to deliver. Number two, he would have stopped the Pitocin.

He would start giving her small doses of morphine to calm her down which would also dilate her blood vessels which would also help her congestive failure. He would give her a large dose of a diuretic which would, within five or ten minutes, start promoting a vigorous diuresis which would start to reduce the amount of blood in her lungs and in her heart.

He might give her some tranquilizers in addition to morphine such as Valium or something like that IV. We're talking about IV administration of drugs so they have an immediate effect.

I think he should have requested that if she didn't improve dramatically, quickly—and by quickly I mean within a very few minutes, by the time people get there—that this lady, from the sounds of her condition, it sounded to me like she was in extreme distress by this time and this lady should have been intubated, ventilated, oxygenated with 100 percent oxygen. And using a bag and mask or—a bag and tube or an anesthesia machine or ventilator, whatever method to not just administer oxygen, but to ventilate the oxygen in and ventilate carbon dioxide out.

If he had sent her blood for any laboratory tests, as was done later on when she was in cardiac arrest, I'm sure he would have found that she was already in some degree of metabolic acidosis though not as severe as she was later on. And he would have administered some bicarbonate or something, to begin to correct this problem as well.

If her blood pressure needed support, then he would have been able to give drugs which would support her blood pressure like Ephedrine which is what he used except he used very massive—in my opinion—very massive doses of Ephedrine IV. They didn't even have an effect on her blood pressure.

But if she had not been in such extreme condition at that time, he could have put her into that extreme condition because he was using a drug to raise her blood pressure which is precisely what she—would precisely harm her cardiac condition, only he didn't realize she had a cardiac condition.

I think there are a number of basic steps, that one does not need to be a highly sophisticated, excessively trained resuscitationist or anesthesiologist or cardiologist, et cetera. Some basic steps that somebody in Dr. Wesley's situation should be able to take care of and, if not, get immediate help from somebody who can take care of it.

Q. Dr. Roberts, do you have an opinion based on your education, experience, and reasonable medical probability, as well as based on your knowledge of the minimal fundamental standards of care which you based your testimony on in this matter, whether or not if Drs. Johnson, Parker, and Wesley had adhered to standards of good medical practice, more probable than not, the baby and Mrs. Lawton would have survived?

A. Yes. I have an opinion.

Q. And what is that opinion?

A. My opinion is that if they had adhered to good or even basic or average medical practice, that both the baby and the mother would have survived intact.

§ 17.5   Cross-Examination of Plaintiff's Obstetrical Expert

The following transcript is from a deposition of an obstetrician/gynecologist who testified as to the standard of care for a person in the same specialty. This transcript shows the cross-examination by the defense attorney, rather than the direct examination of the plaintiff's expert illustrated in § 17.4.

Q. Would you first of all, then, do it this way for me, then, Doctor: Tell me, first of all, after you reviewed all the material that you've listed here, what in general was your understanding of what happened in this case, as far as Dr. Wesley's treatment of Mrs. Lawton was concerned?

A. My understanding?

Q. Just in general. I'm trying to get your understanding of what had occurred as far as Mrs. Lawton is concerned.

A. That she had been a patient of his. That she became pregnant while under his care. That he watched her during this pregnancy. And that she eventually went into labor, was admitted to the hospital, and during the course of that admission the baby died and she died.

Q. And what are your opinions concerning Dr. Wesley's care in this case?

A. The failure to perform a cesarean section; and the failure to diagnose the congestive heart failure led to the death of the mother and the child.

This physician, with the above answer, boiled the entire case down to one that lay people on a jury could readily identify with and understand.

Q. First of all, on what do you base the opinion that congestive heart failure should have been diagnosed by Dr. Wesley?

A. I feel that this patient exhibited a combination of symptoms which should have alerted Dr. Wesley, so that even if he himself did not make the diagnosis by his own hand, that he would have referred the patient where the ultimate diagnosis would have been made. And those particular symptoms—which I think is what you're asking me—would be the combination of edema, paroxysmal nocturnal dyspnea, and severe paroxysmal dyspnea on exertion, combined with a radiologic study which indicated some sort of pulmonary effusion or condition which really didn't go very well with the diagnosis that was established or started. Any patient, and I mean any patient, pregnant or not, who combines severe edema, paroxysmal nocturnal dyspnea, and such dyspnea on exertion that the patient cannot walk 15 or 20 feet without total rest almost should indicate to any physician that that patient needs further workup or consultation.

Q. Isn't it true, that in pregnancy, especially in late pregnancy, it is difficult for women to sleep, and that pillows are recommended for use at that time?

A. The answer is yes. But that is a very general question, yes.

The common difficulty, if I may say, is that the patient is so ungainly she just can't find that particular position in bed that will allow her comfort, and women can go for many nights, as you well know, just almost unable to sleep. It does require the use of pillows, anywhere from three to four pillows.

But those pillows are placed, number one, between the legs with the patient in a position lying usually almost on her side—not quite but almost on her side—with one pillow often underneath her abdomen, which is laying over, and one or more pillows under her head.

I have never had a recent patient, nor do I know of a recent patient of other doctors, who was required to sleep bolt upright in the bed to relieve the ordinary discomfort of later pregnancy. That is unusual.

Q. Have you ever had a woman do that, in your practice?

A. In my current practice, not in my current practice. But I have had patients who did in the past in my training. They all had congestive heart failure.

Q. Is there anything else about the nocturnal paroxysmal dyspnea that we haven't covered, on which you base your opinion?

A. I think other than the fact—what should we say? What I want to tell you is that it is one of the pathonomomic signs in congestive heart failure, and it's commonly seen in that it can be elicited from the very old who have it to the very young who have it, and as I say, I use the word elicit—if the doctor asks the right questions, they'll often get the right answer. Sometimes the patient volunteers. Sometimes the patient doesn't. But it is a sign that you will get. It is a common sign.

Q. Is this by itself specific for congestive heart failure?

A. That by itself with nothing else, not one other thing, would make me send a patient, or any doctor would send a patient to someone who could evaluate her cardiac status. I would be extremely worried about that sign, yes, I would.

Q. Would you diagnose congestive heart failure based on that sign alone?

A. It would have to be disproved to me. I would be extremely worried about that sign, yes, I would. I generally don't diagnose such things, because once I see a sign, I send the patient to a specialist.

Q. How long would that sign have to appear before you would send them to a specialist?

A. Not long.

Q. Well, how long is not long?

A. If the patient came in and I knew about it today, she would be at the specialist today, unless the specialist refused to see her or the specialist was out of town somewhere and she couldn't get there until tomorrow.

Q. Now, what do you base your testimony on, then, given the fact that Dr. Johnson or Dr. Parker are the attending physicians for this illness, on what do you base your testimony that Dr. Wesley should have followed up with other X-rays?

A. To my knowledge, once the patient was discharged, Dr. Wesley, who knew about all of this, followed the patient himself as an obstetrical patient.

Dr. Wesley, in my opinion at that point, should have either gotten clearance from her other physicians—that is, asked Mrs. Lawton what she planned on doing vis-a-vis the other physicians, and gotten whatever plan there was for her further treatment.

She having no plan, he should have either sent her back to her physicians—if you're calling Dr. Johnson her physician for this particular incident, which I think we are—or he should have made some plan for himself.

What apparently occurred was nothing. Nothing occurred. She just kept—she kept coming, and he kept seeing her. She went through her routine obstetrical care.

Q. Now, is it your testimony, then, that Dr. Johnson had no responsibility to follow up after this?

A. I haven't spoken about Dr. Johnson at all. No, I haven't made any statement such as that.

Q. Well, are you testifying, then, that Dr. Wesley is somehow negligent for allowing Dr. Johnson or relying on Dr. Johnson to follow up, as far as this condition is concerned, when he was, after all, her treating physician for this illness at—

A. The only thing that I would say is that Dr. Wesley may not put his head in the sand. He must find out at least what is being intended, or he must at least say to the patient, "Go back to Johnson until you know 100 percent that your chest is fine."

Q. You think that he, knowing that she had a gross abnormality, should have done something?

A. I did not say that he had to take the whole diagnostic question upon his own shoulders. But he should have at least, in his own mind, and with the patient, he together with the patient, should have found out what was the ultimate disposition of her case.

Q. Do you have an opinion, then, that had a C-section been performed when she first came into the hospital as to what the condition of the baby would have been?

A. Oh, I think the baby would have been fine.

Q. Why do you say that? On what do you base that opinion, given the fact that there was probably in her case a chronic insufficiency?

A. Because many, many of the cases that we see are chronic insufficiencies and in fact most of the babies are fine, and because the baby has good reserve.

You can see that the heart rate stays within a normal number, if that's what you want to call it, and that the baby rebounds to, let's say, between 150 and 160, and because the baby had a good beat-to-beat variability.

Q. When, in your opinion, then, is a C-section first indicated in this case? If I understand what you're telling me correctly it would not have been necessary to perform a C-section when she first came in.

A. That is not true. That is not what I said.

Q. Let's do it this way. Why don't you tell me when, in your opinion, it would have been necessary to do a cesarean section?

A. Within 30 minutes when the patient came in with this pattern she should have been sectioned. Any pattern such as this which is not correctable in 30 minutes should be sectioned.

Q. So it's your opinion, then, that a section should be performed within 30 minutes of, say, when the monitor goes on, when you first get a late deceleration; about 30 minutes after the monitor goes on and you note late decelerations, if I understand what you're telling me, if a C-section is not performed within 30 minutes of that point, then the baby is going to be compromised in some manner?

A. I did not say that.

Q. I'm sorry. Then tell me, explain to me again, because I'm obviously not understanding it.

A. Okay. What this indicates is that when the uterus contracts, the baby is deprived of the oxygen and nutrients that it needs.

Q. Right, I understand that.

A. There is some period of time, a finite period of time, which is unknown for each and every baby, during which time if you allow that pattern to continue, the baby will die or be seriously damaged.

For some babies that period may be a few hours. For some babies, that period may be longer, a few more hours.

In this particular case, once the patient began contracting and she was on the monitor, it took eight hours to kill the baby. And that's the finite time you have.

In another case, perhaps, it may have taken 20 hours. In another case, three hours, because you do not know—you must set yourself a guideline. If you see an ominous pattern that you cannot correct, and that ominous pattern would go for 30 minutes, you are obliged to get the patient sectioned.

Q. Now, what would have happened had this lady had a section, but not at 7:30. Say not until 8:30? Would there have been any damage to the baby, in your opinion, at that point?

A. Probably not.

Q. What about at 9:30?

A. Probably not.

Q. Let me put it this way.

A. By damage, you mean, gross abnormalities so that the child was severely retarded, or do you mean in general a salvageable baby?

Q. Let's approach it this way. I think you indicated that the baby died some eight hours after she first came in, so you know at that point that that's too late. Now, is there any point before that point where in your opinion this baby would, even if a C-section had been done at that point, would have, say, suffered from significant brain damage?

A. It's hard to make that statement, so I would rather make the statement that we must consider the baby salvageable as a living human being—if I could say it that way. I would say, well, this monitor strip ends at 10:20 so until that point I think we have to consider the baby a salvageable human.

Q. But you don't feel comfortable about talking about whether or not there would have been any impairment to the baby?

A. Most likely there would have been little, if any, impairment.

Q. If he comes in at 2:15 and he decides to do a C-section, how long would it take to prepare this woman?

A. Well, if I saw this, I had better have her on the table in 30 minutes.

Q. Assuming that was done, in your testimony, would the baby have been normal at that point?

A. Yes.

There is no question that the nurses in this case were grossly negligent in failing to recognize an abnormal fetal heart rate pattern. However, this physician explained quite well the duty that the physician has in making sure that the patient is under the care of competent nurses.

Q. Do you have any indication that there was information that should have indicated to him the nurses' incompetence or that he shouldn't have relied on them to inform him?

A. It is incumbent upon a physician who assigns duties to others to know the quality of those to whom the duties are assigned, that is incumbent upon him.
   This is the hospital's patient, by virtue of the fact that she admitted herself to that hospital. But it is always the obstetrician's patient, and if he chooses to stay home while the patient is in labor, then it is with the clear assumption that he knows, understands, and trusts these nurses' competence, because if he doesn't, he had better spend his nights at the hospital looking at monitor tracings.

Q. I need to know why you feel this was a high-risk patient. And, second, when this patient, in your opinion, was a high risk.

A. When she walked through the door and she was 30 some odd years old, a primigravida. She was an elderly primigravida by definition.

Q. Because she was over 35?

A. 30. We began pushing the age back because—well, the last 10 years we are not so worried about ladies over 30 with their first baby. But they statistically still are problem patients, and she should be considered a problem patient simply by the fact that she is an elderly primigravida.

Q. By that fact alone, is that what you're indicating?

A. Obviously. Absolutely. Positively. A patient over 30, first baby, needs to be watched like a hawk.

Q. And by watching extremely carefully, does that mean that you have to be at her bedside the entire time, or does that mean that she should have been monitored? What do you mean?

A. That means that during her pregnancy she should be watched for signs and symptoms of literally anything, most of which are vascular, in the sense that this is a patient in whom we'll find hypertension in pregnancy, diabetes in pregnancy, some sort of vascular problems, in general, in pregnancy. This is a patient who we'll find intrauterine growth retardation—on top of which she smokes, and that has to be added in. Although, she didn't smoke much. I think she cut it to under a pack.

But all these sorts of things, including such things in older women as abruption—just one thing after another.

Older ladies have problems, and they just need to be watched.

And when she went into labor, I would have monitored her very closely.

Did that make her a high-risk patient? The answer is yes.

She should have and would have been continuously monitored, if she had been my patient, and the first sign that she turned a hair the wrong way, the baby would have been delivered.

And that's the way you've got to do it if you're going to have successful outcomes consistently.

Q. I want to ask you if there is anything else that you want to expand on, other than what we've already gone through.

A. In summary, this patient should have had a cesarean section.

You have not asked me about Mrs. Lawton's death in the sense of the final acts, and that sort of thing.

If you would ask me to expand, I would say simply that we did discuss the baby, and in our discussion you and I, we did—or I did indicate that I thought that the baby would have lived, and indeed by now would probably be getting ready to walk, if not walking, and saying something.

I think it should be noted that the baby came within, at any period of time almost until the very end of its life, within 20 minutes of a life, and that, I guess, made me a little disturbed.

You probably read that in my report.

The other thing which we didn't say anything about was Mrs. Lawton's death.

Q. That's what I was going to ask you about, if there was anything—you said this was a preliminary report.

A. Yes.

Q. And so I assumed there are things that you have considered since you did this.

A. Yes. I would just like to say, in general, that I feel had the cesarean section been done, that Mrs. Lawton would have lived.

You know, for whatever reason she died in the end—let's presume for a minute that it was congestive heart failure and ultimate cardiac collapse.

If this lady had been sectioned, it's my belief that she would be alive today.

Q. That is based on what, Doctor?

A. That is based on the fact that she would not have had to go through any more labor. She would not have had to push. She would have had adequate anesthesia to stop all the pain and anxiety, and that she would have had a therapeutic blood letting, if you would.

After all, before we had fancy drugs how did you treat congestive heart failure? You took a bottle, you took a needle, and you drew blood out of people.

And indeed we know that a cesarean section is a very bloody operation in which the patient loses between two and three units of blood.

And further, that she later would have bled through lochia and other means, so I think taking all and all, I really feel very, very honestly that this patient would not have died had that section been done and the baby delivered.

§ 17.6   Cross-Examination of Internist Testifying as Plaintiff's Expert

The following transcript is from a deposition of an internist taken during the discovery phase of the lawsuit. This internist was viciously attacked by defense counsel because he was a local expert. In the state in which this litigation occurred, physicians do not testify against fellow members of their medical community.

Q. You know there was an X-ray taken, which we had at Dr. Johnson's deposition, among others, back in, I think it was, around May of 1973. Have you seen that X-ray?

A. Yes.

Q. Have you see the X-ray report on it?

A. Yes.

Q. What does that tell you, that X-ray?

A. That X-ray was read and reported as within normal limits, and while I have not had a chance to see the original X-ray—and always reluctant to comment about copies—the copy that I have had a chance to review does seem to be a normal chest X-ray for a woman in her late 20s or early 30s.

Q. Am I correct, you don't feel that that X-ray should have alerted Drs. Porter and Johnson to heart problems in this lady at that time?

A. Not in 1973. There are other things that lead to the suspicion that she might have had heart problems in May of 1973.

Q. What are they?

A. Well, there is the self-history in the medical record and the lady does check off the fact that she had palpitations and some shortness of breath and swelling and so on. And while that is not commented on on the doctor's subsequent physical exam, I believe the self-history is usually given the patient, patient fills it out and hands it to the doctor or office staff, and there is a physical exam where the patient and doctor encounter. And there is no reference made to that.

And I believe Dr. Johnson said in his deposition that he did pursue those issues and discounted them as being not founded on medical fact. But at least she gave a history then that could be interpreted two ways, and I don't mean to say that he should have grasped on those signs or comments and said, ah, this lady must have heart disease. I don't believe that is true at all, but it raised a question. And he says he asked those questions and got negative responses.

There is another issue in office visits subsequent to 1973 and prior to September 1981, where she has swelling and the doctors don't really pursue the cause of her swelling. They treat her with drugs to make her body excrete salt and water, which are diuretics, and this will make swelling go away. And the question wasn't asked why.

I believe early sometime in 1979 there was a question of whether she had some precordial or chest kind of distress. That is not followed up on at all.

There are some little glimpses of information that suggest that she might have had some problem, but they are nonspecific and don't lead you to any conclusion. But in September 1981, things are different.

Q. You say that when she was admitted to the hospital in September of 1981, that she had a complaint of cough and left-sided pleuritic chest pain.

A. Yes.

Q. And then you say neither Dr. Johnson nor Dr. Parker asked for consultation. Why do you feel they should have asked for consultation for some benign findings such as that?

A. I don't believe those are benign. I believe those findings and those complaints are of a serious nature, in anybody, let along a woman who is in the final third of her pregnancy. And given her complaints and her physical examination, the laboratory values that were available and the chest X-ray and the electro-cardiogram, those all point to me to raise my index of suspicion that this lady had a process other than pneumonia, at the root of her complaints of shortness of breath and pain associated with breathing and cough.

Q. What percent of your income last year was earned testifying? All inclusive. I want review of files, depositions, rendering opinions, going to depositions, and testifying.

A. Less than 5 percent.

Q. And the year before?

A. I don't have a recollection. In fact, it's only an estimate for last year, too.

Q. Would you provide your tax returns for an in camera inspection by a court?

PLAINTIFF ATTORNEY: We are not going to provide those without a court order.

DEFENSE ATTORNEY: I appreciate that. Doctor, I want to know what your position is if I would ask for you to provide your tax returns to a court in confidentiality and if the court would read them and decide whether they are relevant to disclose your—

PLAINTIFF ATTORNEY: Would you provide your income tax return statements? The answer is no. If you want to go get a court order, you go get a court order, but this witness is here to render an opinion. If you don't like his opinion, that is fine, but you are not entitled to go into his entire life history and invade the privacy of whatever his financial records are. He has answered the question you asked him.

DEFENSE ATTORNEY: I want to make sure you are finished. Are you done with your speech?

PLAINTIFF ATTORNEY: I may or may not be.

DEFENSE ATTORNEY: Is there a reason why you would not consent to that?

PLAINTIFF ATTORNEY: Because his attorney doesn't believe you have a right to invade the privacy of his financial records when he is here to render an opinion. I consider that harrassment, and I believe it is not justified; and absent a court order, we are not even going to respond to that.

Q. And I gather you consider this gentleman your attorney as opposed—

PLAINTIFF ATTORNEY: You are not going to harrass this witness. Okay? If you want to get an order, go get an order. If you want to find out what his opinions are, get his opinions. The answer is, no, he is not going to produce it and not going to respond to that type of question.

You have asked him a question, he has answered to the best of his ability in regards what amount of money, percentage of his income, as related to defending as well as assisting plaintiffs.

DEFENSE ATTORNEY: Are you done?

PLAINTIFF ATTORNEY: Don't answer any other questions along this line, Dr. Eastland.

Q. Do you consider this gentleman your attorney at these proceedings.

A. No.

Q. And I would assume, then, that you don't feel obligated to take his advice; you may or may not?

A. I have no comment.

Q. Again, sir, is there a reason why you would not provide those tax records, if it's—

PLAINTIFF ATTORNEY: Same reason you wouldn't provide yours.

DEFENSE ATTORNEY: Are you done?

PLAINTIFF ATTORNEY: When you go to the court and you provide yours and let your whole life hang out and all your financial dealings hang out, then we will consider it.

DEFENSE ATTORNEY: I'll stipulate I will give mine to a court, if you will give yours to a court.

PLAINTIFF ATTORNEY: Under court order, we will do that.

Q. Is there a reason, sir, as an impartial expert, why you would not provide your tax records to a court for an in camera inspection and allow the judge to decide whether there is something relevant in there?

A. Yes.

Q. What is the reason for that?

A. They reflect my private life.

This is a standard attack on a physician in an attempt to intimidate him from testifying. No person likes to have a group of strangers have access to private financial dealings. This physician stood up well to this attack, but counsel for both parties should be forewarned that this type of attack can take place.

Q. Does my client malpractice when he doesn't intubate the patient?

A. He did not meet the standard of care when he fails to deliver adequate oxygen by intubating to this patient after having failed with the mask, because she was excited, confused, and pulled the mask off.

Q. Are you saying—

PLAINTIFF ATTORNEY: You go ahead and finish your answer.

A. The exact time when it would have been the most expeditious to intubate this lady would have been after they had observed that they couldn't maintain adequate oxygenation with the systems available. And she is described in the labor flow records from five minutes after 4:30 over the next about 35 minutes, which takes you to 5:10, as being increasingly confused, cyanotic or blue, if you will, and they couldn't keep on a face mask.

    At that point in time it's necessary to ensure ventilation, and the only way to do that is to intubate the patient. Now, the notes aren't complete enough to know just exactly how excited she was, but they do suggest that she was difficult to manage physically.

And when that happens, there is no choice except to intubate the patient. You can paralyze—intubate a cooperative patient by anesthesia of the upper respiratory tract or sometimes even without it, but when a patient is combative, as this lady is described in the records, it is necessary to paralyze.

Sometime between 4:35 and 5:10 would be appropriate. I can't pin it to an exact minute.

Q. And being unable to pin it to anything other than roughly 4:35 to 5:10, would you agree that what you are doing is looking at this case with hindsight?

A. No.

Q. How many patients, in your 18 years of practice, have you administered anectine to and intubated?

A. I always have somebody else do that for me.

Q. So the answer to my question is none?

A. That is correct.

Q. So you have never been placed in the position where you have to make the judgment decision of administering a paralyzing drug, which is going to paralyze the diaphragm, preclude that patient from breathing on their own and administering—and intubating, isn't that correct?

A. No, that isn't true. That isn't what I said. I said I have never done that. I have made that decision, but I always have somebody else actually give the anectine.

Q. You have made the decision before?

A. You bet.

Q. How many times?

A. Several times a year.

Q. And I assume that you could obtain those records, delete the patient's name, and show that to us?

A. I don't think so.

Q. Why not, Doctor?

A. Well, I don't remember the patient names, for one, and I don't remember that I wrote in the chart that I made the decision. But I was at the bedside and made the decision to intubate the patients.

Q. So you could get the name of the doctor who did it so we could talk to him?

A. Like I say, if I don't remember the patient names, I don't think I could remember the doctor's name, and probably it was a resident in anesthesia that did it, and I don't know their names, let alone recognize some of them.

Q. So you don't remember whether it was a doctor or who did it. May have been a resident in anesthesia. You don't remember the patient's name but you feel comfortable testifying that you did it several times last year?

A. Yes, because I tell the truth.

Q. Do you know any way that you could get to some records to support your position, sir, that you made the judgment decision of administering anectine, paralyzing a diaphragm and intubating?

A. No, sir, I don't know how we could find those records.

CHAPTER 18

INTENSIVE CARE: WHAT INTENSIVE CARE IS AND WHO SHOULD GET IT

Steven M. Donn, M.D.

§ 18.1   Historical Perspectives

At birth, a person enters the most perilous segment of his or her life, the neonatal period. Even though neonatal mortality rates have been significantly reduced (see **Appendix 18–1** in **§ 18.17**), they remain higher for infants and newborns than for any other period of life.[1] Much knowledge has been gained from the study of this high-risk situation, knowledge that has evolved into the subspecialty of neonatology. The resulting positive impact of neonatal intensive care on mortality rates is clearly demonstrated in **Appendixes 18–2 (§ 18.18)** and **18–3 (§ 18.19)**.[2] Today, however, survival should not be the only yardstick used to measure success. Intact survival, or survival that is free of serious physical or mental impairment, is the ultimate goal. Fortunately, this is the most frequent outcome for infants graduating from neonatal intensive care.[3]

---

[1] P.R. Swyer, *The Organization of Perinatal Care with Particular Reference to the Newborn, in* Neonatology: Pathophysiology and Management of the Newborn 17–47 (1981); S. Pierog & A. Ferrara, *The Neonate: Problems and Perspectives, in* Approach to the Medical Care of the Sick Newborn 3–13 (1971); S.N. Graven & A.A. Fanaroff, *The Organization of Perinatal Health Services, in* Behrman's Neonatal-perinatal Medicine 4–11 (1983); 1 H.P. Chase, *Perinatal Mortality: Overview and Current Trends,* 1 Clinics Perinatology, no. 1, at 3–17 (1974).

[2] Stahlman, *Newborn Intensive Care: Success or Failure,* J. Pediatr. 105:162–67 (1984); Scott & Stone, *The Unwanted Pregnancy: Inevitable, Burdensome, the Cause of Over Population (abstr.),* 6 Annals Royal C. Physicians Surgeons Can. 51 (1973); Regional Services in Reproductive Medicine, Toronto, The Joint Committee of the Society of Obstetricians and Gynecologists of Canada and the Canadian Pediatric Society 7 (1973); Effer, *Management of High-risk Pregnancy: Report of a Combined Obstetrical and Neonatal Intensive Care Unit,* 101 Canadian Med. A. J. 389–97 (1969); Shennan & Milligan, *Role of Prematurity in Perinatal Mortality,* 47 Ontario Med. Rev. 105 (1979); P. Gosselin, A. Roy, P. Desjardins, A. Deleon & R. Usher, *Perinatal Intensive Care after Integration of Obstetrical Services in Quebec* (quoted in Quebec Perinatal Committee); Quebec City, Quebec Ministry of Social Affairs (1973); Papageorgiou, Masson, Shatz & Gelford, *The Development of Intramural Neonatal and Perinatal Intensive Care Units and Their Impact on Perinatal Mortality (abstr.),* 9 Annals Royal C. Physicians Surgeons Can. 82 (1976).

[3] P.R. Swyer, *The Organization of Perinatal Care with Particular Reference to the Newborn, in* Neonatology: Pathophysiology and Management of the Newborn 17–47 (1981). S.N. Graven & A.A. Fanaroff, *The Organization of Perinatal Health Services, in* Behrman's Neonatal-perinatal Medicine 4–11 (1983); 3 P.M. Fitshardinge, *Follow-up Studies on the Low Birth Weight Infant,* Clinics Perinatology, no. 2, at 503–16 (1976); Department of Health Services and Hospital

Newborns, as individuals or as a group, cannot effectively vocalize complaints and have no innate ability to cause change, traits that make them susceptible to being overlooked. The neonatal intensive care specialty, acting as a neonatal advocate, has developed an aggressive attitude in order to generate appropriate concern and awareness. This approach may account for many of the negative feelings neonatal intensive care has generated in the medical community. Today, great expense of energy continues to be necessary even though, as evidenced by the above statistics, the success of neonatal intensive care has been clearly demonstrated. Today's intensive care graduates have an excellent chance to experience their presumed 70-plus years of life expectancy in an unimpaired fashion. What other field of medicine can offer this to its patients?

Today, improving care for this select patient population is a twofold project. First, research into the pathophysiology and treatment of neonatal diseases must continue to attain the highest possible rate of intact survival. Second, the message must continue to be carried to both providers and consumers of health care in order that what is known can be applied. Only by the education of those individuals most often involved in the care of newborns will the neonate be assured of access to intensive care. It matters very little what state-of-the-art care really is if a newborn does not have the opportunity to experience it.

By understanding the developmental history of newborn care, the reader can better appreciate today's attitudes and their origins. As will be seen, the movement for improved health care for children actually began in other countries and then migrated to the United States. Many of these countries now have better neonatal mortality and morbidity statistics than the United States, a fact indicating that the struggle must continue. Because a complete historical account would be quite lengthy, a brief but revealing summary that encompasses select individuals and events is presented.

§ 18.2   —Founding Fathers

It was not long ago that infants were delivered almost exclusively at home and primarily by midwives. Thus, the infant received little, if any, medical attention in the newborn period. As deliveries moved out of the home and into the hospital, the mother was the favored recipient of medical care. On admission to the hospital, her fetus was usually not considered as a patient but rather as extra baggage. After birth, her newborn continued in this second-class patient status

Insurance, Annual Report from the Registry for Handicapped Children and Adults; Division of Vital Statistics, Health Branch, Department of Health Services and Hospital Insurance, Victoria, British Columbia; Rawlings, Stewart, Reynold, & Strang, *Changing Prognosis for Infants of Very Low Birth Weight,* 1 Lancet 516–19 (1971); Brimblecombe, *A New Approach to Care of Handicapped Children,* 13 J. Royal Physicians London 231–36 (1979); A.W. Brann & J.F. Schwartz, *Central Nervous System Disturbances, in* Behrman's Neonatal-perinatal Medicine 398–400 (1983).

by typically being placed in a makeshift nursery under the care of any available and often untrained staff. Postnatal care was frequently left to the obstetrician until after the mother and infant were discharged.[4] This concept of care by neglect was very eloquently attacked over a century ago by Dr. Andrew Combe in his *Treatise on the Physiological and Moral Management of Infancy:*

> Here, then is unquestionable evidence of the fact that a great mortality prevails in infancy, even among the most civilized communities, and under what are considered the most favorable of circumstances; and the question naturally presents itself, whether this mortality constitutes a necessary part of the arrangements of Divine Providence which men can do nothing to modify, or, on the contrary, proceeds chiefly from secondary causes purposely left, to a considerable extent, under our control, and which we may partially obviate or render innocuous by making ourselves acquainted with the nature of the infant constitution, and carefully adapting our conduct to the laws or conditions under which its different functions are intended to act?
>
> If we consult the past history of mankind, there will be little difficulty in finding the true reply, and proving that the appalling waste of infant life is not a necessary and intentional result of the Divine arrangements, but is produced chiefly by our own ignorance and mismanagement, and consequently may be expected to diminish in proportion as our knowledge and treatment improve, or, in other words, in proportion as we shall discover and fulfill the laws which the Creator has established for our guidance and preservation.[5]

During the late 1900s, Pierre Budin, a French obstetrician destined to be called the Father of Neonatology, supervised a special department for weaklings and authored a very important work, *The Nursling*. This text dealt with newborn infants, both term and preterm, and their subsequent care. Infants who were either large or small for their gestational period and the differences in their clinical presentations were also described. Soon, expanding pediatric interest began to include newborns. Through the efforts of Arvo Ylppo, a Finnish pediatrician, monographs were published that called attention to the special nature of the premature infant. Dr. Albrecht Peiper, from Germany, devoted much effort to the respiratory system. As a result of his work, the respiratory distress syndrome was described. Another German physician, Abraham Jacobi, came to the United States just before the turn of the century and played a leading role in establishing the specialty of pediatrics as a distinct entity. Because of these efforts, medical schools began to establish departments of pediatrics whose existence was to alter the care of all children. Later, Ethel Dunham reached prominence in this

---

[4] S.N. Graven & A.A. Fanaroff, *The Organization of Perinatal Health Services, in* Behrman's Neonatal-Perinatal Medicine 4–11 (1983); H. Abramson, *Foreword, in* Approach to the Medical Care of the Sick Newborn v–vii (1971); S.H. Pierog & A. Ferrara, *Preface, in* Approach to the Medical Care of the Sick Newborn ix, x (1971).

[5] A. Coombe, A Treatise on the Physiological and Moral Management of Infancy, for the Use of Parents (4th ed. 1845).

country by writing *Premature Infants, A Manual For Physicians.* While working at the Children's Bureau in Washington, D.C., Dr. Dunham and associates prepared many articles that served as the basis for the first edition of *Standards and Recommendations for Hospital Care of Newborn Infants, Full Term and Preterm.*[6] It is from here that modern neonatology has developed.

§ 18.3   —Special Care Nurseries

In the past, there was little consideration for the newborn patient during the initial hospital stay. From the standpoint of hospital administration, newborns were seemingly ignored or were treated as second-class patients, as evidenced by their receiving inferior accommodations and less skilled nursing staff. The newborn nursery equated to a warm bed, a rocking chair, and a grandmother-type figure. Essentially the same care was provided to all babies regardless of the fact that some infants were well and others were sick.

Public attention was drawn to the plight of premature infants when fee-for-entrance exhibits of these unfortunate beings were created. Probably the most widely publicized display exhibit was at the Chicago World's Fair in 1914. Whether these exhibits were designed and created in an attempt to provide these unique patients with care, to educate the public, or to feed the morbid curiosity of the onlookers remains a debatable issue.[7]

As the specialty of pediatrics emerged, more concern for the neonatal patient was aroused. The accumulation of new information led to revised caretaking methods that positively affected both mortality and morbidity. Modifications in standard medical treatments began to be implemented and continue as evidenced by the daily infusions of new facilities, staff, and equipment. While the warm bed remains, the rocking chair has been replaced with equipment that would make an astronaut nervous. Likewise, the grandmother figure is no more. In her place is a highly specialized nursing professional whose knowledge of neonatal problems and treatment is quite extensive, frequently to the point of being intimidating to nonneonatal health care professionals.

In the beginning, life support machinery originally designed for adults was modified in the attempt to provide the necessary equipment to treat these

---

[6] H.H. Gordon, *Perspectives in Neonatology, in* Neonatology: Pathophysiology and Management of the Newborn 3–6 (1981); E.H. Waschter & F.G. Blake, *Growth and Development of Health Services, in* Nursing Care of Children 2–9 (1976); H.B.P. Meyer, *Regional Care for Mothers and Their Newborns,* 7 Clinics Perinatology, no. 1, at 205–21 (1980).

[7] H.H. Gordon, *Perspectives in Neonatology, in* Neonatology: Pathophysiology and Management of the Newborn 3–6 (1981); E.H. Waschter & F.G. Blake, *Growth and Development of Health Services, in* Nursing Care of Children 2–9 (1976); American Academy of Pediatrics & The American College of Obstetricians & Gynecologists Committee on Fetus and Newborn, Committee on Obstetrics: Maternal and Fetal Medicine, *Organization of Perinatal Care, in* Guidelines for Perinatal Care. 1–14 (1983).

smaller patients. However, it soon became apparent that these infants were not
miniature adults but rather were physiologically quite different, both in sickness
and in health.[8] When presented with this challenge, the biomedical industry
attacked these problems with the vigor that only exists in a capitalistic society.
The result of this has been an explosion in the development of highly specialized
devices that are now available.[9] The neonatologist has been described as living
in a "sanctum of flashing lights, clicking machines, and hissing vapors."[10] Each
new species of equipment that evolves from this technologic womb is unique;
thus, today's intensive care nursery is a menagerie of these creations giving each
unit its own visual and auditory characteristics.

The cost of this technological explosion has been enormous. It is reflected in
the cost of the basic equipment for an intensive care unit.[11] (See **Appendix
18–4** in **§ 18.20.**) While the human element is the most important part of intensive care, it must be appreciated that adequate equipment is necessary for proper
patient care. It is not a luxury and should not be treated as such by those forces
that control capital expenditure. The dollar value of salvaging these infants has
been the topic of several investigative studies. To date, these analyses indicate
that it is a cost-effective approach, especially for all infants weighing more than
1,000 grams (2.2 pounds) at birth.[12] This type of analysis will likely continue in
the face of rising health care costs.

§ 18.4   Components of Intensive Care

Because the neonatal period does have substantially elevated mortality statistics,
all newborns should be considered high-risk. Therefore, all neonatal care should
be considered as being intensive. As in any field of medicine, there are varying
levels of intensity that may be needed. See **§ 18.11.**

Intensive care is a mixture of several different elements, including doctors,
nurses, respiratory therapists, and hospitals, each making its own contribution.

---

[8] W.E. Nelson, *The Field of Pediatrics: An Introduction to the Medical Problems of Infants and Children, in* Textbook of Pediatrics 1 (1969).

[9] Y.W. Branns, *Equipment Available for Nurseries,* 10 Clinics Perinatology, no. 1, at 263–79 (1983).

[10] Bergman, *Pediatric Education—For What?* 55 Pediatrics 109–13 (1975).

[11] K. Bajo, *Equipment Cost: The Neonatal Intensive Care Unit and the Modern Obstetric Unit,* 10 Clinics Perinatology, no. 1, at 175–187 (1983).

[12] P.R. Swyer, *The Organization of Perinatal Care with Particular Reference of the Newborn, in* Neonatology: Pathophysiology and Management of the Newborn 17–47 (1981); S.H. Pierog & A. Ferrara, *Administration and Organization of Newborn Services, in* Approach to the Medical Care of the Sick Newborn 14–27 (1971); W. Wynn & A. Wynn, Prevention of Handicap of Perinatal Origin: An Introduction to French Policy and Legislation (1976); E.J. Quilligan, A Study on Custodial Care from Connecticut State Hospitals (quoted in P.R. Swyer & J.W. Goodwin, Regional Services in Reproductive Medicine 13 (1973)).

The *Guidelines for Perinatal Care* published by the American Academy of Pediatrics and the American College of Obstetricians and Gynecologists provide a detailed description for each of these areas.[13] Because it is multifactorial, neonatal intensive care exists only when these individual components come together. The resulting care must be appropriate for the particular disease state. The key word in this statement is appropriate, a word whose meaning is in a state of constant change.

In describing the individual components of appropriate neonatal intensive care, each entity should be conceptualized as a player on the health care team. Each has the responsibility to perform certain tasks that, when adequately performed, will result in the best possible opportunity for the patient. A less than desirable outcome is always a possibility in any intensive care setting. Acceptance of human limitations is important when addressing the critically ill patient, for it is only by this approach that the stamina for continuance will be maintained. At times, even when each part of the team has performed its responsibilities well, complete success does not occur. It must be accepted by everyone concerned, including the family, that the patient received the best possible opportunity for an intact survival. If, however, a suboptimal outcome results because the team functioned poorly, then individual performances must be scrutinized and separately judged to determine where the error occurred.

§ 18.5 —Hospitals

When the term intensive care is mentioned, most people immediately think of a physical space inside a health care facility. Hospital corridors are clearly marked with directions to help find intensive care. Thus, it is here that the discussion should begin. As will be demonstrated through the following discussions, it requires more than a name to deliver neonatal intensive care.

§ 18.6 —Space

An *intensive care nursery* (ICN) is a physical space constructed of mortar, bricks, and steel; a space dedicated by the hospital for the provision of intensive care. Inside this shell, the remaining components of the team gather to perform their individual tasks. Without this space the game cannot be played and without the players the space is useless. Underallocation of space or inappropriate design can directly affect health care delivery in a variety of ways and, in so doing, can influence team members as they perform their jobs. Through careful study it has

---

[13] American Academy of Pediatrics & The American College of Obstetricians & Gynecologists Committee on Fetus and Newborn, Committee on Obstetrics: Maternal and Fetal Medicine, Guidelines for Perinatal Care (1983).

been determined that there are square footage and design requirements for appropriate intensive care areas.[14] See **Appendix 18–11** in **§ 18.27.** There is a vast amount of equipment, and personnel must have immediate access to the patient. Failure to appreciate these requirements may seriously limit patient visibility and access which, in turn, can affect the quality of care.

It is imperative that both the mechanical and the electrical designs of the area conform to recognized and published guidelines for ICN facilities. Heating, cooling, electrical power, lighting, and piped-in gases have specific criteria that must be met. For example, if there are not enough electrical outlets, it does not matter how good a piece of equipment really is. If it cannot receive power, it will not work. Additionally, the ICN should be on emergency power so that if the commercial power source is lost, the equipment can continue to provide its life-supporting functions.[15] Two brief experiences will bring this into better prospective. A major hospital was quite proud of its new ICN and the care that was being rendered, until a power failure occurred. When all life-support equipment ceased to function, the infants were placed in a very compromised situation. Respirators, monitors, and infusion pumps all had to be replaced with human power until a mechanism to bring emergency power into the unit could be implemented. Another prominent hospital was under construction when its problems occurred. The ICN was located in a temporary area during the construction of a new multimillion dollar unit. The temporary area had not originally been designed for the electrical workload that an ICN requires. Therefore, multiple-outlet extension cords were used to supply the additional recepticles. One day a nurse became quite excited when her infant's life-support equipment suddenly stopped. Close examination revealed that an extension cord had been moved around the room and someone had actually plugged this cord into its own receptacle box.

[14] D.S. Basler, *Principles of Building a Perinatal Center,* 10 Clinics Perinatology, no. 1, at 9–30 (1983); B.M. Thogmartin, *Major Architectural Considerations in Programming Perinatal Care Facilities,* 3 Clinics Perinatology, no. 2, at 337–48 (1976); American Academy of Pediatrics & The American College of Obstetricians & Gynecologists Committee on Fetus and Newborn, Committee on Obstetrics: Maternal and Fetal Medicine: *Physical Facilities for Perinatal Care, in* Guidelines for Perinatal Care 15–36 (1983); American Academy of Pediatrics Committee on Fetus and Newborn, *Physical Facilities for Care of Newborn Infants, in* Standards and Recommendations for Hospital Care of Newborn Infants 8–29 (1977).

[15] D.S. Basler, *Principles of Building a Perinatal Center,* 10 Clinics Perinatology, no. 1, at 9–30 (1983); B.M. Thogmartin, *Major Architectural Consideration in Programming Perinatal Care Facilities,* 3 Clinics Perinatology, no. 2, at 337–48 (1976); American Academy of Pediatrics & The American College of Obstetricians & Gynecologists Committee on Fetus and Newborn, Committee on Obstetrics: Maternal and Fetal Medicine, *Physical Facilities for Perinatal Care, in* Guidelines for Perinatal Care 15–36 (1983); American Academy of Pediatrics Committee on Fetus and Newborn, *Physical Facilities for Care of Newborn Infants, in* Standards and Recommendations for Hospital Care of Newborn Infants, 8–29 (1977); N.K. Edwards, *Specialized Electrical Grounding Needs,* 3 Clinics Perinatology, no. 2, at 367–74 (1976).

The amount and type of lighting and the colors used in nurseries are quite important. Experience has shown that evaluations of skin color are affected by these factors. For example, if the walls are blue, then the infants may appear to be cyanotic; if, on the other hand, the walls are painted yellow, then the infants may appear jaundiced.[16]

Many additional facets of nursery design are quite important as well. So complex are these areas that architectural specialists in the design of neonatal intensive care units have evolved. The in-depth study of ICN operations has provided these consultants with an abundance of expertise that is not available in any other resource person. To undertake the design of a new unit or the renovation of an existing one without consulting one of these experts is, in most situations, inviting a suboptimal outcome.

§ 18.7   —Equipment and Services

Many types of equipment are necessary adequately to provide the neonatal patient with appropriate intensive care. It may seem absurd to mention that the equipment should do what it is designed to do, but many neonatal equipment systems have been marketed that have subsequently proven to be inadequate.[17]

No nurse can physically perform all the necessary monitoring of vital signs every minute of every shift and accomplish other nursing responsibilities; thus, the importance of adequate monitors and alarms cannot be overstated. Additionally, monitors are not simply a backup system for the nurse; many are also diagnostic devices which allow continual display of important information such as electrical activity of the heart, respirations, and blood pressure.

The specific requirements for each type of equipment is dictated by the number of beds and the nature of the patients' illnesses. At a minimum, each intensive care bed requires the following baseline equipment:

1.   An open bed work surface with a radiant heater or incubator

2.   Cardiopulmonary monitors

---

[16] D.S. Basler, *Principles of Building a Perinatal Center,* 10 Clinics Perinatology, no. 1, at 9–30 (1983). B.M. Thogmartin, *Major Architectural Consideration in Programming Perinatal Care Facilities,* 3 Clinics Perinatology, no. 2, at 337–48 (1976). The American Academy of Pediatrics & The American College of Obstetricians & Gynecologists Committee on Fetus and Newborn, Committee on Obstetrics: Maternal and Fetal Medicine, *Physical Facilities for Perinatal Care, in* Guidelines for Perinatal Care 15–36 (1983); American Academy of Pediatrics Committee on Fetus and Newborn, *Physical Facilities for Care of Newborn Infants, in* Standards and Recommendations for Hospital Care of Newborn Infants 8–29 (1977).

[17] Y.W. Brans, *Planning a Perinatal Center: from Vision to Reality,* 10 Clinics Perinatology, no. 1, at 3–8 (1983); J.J. Pomerance, *Neonatal Intensive Care Unit: Basic Equipment Needs,* 3 Clinics Perinatology, no. 2, at 352–59 (1976); J.J. Pomerance & R.G. Duncan, *Neonatal Intensive Care Unit: Basic Equipment Needs for Neonatal Monitoring,* 10 Clinics Perinatology, no. 1, at 189–94 (1983).

3. Blood pressure monitoring devices (preferably for indwelling vascular lines)

4. Several infusion devices

5. Phototherapy lights

6. Respiratory support equipment including oxygen blender, humidification device, suction equipment, resuscitation bag and mask, oxyhood, devices for continuous positive airway pressure, respirator, and a device for the constant measurement of oxygen (either partial pressure or saturation).

Continuous sampling of end-tidal carbon dioxide, while not currently mandatory for state-of-the-art care, is available and will, in all probability, soon become another necessary item. Other immediately available equipment should include a laryngoscope with properly sized blades, endotracheal tubes of appropriate sizes, and a pair of infant size McGill forceps. Equipment and supplies for the many procedures necessary must also be stocked in the intensive care nursery (ICN) unit. A patient in a life-threatening emergency cannot wait for supplies to arrive from some distant central supply point.[18]

An intermediate care bed would certainly not require all the items listed above. These needs should be individualized for each unit's specific method of functioning as there is far less homogeneity between intermediate care beds from one institution to another. This is because intermediate care beds are used as stepdown beds for the ICN. Depending on the types of illness and number of patients needing admission, varying demands will be placed on the maximum care beds. However, it is not unrealistic to expect that all of the above equipment with the exception of the respiratory assistance devices, the continuous oxygen sampling equipment, and the indwelling blood pressure measuring apparatus should be provided.[19]

---

[18] American Academy of Pediatrics & The American College of Obstetricians & Gynecologists Committee on Fetus & Newborn, Committee on Obstetrics: Maternal and Fetal Medicine, *Physical Facilities for Perinatal Care, in* Guidelines for Perinatal Care 15–36 (1983); American Academy of Pediatrics Committee on Fetus and Newborn, *Physical Facilities for Care of Newborn Infants, in* Standards and Recommendations for Hospital Care of Newborn Infants 8–29 (1977); J.J. Pomerance, *Neonatal Intensive Care Unit: Basic Equipment Needs,* 3 Clinics Perinatology, no. 2, at 352–59 (1976); J.J. Pomerance & R.G. Duncan, *Neonatal Intensive Care Unit: Basic Equipment Needs for Neonatal Monitoring,* 10 Clinics Perinatology, no. 1, at 189–94 (1983).

[19] American Academy of Pediatrics & The American College of Obstetricians & Gynecologists Committee on Fetus and Newborn, Committee on Obstetrics: Maternal and Fetal Medicine, *Physical Facilities for Perinatal Care, in* Guidelines for Perinatal Care 15–36 (1983); American Academy of Pediatrics Committee on Fetus and Newborn, *Physical Facilities for Care of Newborn Infants, in* Standards and Recommendations for Hospital Care of Newborn Infants 8–29 (1977); J.J. Pomerance, *Neonatal Intensive Care Unit: Basic Equipment Needs,* 3 Clinics Perinatology, no. 2, at 352–59 (1976); J.J. Pomerance & R.G. Duncan, *Neonatal Intensive Care Unit: Basic Equipment Needs for Neonatal Monitoring,* 10 Clinics Perinatology, no. 1, at 189–94 (1983).

It is the responsibility of the hospital to provide adequate equipment and to ensure that it is properly maintained. Failure to do so may seriously compromise the ability of the team to perform adequately. Chronic tolerance of inferior performance or refusal to supply the necessary equipment is no less compromising to the patient than inferior medical or nursing care. Keeping the team concept in mind, equipment purchases must be based on evaluations by physicians, nurses, respiratory therapists, biomedical personnel, and administrative representatives rather than solely on input from one or two of these groups.[20]

While the human element of intensive care is the most important, it is highly impractical to assume that either the nurse or the doctor will always be able to compensate for equipment failures. If a bad outcome results from an electro-mechanical failure, who is to blame? To date, no piece of equipment made is perfect; thus, it behooves the staff to be familiar with the known shortcomings of each and to monitor constantly for them.[21] Monitoring the monitors is an important part of appropriate neonatal intensive care. If a system is to be successfully utilized, the staff must be knowledgeable in its use. A system that is inappropriately utilized is a serious problem, perhaps even more serious than not having a monitoring system at all. As a basis for this example, an inventory was conducted of the equipment being utilized on a patient with meconium aspiration syndrome complicated by persistent pulmonary hypertension. The infant's temperature was controlled by a radiant heater with its alarms. The ventilator had low pressure (patient disconnect) alarms, insufficient inspiratory/expiratory time indicators, and electrical failure alarms. The cardiorespiratory monitor had digital and waveform output for heartrate, respirations, and blood pressure. Alarms for low heart rate, high heart rate, *apnea* (cessation of respirations for greater than 15 seconds) and blood pressure were present. The patient was connected to five infusion devices (two arterial, two venous, and one piggyback) each with alarms for the following: device empty, source device empty, obstructed infusion, loss of power, and batteries low.

Appropriate neonatal intensive care lives in this microcosm of flashing lights and noisy alarms. It is a symbiotic relationship designed and proven to positively affect a patient's outcome. A piece of equipment that cannot adequately perform becomes a weak link in the chain, a weakness that must either be compensated or left to whatever consequences might occur.

There are hospital services that are mandatory if the newborn is to receive the best chance for an intact survival. See **Appendix 18–11** in § **18.27.**

---

[20] J.J. Pomerance & R.G. Duncan, *Neonatal Intensive Care Unit: Basic Equipment Needs for Neonatal Monitoring,* 10 Clinics Perinatology, no. 1, at 189–94 (1983); L. McKinnon, *Equipment Maintenance,* 3 Clinics Perinatology, no. 2, at 375–78 (1976).

[21] J.J. Pomerance, *Neonatal Intensive Care Unit: Basic Equipment Needs for Neonatal Monitoring,* 3 Clinics Perinatology, no. 2, at 352–59 (1976); J.J. Pomerance & R.G. Duncan, *Neonatal Intensive Care Unit: Basic Equipment Needs for Neonatal Monitoring,* 10 Clinics Perinatology, no. 1, at 189–94 (1983); L. McKinnon, *Equipment Maintenance,* 10 Clinics Perinatology, no. 2, at 375–78 (1976).

There must be the availability of prompt radiography on a 24-hour-a-day basis. Additionally, there must be the same accessibility to the laboratory for critical tests to be run stat. Blood collection should be performed by personnel trained in the unique problems of the infant as they pertain to phlebotomy. The necessity for around-the-clock blood banking services is also of paramount importance. Failure to have these services represents a serious reduction in the level of care that can be offered to the patient.[22]

§ 18.8   —Policies and Procedures

Another important area of hospital responsibility is the establishment and enforcement of unit policies and procedures. There should be guidelines for virtually every facet of hospital care. Even decisions about housekeeping activities such as how and when the floors are cleaned and what disinfectants to use are extremely important. Infection control policies are mandatory, as are employee health policies concerning working with contagious diseases. Without these standard operational designs and procedures, patient care may be seriously affected.[23] Consider the case when an intensive care nursery patient was exposed to chicken pox by a hospital employee. The individual had been exposed approximately two weeks before and had no knowledge of previously experiencing this disease. When the rash was noted, the individual immediately reported the situation but was instructed to return to work. Over the next 24 hours, the rash progressed and the employee was subsequently sent home. An exposed infant contracted the infection and died.[24] Who should be held accountable in this situation?

---

[22] S.N. Graven & A.A. Fanaroff, *The Organization of Perinatal Health Services, in* Behrman's Neonatal-Perinatal Medicine 4–11 (1983); The American Academy of Pediatrics Committee on Fetus and Newborn, *Personnel for Perinatal Services, in* Standards and Recommendations for Hospital Care of Newborn Infants 30–40 (1977); American Academy of Pediatrics & The American College of Obstetricians & Gynecologists Committee on Fetus and Newborn, Committee on Obstetrics: Maternal Fetal Medicine, *Personnel for Perinatal Services, in* Guidelines for Perinatal Care 37–46 (1983); C.J. Richardson, *Principles of Organization of a Neonatal Intensive Care Unit from Scratch,* 3 Clinics Perinatology, no. 2, at 329–35 (1976).

[23] American Academy of Pediatrics & The American College of Obstetricians & Gynecologists Committee on Fetus and Newborn, Committee on Obstetrics: Maternal and Fetal Medicine, *Control of Infections in Obstetric and Nursery Areas, in* Guidelines for Perinatal Care 106–62 (1983); American Academy of Pediatrics Committee on Fetus and Newborn, *Control of Infection, in* Standards and Recommendations for Hospital Care of Newborn Infants 109–29 (1977).

[24] Gustafson, Shehab & Brunell, *Outbreak of Varicella in a Newborn Intensive Care Nursery,* 138 Am. J. Diseases Children 548–550 (1984).

§ 18.9   —Nursing Staff

The nursing component to intensive care is of such importance that discussions could easily fill a book. The nurse is the glue that bonds the other elements of intensive care together. The nurse is the direct interface between patient and doctor and is also the primary pathway of patient communication with the environment. As the medically trained person who spends the most time with the patient, it is this individual whose observations and skills are so important both to the physician and to the patient. During the work period, not only are routine nursing duties performed (taking vital signs, giving medications, assisting in procedures, and so forth), but also very specialized knowledge and skills must be utilized if the patient is to do well.

Many neonatal problems are quite subtle in the initial presentation and their detection requires someone who has spent considerable time with the patient to notice them. Because some problems and subtle changes are unique to neonates, only someone with training and experience is able to recognize them. Without these nursing observations, the patient may not have a diagnosis made until more concrete signs and symptoms appear. The delay that results from this situation could be the difference between a good and a poor outcome.

Nurses who are pulled from one area of the hospital to another do not have the necessary experience to adequately function in anything more than the most basic level of neonatal care, and certainly should not be placed in a neonatal intensive care area. Another type of administrative device that is used to cover various patient care areas is the nurse who floats from one area to another, depending on the need. While pulls and floats may be necessary, neonatal intensive care is not an area to be staffed with these individuals. If done, this may result in a lower level of care for the patient(s) assigned to this person. Additionally, because of the uniqueness of neonatal intensive care, the regular staff may need to assist in virtually everything that these temporary, inexperienced individuals do, thereby diluting the care given to the other patients in the unit.

The unique nature of neonatal nursing and its specialized requirements are evidenced by the emergence of certifying exams for neonatal nurses and for neonatal nurse practitioners. These exams, which are a tangible sign of a nurse's knowledge, were first administered, respectively, in 1982 and 1983. Entrance to these examinations is gained only after completing the appropriate didactic and practical training.

Current guidelines indicate that an intensive care nursery (ICN) staff nurse should, at a minimum, be a registered nurse with specialized training in neonatology. Unfortunately, there is not a plethora of these individuals from which ICNs can recruit on an as-needed basis. But this scarcity should not be an excuse for accepting inferior nursing. Many units have attempted to fill the void by establishing training programs of their own. By so doing, nurses new to the area can be prepared by didactic and practical sessions for what they will be facing in the ICN.[25]

It is also important to realize that for many months new staff need experienced backup to assist them as they adapt to their new roles. Consider the following real life example. A newly graduated nurse is hired for the ICN. After receiving appropriate orientation, the nurse is assigned to what is classically the least desirable work period, the 11 P.M. to 7 A.M. shift. Traditionally, the night shift usually has the least amount of collective experience. If the new nurse has a question, there may be times when the other nurses will not know the appropriate answer. Therefore, either the question goes unanswered or at 2 A.M. a phone call is made to the only resource person available, the doctor. A question about a rather mundane area of care might precipitate a terse attitude in the doctor. While it is his or her patient and he or she should be concerned, the physician is likely to reject the concept that it is his or her sole responsibility to train nurses at night while the entire administrative nursing staff is sleeping! In the context of the borrowed servant doctrine, the doctor assumes that the hospital is furnishing his or her patient with an adequately trained individual, a point whose importance would be directly proportional to the condition of the patient. Should the doctor interview each nurse concerning the nurse's knowledge and abilities before allowing the nurse to participate in a patient's care? In that regard, does the doctor have the right to remove a nurse from caring for a patient? Does the patient have a right to expect that the patient's health care dollar is buying quality nursing care?

At times, depending on the situation, a nurse must be able to diagnose difficulties as well as initiate emergency treatment. An example of an emergency intervention by a nurse is the case of a patient who experiences sudden respiratory arrest. Another would be a ventilator-dependent patient who either becomes extubated or develops a plugged endotracheal tube. What would be the result if this is in a private hospital and the patient has to wait until the nurse can phone the doctor who must then physically get to the hospital and replace the life-supporting endotracheal tube? What about the infant with respiratory difficulties who, in this same private hospital setting, suddenly develops a spontaneous tension pneumothorax? In this situation, a delay of several minutes could be the difference between life or death. The nurse's ability to perform emergency decompression of this extravasated air is of paramount importance to that patient. These technical skills have been well recognized as falling within the scope of

---

[25] American Academy of Pediatrics Committee on Fetus and Newborn, *Personnel for Perinatal Services, in* Standards and Recommendations for Hospital Care of Newborn Infants 30–40 (1977); American Academy of Pediatrics & The American College of Obstetricians & Gynecologists Committee on Fetus and Newborn, Committee on Obstetrics: Maternal Fetal Medicine, *Personnel for Perinatal Services, in* Guidelines for Perinatal Care 37–46 (1983); S. Strickland, S. Spector, P. Hamlin-Cook, C. Hanna, C. Moore, L. Bellig & A. Fiorato, *Nurse Training and Staffing in the Neonatal Intensive Care Unit,* 7 Clinics Perinatology, no. 1, at 173–86 (1980).

neonatal nursing expertise.[26] If a patient has a suboptimal outcome due to a delay in instituting one of these treatment modalities, where does the fault belong? Should the physician be in the hospital for 24 hours a day while the patient is at risk for one of these complications? Does the hospital have an obligation to the patient and to the doctor to insure that someone on every shift has the necessary skills to stabilize these conditions? In the setting where neonatal physicians or trained neonatal nurse clinicians are not in-house around the clock, should the hospital and the doctor accept and continue to treat patients that require this high degree of sophisticated neonatal intensive care? If this type of intensive support cannot be given, where does the responsibility for this suboptimal approach rest? Is the hospital at fault for not providing the nurses with the necessary expertise? Or, is the doctor at fault for admitting and leaving a patient in an inadequate area? Should the hospital that fails to ensure the presence of these adequate in-house skills be reimbursed the same as one that does provide these resource people?

Another area of major importance concerns the concept of adequate nursing staffing patterns. Even the best nurse can be stretched beyond the point of competence when excessive demands are made. In an understaffed situation, the nurse can actually become a source of problems such as medication errors or failing to detect a subtle change in the patient's condition. References are available that cite the appropriate nurse-to-patient ratios for the various areas.[27] See **Appendix 18–5 in § 18.21.** Attesting to this importance is the fact that Medicaid regulations now determine eligibility for reimbursement as a special care area based on the number of nursing hours per patient day.[28] Where does the fault lie when a nursing error occurs because the nurse is overburdened? Is the nurse at fault for agreeing to work in this situation or is it the responsibility of the hospital for directing the nurse to work in such a situation?

§ 18.10 —Physicians

There is a saying, long used to justify the existence of pediatrics as a specialty— children are not simply small adults. They are physiologically different, both in

[26] L.L., *The Expanded Nursing Role in the Neonatal Intensive Care Unit,* 7 Clinics Perinatology, no. 1, at 159–71 (1980); R.E. Sheldon & P.S. Dominiak, *The Expanding Role of the Neonatal Nurses, in* The Expanding Role of the Nurse in Neonatal Intensive Care 11–15 (1980).

[27] American Academy of Pediatrics Committee on Fetus and Newborn, *Personnel for Perinatal Services, in* Standards and Recommendations for Hospital Care of Newborn Infants 30–40 (1977); American Academy of Pediatrics & The American College of Obstetricians & Gynecologists Committee on Fetus and Newborn, Committee on Obstetrics: Maternal Fetal Medicine, *Personnel for Perinatal Services, in* Guidelines for Perinatal Care 37–46 (1983).

[28] *Special Care Units/Intensive Care Type Units, in* 1 Medicare and Medicaid Guide 2054–56 (1983); R.H. Usher, *The Special Problems of the Premature Infant, in* Neonatology: Pathophysiology and Management of the Newborn 230–61 (1981).

sickness and in health. By paraphrasing this statement, the necessity for neonatology is made quite clear. Infants are not simply small children. However, this statement can again be modified to provide further justification for the existence of neonatology as a subspecialty. A 36-week infant is not the same as a term baby, a 34-week infant is not the same as a 36-week baby, a 32-week infant is not the same as a 34-week baby, and so on down to the limits of viability.[29] At each step along the gestational path there are significant differences in physiology. It is only by thoroughly understanding these differences that a given infant can be offered the best opportunity for intact survival. For example, all neonatologists will agree that it is inappropriate to treat all infants with respiratory distress in the same manner. To do so represents a pigeonhole approach to intensive care, an approach that is not capable of offering the best opportunity for an intact survival. Examples of this philosophy of patient care bring the suboptimal nature of this approach into sharper contrast. In a practitioner's office, the diagnosis of otitis media immediately equates to a certain dose of antibiotics given on a set time schedule. A sore throat that cultures Group A Streptococcus equates to treatment with a certain dose and duraction of penicillin. While this same degree of simplicity would be greatly appreciated by neonatal physicians, it simply is not possible. Each infant's treatment must be custom-tailored to the specific needs of that patient. It is the degree of custom-tailoring that acts as the basis for the three levels of intensive care that are discussed below. See §§ **18.12** to **18.14.**

The subspecialty of neonatology is a newcomer to the list of medical care disciplines. The first certifying exam was in 1975, and since that time exams have been offered every other year. Before there were fellowships and certified specialists, pediatricians with a special interest in the newborn provided care to this patient population. As the field of neonatology grew, fellowships were formalized and training became more uniform. With the establishment of neonatology as a sub-board of pediatrics, a further stimulus for uniform training was applied. Initially, those individuals who had not received formal training but who had spent considerable time in caring for neonates were accepted for testing. This was the grandfather clause method of training; however, that provision was only temporary and no longer exists. Today's certified neonatologist must be a graduate of a neonatal fellowship. This fellowship must be at least a three-year program and must be completed after the pediatric residency.[30] This specialized training provides the opportunity to take the sub-board examination. Additionally, it has been established that after 1985 all neonatal training programs have to be certified by the Residency Review Committee for Pediatrics in order for

---

[29] *Special Care Units/Intensive Care Type Units, in* 1 Medicare and Medicaid Guide 2054—56 (1983).

[30] American Academy of Pediatrics Committee on Fetus and Newborn, *Personnel for Perinatal Services, in* Standards and Recommendations for Hospital Care of Newborn Infants 30—40 (1977).

a graduate to be eligible. This review process represents another major step towards assuring the quality of neonatal training and of the individuals who do become subboard certified.

During the early years of neonatology, the tremendous explosion in the field generated huge demands for physician time spent in direct patient care. As a result, pediatric training programs found much of the resident's time spent in the intensive care nursery (ICN) area. Many individuals graduating from pediatric programs had more months of ICN experience than any other subspecialty. The American Board of Pediatrics has since ruled that no more than six months of a three-year pediatric residency can be spent in any single subspecialty.[31] Thus, the semineonatologists or super-pediatricians who were previously graduated will be no more.

Should every newborn be seen by a neonatologist? The immediate answer to this question is No. The routine newborn can be adequately cared for by the pediatrician or the family practitioner. However, as the newborn infant declares him or herself abnormal, the determination of who should be medically in charge is of paramount importance. In general, the patient who requires maximal intensive care (see § **18.14**) is sick enough to warrant a neonatologist. A baby whose illness is more intermediate (see §§ **18.12** to **18.13**) may require only consultative support to the primary physician. It is important to understand that it is the primary physician who is charged with the responsibility of initiating the referral to the neonatologist.

Many times it is not the limitations in the medical expertise of the physician but rather the limitations of his or her support that dictate the transport of a patient to another facility. A pediatrician with sufficient neonatal training may feel quite comfortable treating a baby with mild respiratory distress; however, if the nursing staff is not adequate, if blood gas analysis or radiology are not readily available, then the physician would be foolish to care for the infant in that facility. What will happen if the patient needs emergency intubation or develops a tension pneumothorax that requires emergency decompression? If the patient were to develop a problem that resulted in a poor outcome and if that problem was due to one of these deficiencies, it would be difficult to find justification for the doctor's failure to move the patient to a more appropriate facility. Most physicians spend the majority of their lives working for the good of patients. Balancing the factors that surround the decision to transfer the care of a patient is not easy. To move an infant away from the family is not without significant emotional cost, not to mention the dollar cost of intensive care. This is a problem in our health care system as it currently exists because not every facility is equipped and staffed to be a full service hospital.[32]

---

[31] American Academy of Pediatrics Task Force on Pediatric Education: The Future of Pediatric Education (1978).

[32] S.N. Graven & A.A. Fanaroff, *The Organization of Perinatal Health Services, in* Behrman's Neonatal-Perinatal Medicine 4–11 (1983); G.B. Avery, *The Morality of Drastic Intervention, in* Neonatology: Pathophysiology and Management of the Newborn 13–16 (1981).

The failure of a timely transfer may be based on medical ignorance, economics, medical politics, or ego, situations that this writer has personally witnessed.[33] To illustrate how medical politics enters the decision-making process, the following true example is used. Pediatricians are dependent on the referral of newborn patients from obstetricians, a fact long appreciated by both groups. If a newborn becomes distressed and the pediatrician feels that better care can be rendered in another facility, he or she may want to transfer the patient. However, the obstetrician, with intense loyalty to his or her hospital, may not want the baby moved. If the pediatrician transports the baby in spite of these feelings, he or she may find that newborn referrals not only from this obstetrician but also from other intensely loyal obstetricians are taken away and given to a pediatrician who is not quite so quick to transfer a baby. The following quote, taken from an obstetrician who shall remain anonymous, was made in just this type of situation and will be of interest: "I giveth, and, by God, I can taketh away!"

Hospitals and physicians must acknowledge their individual and collective deficiencies and must encourage patient transfer if better care is available. Refusal to transfer the patient may not result in a suboptimal outcome for nine cases out of 10, but what about the tenth patient? Neonatology has many procedures and policies that actually matter to only a few patients. However, since infants destined to have the suboptimal outcome often do not announce their intentions, these patient-care techniques are actually preventive measures. The care of any patient is subject to review; therefore, those involved must accept the fact that if a poor outcome results, review by specialists and subspecialists is possible. The more critical the patient's condition, the higher the probability for a poor outcome; and the poorer the outcome, the higher the probability of a critical review of the care. Failure of physicians and hospitals to address these issues internally is an open invitation for an external policing action.[34]

By whatever mechanism, the public has developed the idea that all medical care will yield a perfect result if done correctly. Anything that does not turn out perfectly, according to this logic, must be because of negligence. Neonatology, and medicine in general, are not pure sciences in which A + B = C. In those facets where medicine is a science, there are rules and guidelines that govern care; however, a significant part of this noble profession is still a true art form. As with artists around the world, some providers of medical care are more gifted

---

[33] S.N. Graven & A.A. Fanaroff, *The Organization of Perinatal Health Services, in* Behrman's Neonatal-Perinatal Medicine 4–11 (1983); G.B. Avery, *The Morality of Drastic Intervention, in* Neonatology: Pathophysiology and Management of the Newborn 13–16 (1981).

[34] P.R. Swyer, *The Organization of Perinatal Care with Particular Reference to the Newborn, in* Neonatology: Pathophysiology and Management of the Newborn 17–47 (1981); S.N. Graven & A.A. Fanaroff, *The Organization of Perinatal Health Services, in* Behrman's Neonatal-Perinatal Medicine 4–11 (1983); G.B. Avery, *The Morality of Drastic Intervention, in* Neonatology: Pathophysiology and Management of the Newborn 13–16 (1981); American Academy of Pediatrics Committee on Fetus and Newborn, *Regionalization of Perinatal Services, in* Standards and Recommendations for Hospital Care of Newborn Infants 1–7 (1977).

than others. But who can better appreciate the forces and energies that guide the artist, the critic or a fellow artist? In medicine, one quickly learns that there are several ways to approach a given problem, such as different schools of thought; in neonatology, this is even more true. While treatment differences in neonatal intensive care are very real, the known facts frequently do not demonstrate one approach as being more appropriate than the other. Therefore, only the neonatologist is capable of making the judgment that a given approach is within the scope of acceptable medical practice, even though he or she may not personally use that form of treatment.

§ 18.11   Levels of Neonatal Care

All newborns should be considered high-risk patients because of their elevated mortality rates. As such, they deserve special care. In determining what degree of expertise is required by the patient's problems, it is necessary to understand that health care delivery in this country operates on several different levels. This approach is necessary because not every community is capable of supporting all medical specialties and subspecialties. Because of this fact, a system that screens the patients based on the degree of medical need is the most effective. The term that is used to describe this approach is *regionalization.* In this concept, there are three levels of expertise. (See **Appendix 18–6** in **§ 18.22.**) Level I (primary) care is basic medicine and deals with routine patient problems. The next step on the ladder is Level II (intermediate) care where more skill is gathered to assist in problems not comfortably handled by Level I care. Level III (tertiary) care represents the point of maximal concentration of medical expertise. The Level III facility receives patients that require highly sophisticated care from the surrounding Level I and II units. An overview of these areas is presented in **Appendix 18–7** in **§ 18.23.**[35]

There are many things that intensive care does quite well; however, communication is not one of these. With such intense physical and mental energy being consumed by patient care, doctors and nurses may have difficulty remembering to communicate updates to the patient's family and to the referring physician. To the family, the referring doctor is known and trusted, and the family may continue to use him or her as an information source after the infant has been

---

[35] P.R. Swyer, *The Organization of Perinatal Care with Particular Reference to the Newborn, in* Neonatology: Pathophysiology and Management of the Newborn 17–47 (1981); S.N. Graven & A.A. Fanaroff, *The Organization of Perinatal Health Services, in* Behrman's Neonatal-Perinatal Medicine 4–11 (1983); American Academy of Pediatrics & The American College of Obstetricians & Gynecologists Committee on Fetus and Newborn, Committee on Obstetrics: Maternal and Fetal Medicine, *Organization of Perinatal Care, in* Guidelines for Perinatal Care 1–14 (1983); American Academy of Pediatrics Committee on Fetus and Newborn, *Regionalization of Perinatal Services, in* Standards and Recommendations for Hospital Care of Newborn Infants 1–7 (1977).

transferred to another doctor or facility. It then follows that the doctor needs current information to be successful in his or her interaction. Failure to communicate adequately among the members of this relationship is a problem that can only be solved by close cooperation between the various centers within a given region.

Another problem in communication that not only exists but also plays a major role in determining patient referral is fault finding, also called scape-goating. This is a term used to describe the assignment of blame for the patient's problems. For example, the family may be told that the infant's problems resulted because the obstetrician or the pediatrician did or did not do "such-and-so." In many cases this acts as the initiating event in an adversary relationship among the previous health care providers, the family, and/or the current health care team.[36] While intensive care personnel, both doctors and nurses, have a responsibility to provide the parents with information, it is most important that the information be as correct as possible. Incorrect judgmental information concerning the actions of others is never benign. It is important to realize that as the infant comes to the higher level of care, personnel at that level can only relate to past events through written and oral histories because they were not physically present at the time the events were happening. Thus, as with any event that is conveyed by written or spoken word, there is a possibility for error, omission, and bias. Therefore, judgments made on the basis of these written and spoken facts may not be valid. Whenever parents have questions about previous events, they should be encouraged to return to the physicians involved. In this manner they can ask their questions to those who were physically present. In this author's experience, the degree of fault finding expressed is inversely related to the age and experience of the physicians involved.

The consumer has a major responsibility in our health care system as it currently functions. In the United States, health care delivery is based on patients coming to doctors rather than the other way around. Thus, the timing of a patient's presentation is very important. Each clinical entity has a natural progression that may or may not include a stagnant phase. The physician, therefore, can only treat the problems as they are or will be, not as they were. A primary focus of neonatal medicine today is the prevention of problems. If prevention is not possible, difficulties must then be treated with the best action possible at the time. There is the distinct possibility that the opportunity to use the ideal treatment may be negated by a delay in patient presentation. Consider the situation where a pregnant woman cramps at home for 16 hours. She then presents to the emergency room where premature labor and a fetus in breech presentation are documented. While surgical delivery of this type of pregnancy is ideal, it cannot

---

[36] Freeman, Bostwick, Laros, Roberts & Schuering, *When Birth Injuries Prompt Malpractice Suits,* 24 Contemp. OB/GYN 150–69 (1984).

be performed if the fetal parts are at the introitus at the time the woman seeks medical help.[37]

§ 18.12   —Level I

Level I care is usually the initial point of interface between patients and medicine. This care may be given in a sparsely populated area or it may be in a major metropolitan area. The primary responsibilities of Level I care are the treatment of uncomplicated patients and the identification of high-risk patients by screening for problems, either real or potential. Every newborn is at risk for a potential complication and it is the early identification of this problem that is so important for proper management.

For a newborn, the presence of a nursery admission area is quite important. The newborn should be considered a recovering patient for the first 24 hours of life or until adequately stabilized. The ability to perform an accurate initial assessment of gestational age and to recognize neonatal problems is mandatory. Only by understanding how the newborn adapts to this new extrauterine environment and what problems may be encountered in the transition can the nursing staff adequately address the needs of the patient. **Appendix 18–8** in **§ 18.24** lists disorders that will frequently necessitate transferring the patient to a higher level of care.[38]

Newborn care should be consistent with the recommendations of the American Academy of Pediatrics. Personnel working in the normal newborn area should be skilled in recognizing common problems such as jaundice or cyanosis and should be capable of managing emergencies until assistance can arrive. There must be the capability to resuscitate the infant if needed. Obviously, this resuscitation would require proper equipment for ventilatory support as well as drugs and supplies for the infusion of medications. Staffing guidelines are

---

[37] P.R. Swyer, *The Organization of Perinatal Care with Particular Reference to the Newborn, in* Neonatology: Pathophysiology and Management of the Newborn 17–47 (1981); S.N. Graven & A.A. Fanaroff, *The Organization of Perinatal Health Services, in* Behrman's Neonatal-Perinatal Medicine 4–11 (1983).

[38] American Academy of Pediatrics Committee on Fetus and Newborn, *Personnel for Perinatal Services, in* Standards and Recommendations for Hospital Care of Newborn Infants 30–40 (1977); American Academy of Pediatrics & The American College of Obstetricians & Gynecologists Committee on Fetus and Newborn, Committee on Obstetrics: Maternal Fetal Medicine, Personnel for Perinatal Care 37–46 (1983); American Academy of Pediatrics Committee on Fetus and Newborn, *Interhospital Care of the High-Risk Infant, in* Standards and Recommendations for Hospital Care of Newborn Infants 130–46 (1977); American Academy of Pediatrics & The American College of Obstetricians & Gynecologists Committee on Fetus and Newborn, Committee on Obstetrics: Maternal and Fetal Medicine, *Perinatal Care Services, in* Guidelines for Perinatal Care 47–96 (1983).

shown in **Appendix 18–5** in **§ 18.21** and should usually be based on the ratio of one professional nurse and one nonprofessional staff per 12 to 16 infants.[39]

In order to function properly, certain hospital services must be available. Radiology support is needed on a 24-hour basis and should include portable equipment that can come to the patient rather than vice versa. Laboratory services are needed around the clock to perform bilirubin, glucose, electrolyte, hematocrit, and calcium determinations. The ability to perform blood gas analysis is highly desirable.[40]

At times, it is necessary to deliver a high-risk infant at a Level I facility. In these cases, every effort should be made to have a physician skilled in neonatal resuscitation available for the infant. Because it will not always be possible to have an additional physician present, someone skilled in newborn resuscitation should be present to assist the delivering physician. Additionally, there are times when an unexpected problem arises. Because this situation is not always predictable, standard operational procedures (contingency plans) for prompt action should exist and should be instantly implemented. It would be most naive for a primary care area to suppose that a problem will never happen. By the very nature of a Level I unit, one of limited medical expertise, there will be instances when the patient will require more care than can be provided at that facility. Failure to plan properly for these unexpected situations and to document the effectiveness of the plan is a failure to offer the infant the best chance for intact survival.

Consolidation of Level I health care centers with limited patient activity is advocated, but has not been universally accomplished.[41] Many small units

---

[39] American Academy of Pediatrics Committee on Fetus and Newborn, *Personnel for Perinatal Services, in* Standards and Recommendations for Hospital Care of Newborn Infants 30–40 (1977).

[40] P.R. Swyer, *The Organization of Perinatal Care with Particular Reference to the Newborn, in* Neonatology: Pathophysiology and Management of the Newborn 17–47 (1981); S.N. Graven & A.A. Fanaroff, *The Organization of Perinatal Health Services, in* Behrman's Neonatal-Perinatal Medicine 4–11 (1983); S.H. Peirog & A. Ferrara, *Administration and Organization of Newborn Services, in* Approach to the Medical Care of the Sick Newborn 14–27 (1971); American Academy of Pediatrics Committee on Fetus and Newborn, *Personnel for Perinatal Services, in* Standards and Recommendations for Hospital Care of Newborn Infants 30–40 (1977); American Academy of Pediatrics & The American College of Obstetricians & Gynecologists Committee on Fetus and Newborn, Committee on Obstetrics: Maternal Fetal Medicine, *Personnel for Perinatal Services, in* Guidelines for Perinatal Care 37–46 (1983).

[41] P.R. Swyer, *The Organization of Perinatal Care with Particular Reference to the Newborn, in* Neonatology: Pathophysiology and Management of the Newborn 17–47 (1981); S.N. Graven & A.A. Fanaroff, *The Organization of Perinatal Health Services, in* Behrman's Neonatal-Perinatal Medicine 4–11 (1983); American Academy of Pediatrics & The American College of Obstetricians & Gynecologists Committee on Fetus and Newborn, Committee on Obstetrics: Maternal and Fetal Medicine, *Physical Facilities for Perinatal Care, in* Guidelines for Perinatal Care 15–36 (1983); J.J. Pomerance & R.G. Duncan, *Neonatal Intensive Care Unit: Basic Equipment Needs for Neonatal Monitoring,* 10 Clinics Perinatology, No. 1, at 189–94 (1983).

remain, even in large cities. The reasons for their continued existence include economics, politics, and religion, to list a few. These small and infrequently utilized centers are a source for potential problems if strict attention is not paid to maintaining the standard of care. A portion of health care consumers are medically informed and understand that the mere offering of medical services is not always associated with the same level of care. However, this fact is not always appreciated by the majority of the public when a less expensive alternative is very attractive, especially to those on the lower end of the economic spectrum. These consumers usually do not have the information necessary to judge the care. They merely assume that after presenting themselves to a doctor or a hospital, they will get whatever care they need. As a consumer, one would be wise to remember the old saying, "you get what you pay for." **Appendixes 18–7** in **§ 18.23** and **18–11** in **§ 18.27** summarize the basic requirements for a Level I facility.

§ 18.13   —Level II

Level II care units should have the same capabilities as Level I units and, in addition, they should be able to care for several complicated problems. Because of its position in the health-care pyramid, this unit will have an influx of patients not only from Level I but also from Level III facilities. Those patients returning from Level III care will have successfully traversed their critical period. This extra patient-care responsibility requires that another area be included in the nursery design, the intermediate or continuing care area. The capability to provide continuing care for infants needing to remain in the hospital for further growth and development is a major responsibility. The reason for such a large emphasis being directed towards caring for infants in a feed and grow state is very simple. Most critical and life-threatening neonatal processes are over rather quickly, one way or the other. Thus, there may be a prolonged period between the patient being very seriously ill and being ready for discharge. Additionally, this area should be staffed and equipped to stabilize critically ill newborns prior to their transport to a Level III facility. **Appendixes 18–7** in **§ 18.23** and **18–11** in **§ 18.27** contain a synopsis of the requirements for a Level II facility. **Appendix 18–9** in **§ 18.25** lists those conditions that would typically necessitate transfer from a Level II to a Level III unit.[42]

---

[42] P.R. Swyer, *The Organization of Perinatal Care with Particular Reference to the Newborn, in* Neonatology: Pathophysiology and Management of the Newborn 17–47 (1981); S.N. Graven & A.A. Fanaroff, *The Organization of Perinatal Health Services, in* Behrman's Neonatal-Perinatal Medicine 4–11 (1983); S.H. Peirog & A. Ferrara, *Administration and Organization of Newborn Services, in* Approach to the Medical Care of the Sick Newborn 14–27 (1971); American Academy of Pediatrics Committee on Fetus and Newborn, *Personnel for Perinatal Services, in* Standards and Recommendations for Hospital Care of Newborn Infants 30–40 (1977); American Academy of Pediatrics & The American College of Obstetricians & Gynecologists Committee on Fetus and Newborn, Committee on Obstetrics: Maternal Fetal Medicine,

The organizational and operational design of the nursing service is very important to a unit functioning adequately as a Level II facility. The staff should include a head professional nurse, preferably one with an advanced degree in pediatric or neonatal nursing, who has a great deal of experience and training in the care of sick infants. The personnel working in the Level II unit should be knowledgeable in the observation and treatment of moderately severe neonatal problems. In addition to the skills listed under Level I, these nurses should be trained in the provision of cardiorespiratory monitoring, in providing assisted ventilation, and in the infusion of fluids and medications. Additionally, these nurses must be able to adequately assist, and sometimes perform, certain procedures, especially those that pertain to life-threatening conditions. These skills are very important in the Level II setting where constant physician presence is unlikely. In many situations it may be necessary for these nurses to be skilled in transport because they may be required to participate in the movement of infants among the various units within the referral system. Acquisition of these skills can only come from advanced didactic training and practical experience. Staffing numbers should conform to published guidelines (see **Appendix 18–5** in **§ 18.21**) which in most situations will equate to one professional nurse for every two to four infants.[43]

The unit should have a physician who serves as the medical director of that facility. This individual should be a board-certified pediatrician with special interest, experience, and, in some situations, subspecialty certification in neonatal medicine.[44] Administrative functions of the medical director should include working with the hospital and medical staff to develop policies concerning equipment, supplies, and procedures for the unit. In addition to caring for his or her own patients, the medical director should also be available for consultation with other physicians whose patients are admitted to the area.[45]

Personnel for Perinatal Services, in Guidelines for Perinatal Care 37–46 (1983); American Academy of Pediatrics Committee on Fetus and Newborn, *Interhospital Care of the High-risk Infant, in* Standards and Recommendations for Hospital Care of Newborn Infants 130–46 (1977); American Academy of Pediatrics & The American College of Obstetricians & Gynecologists Committee on Fetus and Newborn, Committee on Obstetrics: Maternal and Fetal Medicine, Perinatal Care 47–96 (1983).

[43] American Academy of Pediatrics Committee on Fetus and Newborn, *Personnel for Perinatal Services, in* Standards and Recommendations for Hospital Care of Newborn Infants 30–40 (1977); American Academy of Pediatrics & The American College of Obstetricians & Gynecologists Committee on Fetus and Newborn, Committee on Obstetrics: Maternal Fetal Medicine, *Personnel for Perinatal Services, in* Guidelines for Perinatal Care 37–46 (1983).

[44] American Academy of Pediatrics & The American College of Obstetricians & Gynecologists Committee on Fetus and Newborn, Committee on Obstetrics: Maternal Fetal Medicine, *Personnel for Perinatal Services, in* Guidelines for Perinatal Care 37–46 (1983).

[45] American Academy of Pediatrics Committee on Fetus and Newborn, *Personnel for Perinatal Services, in* Standards and Recommendations for Hospital Care of Newborn Infants 30–40 (1977); American Academy of Pediatrics & The American College of Obstetricians & Gynecologists Committee on Fetus and Newborn, Committee on Obstetrics: Maternal Fetal Medicine, Personnel for Perinatal Care 37–46 (1983).

Support of the more sophisticated problems encountered in a Level II nursery requires additional capabilities besides those listed for the Level I unit. The more important of these include:

1. 24-hour capability to provide an enriched oxygen environment to the patient and to measure the amount of oxygen being administered
2. 24-hour capability to monitor the patient's blood gases
3. 24-hour capability for short-term respiratory assistance
4. The ability to administer intravascular fluids by controlled infusion devices
5. The ability to monitor cardiopulmonary functions with appropriate equipment
6. The ability to monitor blood pressure
7. The ability to monitor and maintain surface and core body temperature
8. The ability to perform exchange transfusions

By necessity, Level II units will have individual areas of expertise. Thus, the supporting capabilities will need to be adapted to the unique nature of that particular unit.[46]

The Level II unit has great potential for major problems and difficulties. Because the Level II unit is accustomed to caring for less than routine infants, there is the possibility that inordinate delays in transferring the patient to a Level III unit may occur. One reason for this is that many neonatal conditions are transient in nature. If a patient can be spared the ordeal of transport, then the patient, the family, the hospital, and the doctor are winners physically, emotionally, and financially.[47] But, in those situations in which the disease is not transient but rather is progressive, this delay might result in the transport of a more critically ill patient whose outcome may not be optimal. As an example, the following case will be useful. A patient was transferred from a Level II to a Level III facility at two days of age. At the Level II unit the infant was initially felt to be slightly premature and to be experiencing transient tachypnea of the newborn. This is a respiratory condition characterized by mild difficulties and generally requires only supplemental oxygen therapy for 24 hours or less. When the infant

---

[46] American Academy of Pediatrics Committee on Fetus and Newborn, *Personnel for Perinatal Services, in* Standards and Recommendations for Hospital Care of Newborn Infants 30–40 (1977); American Academy of Pediatrics & The American College of Obstetricians & Gynecologists Committee on Fetus and Newborn, Committee on Obstetrics: Maternal Fetal Medicine, Personnel for Perinatal Care 37–46 (1983).

[47] S.N. Graven & A.A. Fanaroff, *The Organization of Perinatal Health Services, in* Behrman's Neonatal-Perinatal Medicine 4–11 (1983); R.G. Harper, M.M. Sokal, & C.G. Sia, *Mothers in the Neonatal Intensive Care Unit: An Examination of Some Problems and Consequences of Modern Intensive Care on Mother-Infant Interaction,* 3 Clinics Perinatology, no. 2, at 441–46 (1976).

developed complicating bilateral pneumothoraces and had severe clinical deterioration, he was transferred to a Level III unit. In the Level III unit, the infant was noted to be suffering from severe respiratory distress syndrome and could not be stabilized even with the use of a ventilator and 100 percent oxygen. After a short period of time, the patient expired. Perhaps earlier transport would have altered the disease course and the outcome.

§ 18.14   —Level III

The Level III unit represents the top of the pyramid in the concept of regionalization. It is here that the resources should be available to manage any neonatal conditions that may arise. Many articles have been written about the requirements of a Level III facility, and these criteria are summarized in **Appendixes 18–7** in **§ 18.23** and **18–11** in **§ 18.27**.[48] Indeed, the proper functioning of this facility does require a tremendous amount of effort from physicians, nurses, paraprofessionals, and administrative personnel.

Physician involvement is both health care and administrative in nature. The regional intensive care unit

> should be directed by a full-time, board-certified pediatrician with special competence and, in most cases, subspecialty certification in neonatal medicine . . . [T]hese physicians are responsible for maintenance of standards of patient care, development of the operating budget, equipment evaluation and purchase, planning and development of . . . educational programs, and evaluation of the effectiveness of perinatal care in the region.[49]

Other physicians with similar training and experience may be needed to assist the medical director in either patient care or in administrative duties. In addition to a full complement of pediatric subspecialists, consultative support from the various subspecialty areas of anesthesia, surgery, internal medicine, and genetics must also be obtainable.[50]

---

[48] P.R. Swyer, *The Organization of Perinatal Care with Particular Reference to the Newborn, in* Neonatology: Pathophysiology and Management of the Newborn 17–47 B. (1981). S.N. Graven & A.A. Fanaroff, *The Organization of Perinatal Health Services, in* Behrman's Neonatal-Perinatal Medicine 4–11 (1983). American Academy of Pediatrics Committee on Fetus and Newborn, *Personnel for Perinatal Services, in* Standards and Recommendations for Hospital Care of Newborn Infants 30–40 (1977); American Academy of Pediatrics & The American College of Obstetricians & Gynecologists Committee on Fetus and Newborn, Committee on Obstetrics: Maternal Fetal Medicine, *Personnel for Perinatal Services, in* Guidelines for Perinatal Care 37–46 (1983).

[49] American Academy of Pediatrics & The American College of Obstetricians & Gynecologists Committee on Fetus and Newborn, Committee on Obstetrics: Maternal Fetal Medicine, *Personnel for Perinatal Services, in* Guidelines for Perinatal Care 37–46 (1983).

[50] P.R. Swyer, *The Organization of Perinatal Care with Particular Reference to the Newborn, in* Neonatology: Pathophysiology and Management of the Newborn 17–47 (1981); S.N. Graven

Nursing service support should begin with a supervisor of nurses who has obtained an advanced degree that satisfies the qualifications for a designation of clinical nurse specialist. Staff nurses in the intensive care nursery (ICN) should be baccalaureate degree recipients who have received additional didactic training and practical experience. Abilities that are required include those previously described under Level II care plus highly developed skills in:

1. Cardiopulmonary monitoring
2. The equipment and techniques of respiratory support
3. The equipment and techniques for administering fluids and medications
4. The equipment and techniques for dealing with intravenous and intra-arterial catheters
5. The diagnosis and treatment of life-threatening conditions such as seizures, apnea, extubation, and pulmonary air leaks
6. The preoperative stabilization and postoperative recovery of neonatal patients.

Staffing patterns should be consistent with those guidelines previously established as necessary for good patient care. See **Appendix 18–5** in **§ 18.21.** This usually equates to one nurse for every one to two infants.[51] In addition to the doctors and nurses, many other areas of expertise are needed in the Level III facility. Respiratory therapists skilled in caring for infants who are experiencing respiratory difficulties should be present in the unit. Staffing must be adjusted depending on the number of infants and their individual needs. However, it is recommended that there be one therapist for every four infants who are receiving respiratory assistance. Additional support should include support from social services, a nutritionist, and clerical staff to accommodate the abundance of paperwork that a busy ICN generates.[52]

& A.A. Fanaroff, *The Organization of Perinatal Health Services, in* Behrman's Neonatal-Perinatal Medicine 4–11 (1983); S.H. Pierog & A. Ferrara, *Administration and Organization of Newborn Services, in* Approach to the Medical Care of the Sick Newborn 14–27 (1971); American Academy of Pediatrics Committee on Fetus and Newborn, *Personnel for Perinatal Services, in* Standards and Recommendations for Hospital Care of Newborn Infants 30–40 (1977); American Academy of Pediatrics & The American College of Obstetricians & Gynecologists Committee on Fetus and Newborn, Committee on Obstetrics: Maternal Fetal Medicine, *Personnel for Perinatal Services, in* Guidelines for Perinatal Care 37–46 (1983).

[51] American Academy of Pediatrics Committee on Fetus and Newborn, *Personnel for Perinatal Services, in* Standards and Recommendations for Hospital Care of Newborn Infants 30–40 (1977); American Academy of Pediatrics & The American College of Obstetricians & Gynecologists Committee on Fetus and Newborn, Committee on Obstetrics: Maternal Fetal Medicine, *Personnel for Perinatal Services, in* Guidelines for Perinatal Care 37–46 (1983).

[52] P.R. Swyer, *The Organization of Perinatal Care with Particular Reference to the Newborn, in* Neonatology: Pathophysiology and Management of the Newborn 17–47 (1981); S.N. Graven & A.A. Fanaroff, *The Organization of Perinatal Health Services, in* Behrman's Neonatal-Perinatal Medicine 4–11 (1983); S.H. Pierog & A. Ferrara, *Administration and Organization of*

An additional area that deserves special discussion is the psychological support of the staff. A major focus of this support is to prevent situations that lead to burnout. This is a syndrome characterized by both emotional and physical exhaustion. While burnout can be seen in many professions, it occurs with great frequency and is very familiar to those individuals working in intensive care. Doctors, nurses, and all support personnel involved with patients and their families are targets.

There are multiple factors that contribute to this problem. A major contributor to the stress of working in intensive care is the emotional factor. Life in the ICN is quite literally an emotional roller coaster. Patients and staff may experience life and death situations several times a day that, depending on the outcome, can precipitate feelings of joy or inadequacy. Also, ethical issues are faced on a recurring basis and represent additional stress factors. Making decisions about whether or not to resuscitate a severely brain damaged infant or about offering advanced life support techniques to a severely immature infant are quite difficult.

Interacting with families of ICN patients is another major source of stress. As the family attempts to cope with the problem of having a critically ill infant, family members may handle their stress in different ways. They may completely resist becoming involved with the infant or they may express their frustrations and fear by abusing staff members.

Whenever the ICN staff must deal with other support areas of the hospital, this can also be stressful. Because these support areas may not be immediately available or may not respond exactly as the ICN demands, staff members may feel isolated or discriminated against, a situation that adds stress to their lives.

The problem of burnout can be reflected in both interpersonal relations and patient care. The following list of characteristics is quoted from a discussion related to nursing personnel but is equally applicable to all members of the intensive care team:

1. Feeling helpless, impotent, and unable to cope
2. Suffering from exhaustion, fatigue, and becoming physically rundown
3. Manifesting frequent physical symptoms, such as headaches, gastrointestinal upsets, weight loss, sleeplessness, depression, and shortness of breath

---

Newborn Services, in Approach to the Medical Care of the Sick Newborn 14–27 (1971); American Academy of Pediatrics Committee on Fetus and Newborn, *Personnel for Perinatal Services, in* Standards and Recommendations for Hospital Care of Newborn Infants 30–40 (1977); American Academy of Pediatrics & The American College of Obstetricians & Gynecologists Committee on Fetus and Newborn, Committee on Obstetrics: Maternal Fetal Medicine, *Personnel for Perinatal Services, in* Guidelines for Perinatal Care 37–46 (1983); J.E. Wimmer & D.G. Parsons, *Respiratory Therapy in the Neonatal Intensive Care Unit,* 3 Clinics Perinatology, no. 2, at 379–90 (1976); M. Sherman, *Psychiatry in the Neonatal Intensive Care Unit,* 7 Clinics Perinatology, no. 1, at 33–46.

4. Becoming silent, a noncontributor at staff meetings; this applies especially to someone who is ordinarily talkative

5. Exhibiting a quick temper, instant irritation, and frustration

6. Demonstrating suspicious attitudes from which paranoia may evolve

7. Becoming rigid and closed; the nurse's thinking is inflexible and change becomes impossible

8. Exhibiting a decrease in risk-taking behavior or exhibiting an increase in risk-taking; he or she may act without regard to the consequences

9. Developing a negative attitude; he or she becomes the staff cynic

10. Becoming disagreeable; someone who bad-mouths any creative ideas

11. Becoming cynical regarding his or her own work and organization

12. Fighting the system in an unproductive manner

13. Manifesting an increase in personal problems including alcoholism or drug abuse, mental illness, family conflict, and suicide

14. Being unable to relax

15. Moving away from others and problems in the following ways: moving away from clinical practice into an administrative or teaching position, reducing personal involvement with clients and others, diminishing socialization with other staff members, and minimizing physical contact

16. Manifesting reduction in initiative so that his or her work becomes less efficient, particularly in times of stress.[53]

As the personnel are affected, the operation of the ICN is also compromised by the emergence of problems directly related to burnout. There can be an increase in the amount of interpersonal problems in the unit and between other service areas. The amount of time spent away in sick time may leave the unit short on staff. The number of accidents and judgmental errors can increase. The possibility of difficulties with the family is also very real, a factor that can be the cornerstone for future anger and hostility on the part of the parents.[54]

Only by having an appreciation of this complex and important syndrome can one adequately relate to the ICN staff. This is especially true if the question of medical negligence is involved. Because the intensive care team is usually deeply involved with being neonatal advocates, a challenge concerning the quality of patient care will probably be a very emotional issue. For the person experiencing, or close to experiencing, burnout, this additional stress may precipitate the full-blown clinical syndrome. Therefore, as the question of negligence is

---

[53] M.L. Duxbury, *The Role of the Nurse in Neonatology: Theoretical and Administrative Considerations, in* Neonatology: Pathophysiology and Management of the Newborn 50–51 (1981).

[54] S.N. Graven & A.A. Fanaroff, *The Organization of Perinatal Health Services, in* Behrman's Neonatal-Perinatal Medicine 4–11 (1971); M.L. Duxbury, *The Role of the Nurse in Neonatology: Theoretical and Administrative Considerations, in* Neonatology: Pathophysiology and Management of the Newborn 50–51 (1981).

addressed, bizarre behavior may occur. In these situations, it may be necessary
to perform substantial background research before there can be an appreciation
of the current events. Failure to obtain this information can be a major mistake.

§ 18.15   Gaining Access to Intensive Care

A statement commonly made by visitors to intensive care nursery units is that
they had no idea such a place existed. This is not surprising in view of the relatively young age of neonatal intensive care. While there has been a recent
increase in media attention to the fetus and newborn, there are still large segments of the population that have not been enlightened. Because of this fact,
there is a very real possibility that a newborn's family will lack the knowledge to
judge how severe a problem is and what degree of expertise is needed to provide
adequate care. Typically, the family presents itself for medical care to a person
or to a place it knows and trusts; it places its care in the hands of the physician
and the hospital that will, it assumes, do all that is necessary to deal with the
problem.

It is the health care providers who are saddled with the responsibility of
deciding what type of patient can be treated and which ones should be transferred to another facility or to another physician's care. Each decision must be
carefully considered before reaching a conclusion. Bringing in a new physician
or moving the patient to another facility is an enormous emotional experience
for everyone concerned. However, failure to consult or transfer the patient must
be accompanied by the acceptance of the position taken. The unstated position
of failure to transfer is that no better care is immediately available. In critical situations just as in routine ones, all members of the health care team must expect
and accept that their care may be closely scrutinized and must be comfortable
that it will pass such a review.

Because the burden of referral usually does rest with health care providers
(doctors and hospitals), the attempt to make referral within a given region should
be virtually automatic. All Level I and II units, by reason of their designations,
can expect that some patients will require medical care exceeding their capabilities. It then follows that a clear line of referral should exist so that when these
patients present themselves, their transport will be accomplished smoothly and
without delay. By not having this pattern established, patients with severe and
potentially life-threatening conditions may be delayed in receiving appropriate
care.[55] Failure to have solid lines of consultation and referral by the Level I and
Level II units could be construed as an attitude that it is the patient's bad luck to

---

[55] S.N. Graven & A.A. Fanaroff, *The Organization of Perinatal Health Services, in* Behrman's
Neonatal-Perinatal Medicine 4–11 (1983); Freeman, Bostwick, Laros, Roberts & Schuering,
When Birth Injuries Prompt Malpractice Suits, 24 Contemp. OB/GYN 150–69 (1984); R.E.
Marshall & C. Kasman, *Burnout, in* Coping with Caring for Sick Newborns 5–14 (1982).

exceed their capabilities and that the patient will just have to take whatever care is available until referral can be arranged.

§ 18.16   —Transport to Intensive Care

Initially, infant transport consisted of an ambulance rushing to pick up a patient at a referring hospital and then rushing to get the patient back to intensive care. This method of transport is based on the concept of getting the patient to intensive care as rapidly as possible. In recent years this concept has undergone a philosophical metamorphosis. Currently, the thrust of transport is to get intensive care to the patient as soon as possible. The change in approach evolved in an effort to prevent many of the problems and complications experienced while the infants were physically en route to the Level III unit.[56] The best mechanism for transport is the intrauterine method, maternal transport.[57] When this is not possible, today's neonatal transport team should bring with it all the specialized equipment, supplies, and skills to handle virtually any emergency situation. In this way the infant is stabilized prior to leaving the referral hospital, a procedure that minimizes the risks of problems during the actual transport.

The composition of the transport team varies depending upon the setting. Some centers feel that physicians should be present on every transport. However, many Level III units use trained neonatal nurses or neonatal nurse practitioners for their transports with physicians accompanying the patient only on selected trips. Additional personnel such as a respiratory therapist may be necessary if the infant has a specific type of problem such as respiratory distress. The team should be specially trained in neonatal transport, as it has been proven that undereducated personnel are a potential risk to the patient.[58]

The equipment for transport has special needs because of the unique situations that it will face. It must be reliable and capable of safe and easy movement. Typically, a commercially available transporter serves as the transport incubator. To this are added monitors, a respirator, and infusion pumps, all of which must

---

[56] J.A. Cannon, *Neonatal Transport, in* Neonatology: Pathophysiology and Management of the Newborn 53–59 (1981); W.T. Greene, *Organization of Neonatal Transport Services in Support of a Regional Referral Center,* 7 Clinics Perinatology, no. 1, at 187–95 (1980).

[67] S.N. Graven & A.A. Fanaroff, *The Organization of Perinatal Health Services, in* Behrman's Neonatal-Perinatal Medicine 4–11 (1983).

[58] S.M. Donn et al., *Emergency Transport of the Critically Ill Newborn, in* 58 Neonatal Emergencies 75–86 (S.M. Donn & R.G. Faix eds., 1991); Freeman, Bostwick, Laros, Roberts & Schuering, *When Birth Injuries Prompt Malpractice Suits,* 24 Contemp. OB/GYN 150–69 (1984). J.A. Cannon, Neonatology: Pathophysiology and Management of the Newborn 50–51 (1981); B.H. Feldman & R.S. Sauve, *The Infant Transport Service,* 3 Clinics Perinatology, no. 2, at 469–78 (1976); American Academy of Pediatrics & The American College of Obstetricians & Gynecologists Committee on Fetus and Newborn, Committee on Obstetrics: Maternal and Fetal Medicine, *Interhospital Care of the Perinatal Patient, in* Guidelines for Perinatal Care 185–98 (1983).

be securely fastened to the unit. Battery power must be reliably present to allow the equipment to operate. Emergency medications and supplies are also carried. See **Appendix 18–10** in § **18.26.** Thus, the neonatal transport team and equipment are quite literally a portable intensive care nursery (ICN) work station.[59]

The vehicles utilized for transport must be individualized for the separate Level III units and the surrounding region. Helicopters, fixed-wing aircraft, and ground units have all been used with success. In determining the type of vehicle to be used, it would be optimal to have capability for all three types; however, this is not a very common finding. For the patient, the *response time*—the interval between initiating a request for transport and the arrival of the team—is very important. For example, if a referring unit has minimal ability to stabilize a given patient's problem, quick response is necessary. If this were a transport from a long distance, fixed-wing or helicopter would be indicated. If the distance were short but traffic made prompt response impossible, the helicopter would be most effective. For most situations, ground transport is the best option.[60]

There are several medicolegal concerns relative to neonatal transport. The crossing of state lines and the subsequent unlicensed performance of medicine and nursing services is certainly of concern. Additionally, there are times when transport personnel perform in hospitals where no privileges have been granted. These difficult issues are joined by several others. If the team originates from the referring institution, when does the responsibility for the infant shift from the sending to the accepting hospital? When the team comes from the receiving hospital to pick up the baby, certain issues become cloudy. If the transport team does not include a physician, to whom is the transport team responsible while at the referring unit? Without a precise chain of command to follow, neither the

[59] American Academy of Pediatrics Committee on Fetus and Newborn, *Interhospital Care of the High-risk Infant, in* Standards and Recommendations for Hospital Care of Newborn Infants 130–46 (1977); J.A. Cannon, Neonatology: Pathophysiology and Management of the Newborn 53–59 (1981); W.T. Greene, *Organization of Neonatal Transport Services in Support of a Regional Referral Center,* 7 Clinics Perinatology no. 1, at 187–95 (1980); B.H. Feldman & R.S. Sauve, *The Infant Transport Service,* 3 Clinics Perinatology, no. 2, at 469–78 (1976); American Academy of Pediatrics & The American College of Obstetricians & Gynecologists Committee on Fetus and Newborn, Committee on Obstetrics: Maternal and Fetal Medicine, *Interhospital Care of the Perinatal Patient, in* Guidelines for Perinatal Care 185–98 (1983).

[60] American Academy of Pediatrics Committee on Fetus and Newborn, *Interhospital Care of the High-risk Infant, in* Standards and Recommendations for Hospital Care of Newborn Infants 130–46 (1977); J.A. Cannon, Neonatology: Pathophysiology and Management of the Newborn 53–59 (G. Avery ed 1981); W.T. Greene, *Organization of Neonatal Transport Services in Support of a Regional Referral Center,* 7 Clinics Perinatology no. 1, at 187–95 (1980); B.H. Feldman & R.S. Sauve, *The Infant Transport Service,* 3 Clinics Perinatology, no. 2, at 469–78 (1976); American Academy of Pediatrics & The American College of Obstetricians & Gynecologists Committee on Fetus and Newborn, Committee on Obstetrics: Maternal and Fetal Medicine, *Interhospital Care of the Perinatal Patient, in* Guidelines for Perinatal Care 185–98 (1983).

team nor the referring and receiving physicians know who is in charge. Currently, most Level III centers with a transport team operate on the concept that the patient is admitted to their hospital when the transport team arrives. This gives the transport team a very clear path to follow for communications and questions. It is highly desirable to have the referring physician present at the time of transport. This frees him or her of concern about responsibility for the team.[61]

Through close cooperation between all levels of care, a mechanism for referring patients can be devised. Each Level III unit should have a protocol for processing an incoming call for assistance, be it a call for consultation or for patient transfer. In determining if a unit can receive a patient, the medical assessment requires only a brief period. The neonatal physician should speak with the referring doctor to determine if the patient needs to be transferred. If the patient does require transport, the next step is to determine if there is an available bed in the unit. If there is an open ICN bed, then, from the doctor's standpoint, the answer concerning acceptance of the patient is immediately available. However, hospital administrations sometimes desire to know more about the patient before granting the admission, such as whether the patient has insurance. If not, the hospital may refuse the admission. This brings into focus the need for each regional system to know its limitations and constraints. It is far better for health care within the region to be planned in a calm manner rather than in the anxious state that surrounds an emergency transfer.

While cooperation between units in the referral system works for the benefit of the patient, it is not a universally accepted necessity.[62] Consider the following situation. In many states a hospital cannot be forced to care for a patient; therefore, from an administrative standpoint, some of the Level III units may not feel the need to work closely with surrounding institutions. This noncooperation is usually based on two reasons. First, if transfer from a hospital is difficult, some of the doctors might be influenced to move some or all of their paying deliveries to that facility. Second, it keeps indigent patients to a minimum. While this may represent an acceptable method of operation, the morality of this issue is a highly emotional and debatable topic.

As a worse-case scenario, consider the plight of a distressed newborn who has been delivered in a Level I or Level II setting. No standard referral for ill newborns has been previously established. The referring physician must attempt to render care to the baby while at the same time making arrangements for transfer. Because the family does not have health insurance, the private Level III hospitals refuse admission and the charity hospital has no beds. Is this another example

---

[61] American Academy of Pediatrics & The American College of Obstetricians & Gynecologists Committee on Fetus and Newborn, Committee on Obstetrics: Maternal and Fetal Medicine, *Interhospital Care of the Perinatal Patient, in* Guidelines for Perinatal Care 185–98 (1983).

[62] S.N. Graven & A.A. Fanaroff, *The Organization of Perinatal Health Services, in* Behrman's Neonatal-Perinatal Medicine 4–11 (1983).

of "divine arrangements" or does it represent "our own ignorance and misman-agement"?[63]

Outreach Education and Quality Assurance

A strong working relationship between the Level III hospital and its referral institutions can do much to improve the quality of perinatal and neonatal health care. In addition to providing invaluable clinical service, the Level III center must also serve as an educational resource to its region. Many avenues for these activities can be utilized, including didactic conferences held either at the Level III center or at one of the referral hospitals, preparation of written or audiovisual educational materials, visiting fellowships at the Level III center (where physi-cians can retrain or refresh old skills that were not frequently utilized in the community hospital setting), and availability for advice or consultation by tele-phone, facsimile, or electronic mail. It is also incumbent upon the Level III cen-ter to provide quality assurance activities designed to critique not only its own clinical performance but also that of its referral hospitals. Joint problem solving based on an objective analysis, performed under collegial peer review, can go a long way in improving interinstitutional relationships and the quality of care delivered to these shared patients.[64]

---

[63] A. Coombe, A Treatise on the Physiological and Moral Management of Infancy, for the Use of Parents (4th ed. 1845).

[64] S.M. Donn et al., *User-Friendly Computerized Quality Assurance Program for Regionalized Neonatal Care*, 13 J. Perinatology 72–75 (1993).

§ 18.17   Appendix 18–1: Neonatal and Infant Mortality in the United States Since 1950

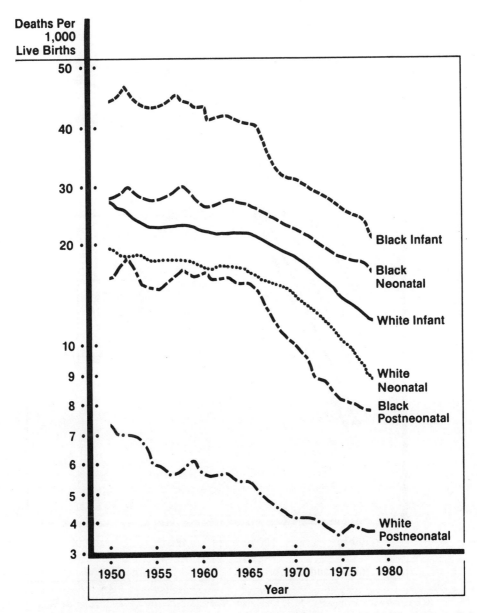

Source: National Center for Health Statistics. Computed by the Division of Analysis from data compiled by the Division of Vital Statistics.

§ 18.18   Appendix 18–2: Infant Survival

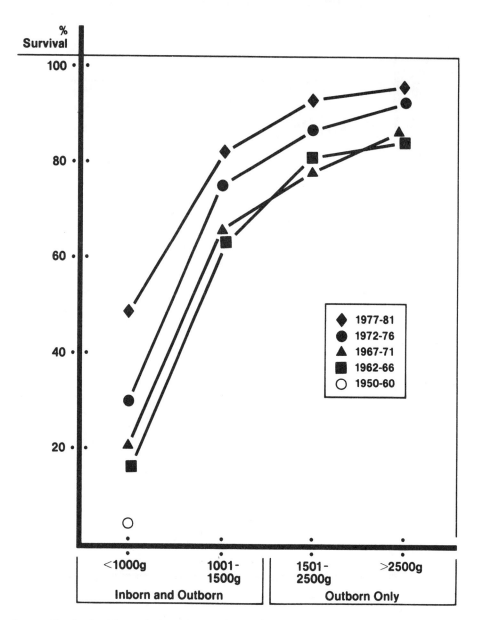

Source: Reprinted with permission: M.T. Stahlman, *Newborn Intensive Care: Success or Failure,* J. Pediatr. 105:163 (1984).

§ 18.19   Appendix 18–3: Impact of Intensive Care (IC)

	Hospital	Before IC	After IC		
Stillbirth Rate	St. Boniface,	8.8	3.5	1973	
(SB/1000 births)	Winnipeg				
	St. Joseph's	10.4	7.3	1969	
	London				
	Women's College,	—	8.3	1978	
	Toronto				
	Royal Victoria,	—	6.9	1970–72	Fetal and
	Montreal				neonatal IC
	Queen's Halifax	20.8	12.0	1965–68	
Neonatal	St. Boniface,	5.0	3.5	1973	> 1000 g
Mortality Rate	Winnipeg				
(0–6 days:	Women's College,	10.6	6.2	1791	
rate per 1000	Toronto				
live births)	Women's College,	–	5.6	1978	
	Toronto				
	Jewish General,	7.6	6.4	1973	
	Montreal				
	Jewish General,	—	3.7	1974	
	Montreal				
	Jewish General,	—	3.4	1975	
	Montreal				
	Queen's, Halifax	17.0	9.9	1965–68	> 500 g
Perinatal	St. Boniface,	13.9	7.0	1973	> 1000 g
Mortality Rate	Winnipeg				
(per 1000	St. Joseph's,	21.6	19.0	1969	> 500 g + SB
live births)	London				
	Women's College,	20.5	14.8	1971	Neonatal IC
	Toronto				
	Women's College,	—	13.9	1978	Fetal and
	Toronto				neonatal IC
	Royal Victoria,	19.1	15.2	1970–72	Neonatal IC
	Montreal				
	Royal Victoria,	—	11.6	1970–72	Fetal and
	Montreal				neonatal IC
	Jewish General,	20.9	14.9	1973	
	Montreal				
	Jewish General,	—	9.0	1974	
	Montreal				
	Queen's, Halifax	—	8.9	1975	
	Grace, Halifax	12.5	7.7		Before and
					after fetal IC

Source: Reprinted with permission. P.R. Swyer, *The Organization of Perinatal Care with Particular Reference to the Newborn, in* Neonatology: Pathophysiology and Management of the Newborn 27 (G.B. Avery ed., J.B. Lippincott Co. 1981).

§ 18.20 Appendix 18–4: Average Number of Pieces of Equipment by Class, Type, and Cost (21-bed Unit)

Class and Type of Equipment	Average No. Piece Equipment/unit	Least No. Piece Equipment/unit	Maximal No. Piece Equipment/unit	Average No. Piece Equipment/bed	Cost Range Studied	Total Cost Range/Unit
Respiratory						
Respirators	9.07	1	45	0.43	$3,600–$4,500	$32,652–$40,815
Hoods	10.5	3	100	0.49	150– 315	1,575– 3,308
Respiratory paraphernalia Humidifiers & Blenders	11.13	1	47	0.52	— —	— —
Infusion Pumps	21.9	1	76	1.03	2,000– 2,557	43,800– 55,996
Cardiorespiratory Monitors						
Cardiac Monitors	10.6	1	43	0.5	1,950– 5,900	20,670– 62,540
Blood Pressure Monitors	1.6	1	8	0.08	1,950– 9,000	3,120– 14,400
Po_2 Monitors	3.0	1	18	0.14	6,300– 7,900	18,900– 23,700
Incubators	24.8	7	124	1.18	2,100– 5,700	52,080–141,360
Lights						
Bilights	8.5	3	20	0.4	2,000–	17,000– 17,000
Exam lights	3.4	1	18	0.16	710–	2,414– 2,414
Warmers	0.68	1	13	0.032	3,250– 4,300	2,210– 2,924
Computer Terminals	0.7	1	6	0.04	Variable	$194,421–364,299

Source: Reprinted with permission. K. Bajo, Equipment Cost: The Neonatal Intensive Care Unit and the Modern Obstetric Unit, 10 Clinics Perinatology, no. 1, 177 (1983).

§ 18.21   Appendix 18–5: Recommended Nurse/Patient Ratios for Perinatal Care Services

Staffing Ratio	Care Provided
1:1-2	Antepartum testing
1:2	Laboring patients
1:1	Patients in second stage of labor
1:1	Ill patients with complications
1:2	Oxytocin induction or augmentation of labor
1:1	Coverage for initiating epidural anesthesia
1:1	Circulation for cesarean delivery
1:6	Antepartum/postpartum patients without complications
1:2	Postoperative recovery
1:3	Patients with complications, but in stable condition
1:4	Recently born infants and those needing close observation
1:6-8	Newborns needing only routine care
1:3-4	Normal mother-newborn couplet care
1:3-4	Newborns requiring continuing care
1:2-3	Newborns requiring intermediate care
1:1-2	Newborns needing intensive care
1:1	Newborns requiring multisystem support
>1:1	Unstable newborns requiring complex critical care

Source: Reproduced with permission. American College of Obstetricians & Gynecologists: Guidelines to Perinatal Care, 3rd ed. Washington, DC, ACOG © 1992.

§ 18.22 Appendix 18–6: Levels of Program Development (I, II, III)

Levels of perinatal network	Activity	Locations	Usual Physician leadership
I I I I	Usual focus of patient entry into system Risk assessment Uncomplicated perinatal care Stabilization of unexpected problems Data collection Sponsor of local education	Community hospital or colocated at level II or level III facility	Primary care physician or specialist
II II	Level I activities, plus: Diagnosis and treatment of selected high-risk pregnancies and neonatal problems Patient transport Education efforts for part of network	Large community hospitals with many support services or colocated at level III facility	Specialist or subspecialist
III	Usually level I and level II activities,[a] plus: Diagnosis and treatment of most perinatal problems Research and outcome surveillance Regional education Regional administration	Large medical centers with comprehensive academic programs	Subspecialist

Source: Reproduced with permission of PEDIATRICS. Committee on Fetus and Newborn, Committee on Obstetrics: Maternal and Fetal Medicine, *Organization of Perinatal Care, in* Guidelines for Perinatal Care 5 (1983).

[a]Some level III facilities, such as level III neonatal units in children's hospitals, may not provide level I and level II services. Regional Resource Centers provide specialized knowledge and skills in academic medical centers (level III) at a subspecialty (academic) level.

§ 18.23   Appendix 18–7: Services Provided by Perinatal Facilities

Services	Level I	Level II	Level III
Complete prenatal care for maternity patient with no complications or with minor complications	X	X	X
Complete prenatal care for maternity patients with most complications		X	X
A special diagnostic and management clinic for high-risk prenatal patients			X
Risk identification scoring system	X	X	X
Management of uncomplicated labor and delivery of normal term fetus	X	X	X
Prompt management of unexpected complications occurring during labor and delivery, including anesthesia, cesarean section, and blood administration	X	X	X
Management of complicated labor and delivery		X	X
Intrapartum intensive care			X
In-house anesthesia service		X	X
Electronic fetal monitoring	±	X	X
Physically separated facilities for obstetrics	X	X	X
Capability for resuscitation of depressed neonate at every delivery	X	X	X
Care for the healthy newborn	X	X	X
Stabilization and risk assessment of all neonates	X	X	X
Intravenous fluid administration to neonates	X	X	X
Management of most neonates who have complications up to short-term assisted ventilation		X	X
Continuous neonatal monitoring capability		X	X
Blood gases available on 24-hour basis		X	X
Neonatal intensive care including assisted ventilation and hyperalimentation			X
Neonatal surgical capability			X
Availability of pediatric subspecialists in cardiology genetics and hematology			X
Care of mothers with no postpartum complications	X	X	X
Management of unexpected postpartum complications including hemorrhage and sepsis	X	X	X

Services	Level I	Level II	Level III
Management of most postpartum complications		X	X
Data collection on performance and outcome	X	X	X
Laboratory services for electrolytes, bilirubin, blood glucose, calcium on 24-hour basis	X	X	X
X-ray services with portable film capability on 24-hour basis	X	X	X
Laboratory services to assess fetal well-being and maturity		X	X
Diagnostic x-ray and ultrasound facilities		X	X
Nutritional consultation		X	X
Social service		X	X
Respiratory therapy consultation		X	X
Sterilization and family planning services	X	X	X
Follow-up developmental assessment clinic			X

Source: Reprinted with permission. S.N. Graven & A.A. Fanaroff, *The Organization of Perinatal Health Services, in* Behrman's Neonatal-Perinatal Medicine 10 (S. Bircher ed., C.V. Mosby Co., 4th ed. 1987).

§ 18.24   Appendix 18–8: Criteria for Consultation and Possible Transfer of Infants from a Level I Unit to a Level II or Level III Unit*

1. Gestation less than 35 weeks or weight less than 2,500 gm.
2. Neonatal sepsis or severe infection
3. Respiratory distress persisting for longer than 2 hours
4. Significant neonatal blood loss
5. Hypoglycemia
6. Hemolytic disease of the newborn
7. Infants whose mothers were taking hazardous drugs
8. Infants needing special observation.

Source: Reproduced with permission of PEDIATRICS. Adapted from American Academy of Pediatrics Committee on Fetus and Newborn, *Regionalization of Perinatal Services, in* Standards and Recommendations for Hospital Care of Newborn Infants, 144 (1977).

§ 18.25   Appendix 18–9: Criteria for Consultation and Possible Transfer of Infants to a Level III Unit*

1. Any criteria listed in Table 24-6
2. Infants of diabetic mothers
3. Neonatal seizures
4. Sepsis and/or meningitis
5. Significant congenital malformations
6. Infants requiring surgical correction of a problem
7. Severe neonatal asphyxia
8. Hypoglycemia, persistent or recurrent
9. Progressive respiratory distress
10. Any neonatal condition requiring ventilator support for longer than one hour.

§ 18.26   Appendix 18–10: Equipment of Neonatal Transport**

Respiratory Therapy Equipment for Neonatal Transport

Mechanical ventilator

Sterile ventilator tubing and water traps

Full (2,000 psi) E-tanks of oxygen and air; flow regulators

Wrenches for E-tanks

Low-flow blender

Air/oxygen high-pressure hoses to blender

---

*Source: Reproduced with permission of PEDIATRICS. Adapted from American Academy of Pediatrics Committee on Fetus and Newborn, *Regionalization of Perinatal Services, in* Standards and Recommendations for Hospital Care of Newborn Infants, 144 (1977).

**S.M. Donn et al., Neonatal transport, Curr Probl Pediatr 1985; 15:1–65, copyright Year Book Medical Publishers, Chicago.

Air/oxygen quick disconnect adaptors to high-pressure hoses

Oxygen tubing/connectors

Oxygen hood/aerosol tubing

Resuscitation bag/variable PEEP attachment/1.0 FiO_2 adaptor

Manometer/bifurcation tubing to resuscitation bag

Resuscitation masks/variable sizes

Stethoscopes

All-purpose nebulizer with plugs

Nonimmersion heater

Tape

Miscellaneous: hemostat; flow meter nipple; wrenches; infant and small child oral airways

Intubation set: laryngoscope handle, blades (nos. 0, 1) and bulb (with spare); batteries; adhesive; adhesive remover; cotton swabs; uncuffed endotracheal tubes (2.5 to 4.0 mm I.D.); DeLee suction catheters

Continuous positive airway pressure set: nasal prongs, variable sizes; headbands; nasal lubricant; elastic bandage; tape

Essential Medications for Neonatal Transport

Lidocaine 1% (local anesthesia)

Lidocaine 2% without epinephrine (arrhythmias)

Albumin/Plasmanate

Dextrose 50% in water

Dextrose 10% in water, 500 mL

Dextrose 5% in water

Pancuronium

Ampicillin

Gentamicin

Normal saline for injection

Vitamin K

Phenobarbital

Heparin

Sodium bicarbonate

Epinephrine 1:10,000

Atropine

Calcium gluconate 10%

Sterile water for injection

Naloxone

Isoproterenol

Dopamine

Tolazoline

Glucagon

Prostaglandin E_1

Furosemide

Dexamethasone

Essential Medical and Nursing Equipment for Neonatal Transport

Iodophor; swabs, ointment, solution

Alcohol wipes

Sutures, 4.0 silk with needle

Umbilical tape, clamp

Labels

Safety pins

Rubber bands

Infant restraints

Tourniquet

Tape

Blood culture tubes

Rubber bulb syringe

Cotton balls

Lancets

Needles; 18-gauge, 22-gauge, 25-gauge

Lubricant gel

Blood tubes; plain, EDTA, citrate

Scalp vein needles; 23-gauge, 25-gauge

Syringes; 1–60 cc

Sterile instruments;

    Forceps

    Iris forceps

    Hemostat-straight, curved

    Scissors

    Dilator probe

    Tape measure

Infusion pump tubing

Feeding tubes; 5 French, 8 French

Sump tube

Sterile gauze; $2 \times 2, 4 \times 4$ in.

T-connectors

IV catheters; 22-gauge, 24-gauge

Armboard, locking stopcocks, extension sets

Stethoscopes

Polaroid® camera, film, flash

Umbilical catheter set

Blunt needles

Buretrol with microdrip chamber

Tubing for IV fluids

Sterile gloves; $6^1/_2$, 7, $7^1/_2$, 8

Thoracostomy tube drainage kit

Latex suction catheters

Glucose test strips

DeLee suction apparatus

Stopcocks and plugs

McSwain darts/Heimlich valves

Thermometers

§ 18.27   Appendix 18–11: Perinatal Care Programs

	Level I	Level II	Level III
General Function	Risk assessment Management of uncomplicated perinatal care Stabilization of unexpected problems Initiation of maternal and neonatal transports Patient and community education Data collection and evaluation	Level I plus: Diagnosis and treatment of selected high-risk pregnancies and neonatal problems Initiation and acceptance of maternal-fetal and neonatal transports Education of allied health personnel Residency education (affiliation)	Levels I and II plus: Diagnosis and treatment of all perinatal problems Acceptance and direction of maternal-fetal and neonatal transports Research and outcome surveillance Graduate and postgraduate education System management
Types of patients	Uncomplicated, emergency, and remedial problems such as lack of progress, immediate resuscitation of asphyxiated neonates, uterine atony, nursery care of large premature neonates (>2000 g) without risk factors, physiologic jaundice	Level I plus: Selected problems such as preeclampsia, premature labor at 32 weeks and later, mild to moderate respiratory distress syndrome, suspected neonatal sepsis, hypoglycemia, neonates of diabetic mothers, postasphyxia without life-threatening sequaise	Levels I and II plus: Premature rupture of membranes at 24–26 weeks, severe maternal medical complications, pregnancy with concurrent cancer, complicated antenatal genetic problems, prematurity at 26–32 weeks (500–1250 g), severe respiratory distress syndrome, sepels, severe postasphyxia, symptomatic congenital cardiac and other

	Level I	Level II	Level III
			systems disease, neonates with special needs such as hyperalimentation, prolonged mechanical ventilation.
Location and number of births, neonatal beds	Located within Level II or III hospital or in sparsely populated or isolated areas; at least 1 birth/day unless in isolated area	Medium and large communities, may be part of Level III facility, several births/day, 3–4 neonatal beds/1000 births served	Medium and large communities, usually in academic centers, several births/day, 1 intensive care neonatal bed/1000 births served in addition to Level II
Space Sq ft/bed	Delivery/resuscitation 120 Admission/observation 40 Newborn nursery 20 Postpartum unit 100	Level I plus: Intermediate nursery 50 Continuous/convalescent nursery 30	Levels I and II plus: Intensive neonatal 80–100
Ancillary Support Operating room	Technicians on call 24 h./day available within 15–30 min	Technicians immediately available for emergency situations	Level II, may be in delivery room area
Laboratory (microtechnique for neonates) Within 16 min Within 1 h	Hematocrit Glucose, BUN, creatinine, blood gases, routine urinalysis	Blood gases, blood type and Rh Level 1 plus: Electrolytes, coagulation studies, blood available from Type and Screen program	Level II Levels I and II plus: Special blood and amniotic fluid tests

	Level I	Level II	Level III
Within 1–6 hr	CBC, platelet appearance on smear, blood chemistries, blood type and cross-matched Coombs' test, bacterial smear	Level I plus: Coagulation studies magnesium, urine, electrolytes, and chemistries	Levels I and II
Within 24–48 hr	Bacterial cultures and antibotic sensitivity	Level I plus: Liver function test, Metabolic screening	Levels I and II
Within hospital or facilities available	Viral cultures	Level I	Level I plus: Laboratory facilities available
Radiography and ultrasound	Technicians on call 24 hr/day, available in 30 min Technicians experienced in performing abdominal, pelvic and OB ultrasound examinations Professional interpretation available on 24-hr basis Portable X-ray and ultrasound equipment available to labor and delivery rooms and to nurseries	Experienced radiology technicians immediately available in hospital (ultrasound on call) Professional interpretation immediately available Portable X-ray equipment Ultrasound equipment may be in labor or delivery or nursery area Sophisticated equipment for emergency GI, GU or CNS studies available 24 hr/day	Level II plus: Computerized axial tomography
Blood bank	Technicians on call 24 hr/day, available in 30 min. performing routine blood banking procedures	Experienced technicians immediately available in hospital for blood banking procedures and identification of irregular antibodies	Levels II plus: Resource center for network Direct line communication to labs and delivery area and nurseries

	Level I	Level II	Level III
Examination and treatment room	Pelvic examination Culture of cervix and uterus	Blood component therapy readily available Level I plus: Amniocentesis Equipment for removal of suture for cerclage	Levels I and II plus: Services within unit
Auxiliary areas	Parent education Conference room Locker room (may be remote) Physician on-call room near-by	Level I plus: Breast-feeding area within unit Parent waiting room for intensive care	Levels I and II plus: All areas within unit Conference/lecture rooms as necessary for professional/regional education commitment
	Laboratory within unit for hematocrit, centrifuge for dip stick for urine, albumin, glucose, microscope	Level I plus: Refrigerator to hold cultures, materials Gram's stain material	Levels I and II
Personnel Chief of service	One physician responsible for perinatal care (or co-directors from obstetrics and pediatrics)	Joint planning: *Ob*: Board-certified obstetrician with certification, special interest, experience or training in maternal-fetal medicine *Peds*: Board-certified pediatrician with certification, special interest, experience, or training in neonatology	Codirectors: *Ob*: Full-time board-certified obstetrician with special competence in maternal-fetal medicine *Peds*: Full-time board-certified pediatrician with special competence in neonatal medicine

	Level I	Level II	Level III
Other physicians	Physician (or certified nurse-midwife) at all deliveries Anesthesia services Physician care for neonates	Level I plus: Board-certified director or anesthesia services Medical, surgical, radiology, pathology consultation	Levels I and II plus: Anesthesiologists with special training or experience in perinatal and pediatric anesthesia Obstetric and pediatric subspecialists
Supervisory nurse	RN in charge of perinatal facilities	*Ob:* RN with education and experience in normal and high-risk pregnancy only responsible *Peds:* RN with education and experience in treatment of sick neonates only responsible	Supervisor of perinatal with advanced skills Separate head nurses for maternal-fetal and neonatal services
Staff nurse/patient ratio	Normal labor 1:2 Delivery in second stage 1:1 Oxytocin inductions 1:2 Cesarean delivery 2:1 Normal nursery 1:6–8	Level I plus: Complicated labor/delivery 1:1 Intermediate nursery 1:3–4	Levels I and II plus: Intensive neonatal care 1:1–2 Critical care of unstable neonate 2:1
Other personnel	LPN, assistants under direction of head nurse	Level I plus: Social service, biomedical, respiratory, therapy, laboratory as needed	Levels I plus: Designated and often full-time social service, respiratory therapy, biomedical engineering, laboratory technician Nurse-clinician and specialists Nurse program and education coordinators

	Level I	Level II	Level III
Obstetric Units			
Admission/observation	Close to labor and delivery comfortable, room to ambulate	Level I plus: Beds, space for diagnostic procedures, possible emergency delivery	Levels I and II plus: Other bed designated for observation
Family waiting	Nearby/adjacent	Level I	Level I
Labor	Single: 140 sq ft multiple, 80 sq ft/patient. Beds adjustable and moveable to delivery, may be used as birthing bed. Full utilities, including auxiliary electrical, oxygen, suction. Communication system. Full routine patient care and CPR equipment. Secure medication area. Monitoring capabilities	Level I	Level I
Birthing (labor/delivery/recovery)	Combined equipment for labor and delivery, may be concealed. Adequate space, equipment for ambulation, support person	Level I	Level I
Delivery (vaginal and operative	Contiguous to labor; at least two available, with one equipped for cesarean delivery	Level I (Actual number of delivery rooms depends on total births) plus:	Levels I and II plus: intensive care area

	Level I	Level II	Level III
	Operating room in design Equipment/supplies necessary for normal delivery and management of complications, including surgical intervention	Intensive care room in labor/delivery area for patients with significant complication	
Antepartum and postpartum area	Contiguous with nursery Large enough to accommodate mother, baby, visitors Maximum two mothers/room 100 sq ft/patient in multiple rooms Communication system Hospital standard utilities	Level I	
Nursery Resuscitation	100 foot-candles illumination Overhead radiant heat Heating pad Wall clock Resuscitation and stabilization equipment Designated area (40 sq ft) or room (120 sq ft) Full utilities, including suction, oxygen, compressed air, electrical outlets	Level I	

	Level I	Level II	Level III
Admission/ observation	Near adjacent to delivery/ cesarean birth room, may be part of maternal recovery area 40 sq ft/neonate Equipment as in resuscitation area	May be located in newborn or continuing care area	Level II
Newborn nursery	Close to postpartum area Beds and equipment to exceed obstetric beds by 20%–30% 20 sq ft/neonate Resuscitation equipment 1 electrical outlet/2 beds 1 O_2, air suction/5–6 beds	Level I	Level I
Continuing care	Usually not located in Level I	Near intermediate nursery. 30 sq ft/neonate Resuscitation equipment 4 electrical outlets 1 O_2, 1 air, 1 suction/neonate	Level II
Intermediate care	Not present	Near delivery and intensive care nurseries Full life support and monitoring in addition to resuscitation equipment 50 sq ft/neonate 8 electrical, 2 O_2, 2 compressed air, 2 suction outlets/neonate	Level II

WHAT INTENSIVE CARE IS

	Level I	Level II	Level III
Intensive care	Not present	Present in some hospitals	Near delivery/cesarean birth rooms 80–100 sq ft/neonate 12 electrical, 2 O_2, 2 compressed air, 2 suction outlets/neonate Full life support, monitoring and resuscitation equipment

Source: Reproduced with permission of PEDIATRICS. Committee on Fetus and Newborn, Committee on Obstetrics: Maternal and Fetal Medicine, Guidelines for Perinatal Care 247–53 (1983).